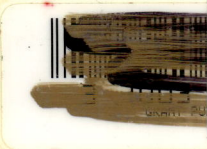

Breast Cancer
SOURCEBOOK

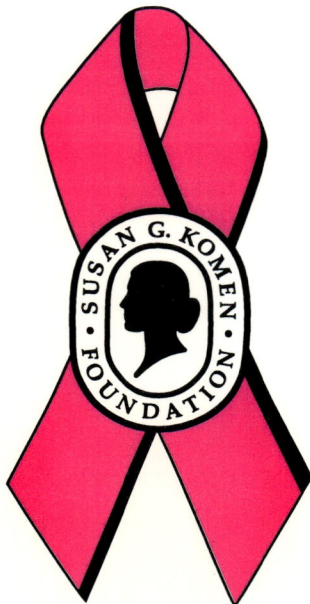

This resource was
funded by a grant
from the
**Grand Rapids
Susan G. Komen
Breast Cancer
Foundation**

P.O. Box 1053
Grand Rapids, MI
49501
616.752.8262

For more information
on Breast Health call
1-800-I'M-AWARE

Health Reference Series

First Edition

Breast Cancer
SOURCEBOOK

*Basic Consumer Health Information about
Breast Cancer, Including Diagnostic Methods,
Treatment Options, Alternative Therapies,
Self-Help Information, Statistical and
Demographic Data, and Facts for Men
with Breast Cancer*

*Along with Reports on Current Research
Initiatives, a Glossary of Related Medical
Terms, and a Directory of Sources for Further
Help and Information*

Edited by
Edward J. Prucha and Karen Bellenir

Omnigraphics

615 Griswold Street • Detroit, MI 48226

Bibliographic Note

Because this page cannot legibly accommodate all the copyright notices, the Bibliographic Note portion of the Preface constitutes an extension of the copyright notice.

Each new volume of the *Health Reference Series* is individually titled and called a "First Edition." Subsequent updates will carry sequential edition numbers. To help avoid confusion and to provide maximum flexibility in our ability to respond to informational needs, the practice of consecutively numbering each volume has been discontinued.

Edited by Edward J. Prucha and Karen Bellenir

Health Reference Series

Karen Bellenir, *Series Editor*
Peter D. Dresser, *Managing Editor*
Maria Franklin, *Permissions Assistant*
Joan Margeson, *Research Associate*
Dawn Matthews, *Verification Assistant*
Carol Munson, *Permissions Assistant*
Jenifer Swanson, *Research Associate*

Omnigraphics, Inc.

Matthew P. Barbour, *Vice President, Operations*
Laurie Lanzen Harris, *Vice President, Editorial Director*
Kevin Hayes, *Production Coordinator*
Thomas J. Murphy, *Vice President, Finance and Controller*
Peter E. Ruffner, *Senior Vice President*
Jane J. Steele, *Marketing Coordinator*

Frederick G. Ruffner, Jr., Publisher

© 2001, Omnigraphics, Inc.

Library of Congress Cataloging-in-Publication Data

Breast cancer sourcebook / edited by Edward J. Prucha and Karen Bellenir.-- 1st Ed.
    p. cm.-- (Health reference series)
    Subtitle: Basic consumer health information about breast cancer, including diagnostic methods, treatment options, alternative therapies, self-help information, statistical and demographic data, and facts for men with breast cancer; along with reports on current research initiatives, a glossary of related medical terms, and a directory of sources for further help and information.
    Includes bibliographical references and index.
    ISBN 0-7808-0244-6
    1. Breast--Cancer--Popular works. I. Prucha, Edward J. II. Bellenir, Karen. III. Series.
RC280.B8 B6887 2001
616.99'449—dc21

        2001036253

∞

Table of Contents

Part IV: Mammograms and Other Screening Tools

Part V: Treatment Options

Part VI: Clinical Trials and Other Research

Part VII: Coping with Breast Cancer

Part VIII: Additional Help and Information

Preface

About This Book

Each year in the United States, more than 180,000 women (and 1,400 men) are diagnosed with breast cancer. Although the exact causes of breast cancer are not known, studies have identified several risk factors that increase a woman's chance of developing breast cancer, including:

- A personal history of previous breast cancer.

- A family history of breast cancer, especially if a woman's mother, sister, or daughter developed breast cancer at a young age.

- Breast changes, such as atypical hyperplasia (a condition in which the cells have abnormal features and are increased in number) or lobular carcinoma *in situ* (a condition in which abnormal cells are found in the lobules of the breast).

- Changes in certain genes, two of which have been identified as BRCA1 and BRCA2.

- Exposure to elevated levels of estrogen.

- Having a first child after the age of 30.

- Having breasts with a high proportion of dense tissue.

- Being exposed to radiation therapy before age 30.

- Alcohol consumption.

Improved screening methods for early detection mean that most women with breast cancer are diagnosed at an early stage and are able to benefit from newer, more effective treatments. According to the National Cancer Institute, most women who are treated for early breast cancer go on to live healthy, active lives.

Breast Cancer Sourcebook provides information about breast health, normal breast changes, and symptoms that may indicate cancer. It offers facts about early screening methods, diagnostic procedures, and treatment options. It reports on current research initiatives and clinical trials in breast cancer treatment and prevention. A glossary of breast and cancer terms, directories of informational and support organizations, and a list of additional resources guide readers to sources of further help and information.

How to Use This Book

This book is divided into parts and chapters. Parts focus on broad areas of interest. Chapters are devoted to single topics within a part.

Part I: Assessing Breast Health provides women with information about maintaining breast health and understanding normal breast changes that occur during the menstrual cycle, through the childbearing years, during menopause, and beyond. Facts about breast self-examination and tips for avoiding breast cancer risk factors are also included.

Part II: Breast Cancer Fundamentals explains how different types of breast cancer develop and progress. A chapter on male breast cancer addresses concerns specific to men, and a chapter on metastatic cancer explains what happens when breast cancer spreads to other parts of the body.

Part III: Evaluating Breast Cancer Risk Factors describes some known risk factors for developing breast cancer, including genetic risks, hormonal risks, and risks associated with dietary choices and other lifestyle decisions. Controversies about unknown risks and studies challenging some reports in the popular media are also presented.

Part IV: Mammograms and Other Screening Tools offers facts about mammography and other screening tools for early detection of breast cancer. Difficulties sometimes associated with mammography, including the possibility of false results, are outlined, and federal initiatives to improve mammography standards are explained.

Part V: Treatment Options helps women with breast cancer under-stand the choices surrounding their treatment. It includes facts about surgery, radiation therapy, chemotherapy, hormonal therapy, and complementary and alternative therapies.

Part VI: Clinical Trials and Other Research provides details about current research initiatives in breast cancer prevention and treat-ment. Information about taking part in clinical trials and reports about new genetic discoveries are also included.

Part VII: Coping with Breast Cancer provides information about psycho-logical, family, and legal issues surrounding a breast cancer diagnosis.

Part VIII: Additional Help and Information provides a glossary of breast and cancer terms, directories of organizations able to provide cancer information and support, and a chapter with suggested addi-tional reading and internet sources.

Bibliographic Note

This volume contains documents and excerpts from publications issued by the following government agencies: Agency for Healthcare Research and Quality (AHRQ), Centers for Disease Control and Pre-vention (CDC), National Cancer Institute (NCI), National Institutes of Health (NIH), U.S. Department of Health and Human Services (DHHS), U.S. Department of Labor (DoL), and the U.S. Food and Drug Administration (FDA).

In addition, this volume contains copyrighted articles from the American Psychological Association, Community Breast Health Pro-ject, Cornell University's Program on Breast Cancer and Environmen-tal Risk Factors, Jeanne Fournier, Susan G. Komen Breast Cancer Foundation, Dr. Ellen Mahoney, Massachusetts Medical Society, New York State Department of Health, and the University of Wisconsin Medical School's Breast Problem Clinic.

Full citation information is provided on the first page of each chap-ter. Every effort has been made to secure all necessary rights to re-print the copyrighted material. If any omissions have been made, please contact Omnigraphics to make corrections for future editions.

Acknowledgements

In addition to the organizations listed above, special thanks are due to researchers Jenifer Swanson and Joan Margeson, verification assistant Dawn Matthews, permissions specialists Maria Franklin and Carol Munson, and editorial assistants Michael Bellenir and Buffy Bellenir.

Note from the Editor

This book is part of Omnigraphics' *Health Reference Series*. The series provides basic information about a broad range of medical concerns. It is not intended to serve as a tool for diagnosing illness, in prescribing treatments, or as a substitute for the physician/patient relationship. All persons concerned about medical symptoms or the possibility of disease are encouraged to seek professional care from an appropriate health care provider.

Our Advisory Board

The *Health Reference Series* is reviewed by an Advisory Board comprised of librarians from public, academic, and medical libraries. We would like to thank the following board members for providing guidance to the development of this series:

Dr. Lynda Baker,
Associate Professor of Library and Information Science,
Wayne State University, Detroit, MI

Nancy Bulgarelli,
William Beaumont Hospital Library, Royal Oak, MI

Karen Imarasio,
Bloomfield Township Public Library, Bloomfield Hills, MI

Karen Morgan,
Mardigian Library, University of Michigan-Dearborn,
Dearborn, MI

Rosemary Orlando,
St. Clair Shores Public Library, St. Clair Shores, MI

Health Reference Series *Update Policy*

The inaugural book in the *Health Reference Series* was the first edition of *Cancer Sourcebook* published in 1990. Since then, the Series has been enthusiastically received by librarians and in the medical community. In order to maintain the standard of providing high-quality health information for the layperson the editorial staff at Omnigraphics felt it was necessary to implement a policy of updating volumes when warranted.

Medical researchers have been making tremendous strides, and it is the purpose of the *Health Reference Series* to stay current with the most recent advances. Each decision to update a volume will be made on an individual basis. Some of the considerations will include how much new information is available and the feedback we receive from people who use the books. If there is a topic you would like to see added to the update list, or an area of medical concern you feel has not been adequately addressed, please write to:

Editor
Health Reference Series
Omnigraphics, Inc.
615 Griswold Street
Detroit, MI 48226

The commitment to providing on-going coverage of important medical developments has also led to some format changes in the *Health Reference Series*. Each new volume on a topic is individually titled and called a "First Edition." Subsequent updates will carry sequential edition numbers. To help avoid confusion and to provide maximum flexibility in our ability to respond to informational needs, the practice of consecutively numbering each volume has been discontinued.

Part One

Assessing Breast Health

Chapter 1

Understanding Breast Changes

Breast cancer is hard to ignore. It is the most common form of cancer among American women, and almost everyone knows at least one person who has been treated for it.

Understandably, women are concerned about getting breast cancer, and this concern prompts them to watch for breast changes. Breast changes are common. Even though most are not cancer, they can be worrisome.

This information is designed to help you with these concerns. It describes screening for the early detection of breast cancer, explains the various types of breast changes that women experience, and outlines methods that doctors use to distinguish between benign (noncancerous) changes and cancer. It reviews factors that can increase a woman's cancer risk and reports on current approaches to breast cancer prevention.

Breast Cancer: Status Report

This year in the United States an estimated 180,000 women will learn they have breast cancer. Three-fourths of the cases of breast cancer occur in women ages 50 or older, but it affects younger women, too (and about 1,400 men a year).

More women are getting breast cancer, but no one yet knows all the reasons why. Some of the increase can be traced to better ways of

National Institutes of Health, National Cancer Institute, NIH Pub. No. 98-3536, September 1998.

recognizing cancer and detecting cancers in an early stage. The increase also may be the result of changes in the way we live—postponing child-birth, taking replacement hormones and oral contraceptives, eating high-fat foods, or drinking more alcohol.

The encouraging news is that, more and more, breast cancer is being detected early, while the tumor is limited to the breast and very small. Currently, two-thirds of newly diagnosed breast cancers show no signs that the cancer has spread beyond the breast.

With prompt and appropriate treatment, the outlook for women with breast cancer is good. Moreover, a majority of women diagnosed with early stage breast cancer are candidates for treatment that saves the breast.

The Key: Early Detection

The key to finding breast cancer is early detection, and the key to early detection is screening: looking for cancer in women who have no symptoms of disease. The best available tool is a regular screen-ing mammogram—x-ray of the breast—coupled with a clinical breast exam—by a doctor or nurse.

Mammography

A mammogram is an x-ray of the breast. Cancers that are found on mammograms but that cannot be felt (nonpalpable cancers) usu-ally are smaller than cancers that can be felt, and they are less likely to have spread.

Mammography is not foolproof. Some breast changes, including lumps that can be felt, do not show up on a mammogram. Changes can be especially difficult to spot in the dense, glandular breasts of younger women. This is why women of all ages should have their breasts examined every year by a physician or trained health profes-sional.

A lump should never be ignored just because it is not visible on a mammogram.

Two Kinds of Mammography: Diagnostic and Screening

If a woman visits her doctor because of unusual breast changes such as a lump, pain, nipple thickening or discharge, or changes in breast size or shape, or has a suspicious screening mammogram, the doctor often asks her to have a diagnostic mammogram: an x-ray of the breast to help assess her symptoms. A diagnostic mammogram is a basic medical tool, and it is appropriate for women of any age.

This chapter discusses screening mammograms: x-rays that are used to look for breast changes in women who have no signs of breast cancer. (Even though the woman has no symptoms of breast disease, a diagnosis of breast cancer can begin with a doctor checking a screening mammogram.)

What Are the Benefits of Screening Mammography?

High-quality mammography is the most effective tool now available to detect breast cancer early, before symptoms appear—often before a breast lump can even be felt. Regularly scheduled mammograms can decrease a woman's chance of dying from breast cancer. For some women, early detection may prevent the need to remove the entire breast or receive chemotherapy.

Who Benefits from Screening Mammography?

Studies done over the past 30 years clearly show that regular screening mammography significantly reduces the death rate from breast cancer in women over the age of 50. Recent results from studies show that regular mammography also reduces death rates from breast cancer in women who begin screening in their forties.

The effectiveness of mammography seems to increase as a woman ages, and the time it takes for benefits to emerge appears to take longer in younger women.

New guidelines have been developed based on the recent research data. The National cancer Institute (NCI) now recommends that:

- All women in their forties or older who are at *average* risk for breast cancer should have screening mammograms every 1 to 2 years.

- All women who are at *higher* risk for breast cancer should ask their doctors about when and how often to schedule screening mmmograms.

Who Is at Average Risk for Breast Cancer?

Simply being a woman and getting older puts you at average risk for developing breast cancer. The older you are, the greater your chance of getting breast cancer. No woman should consider herself too old to need regular screening mammograms.

Table 1.1. *What are a woman's chances of getting breast cancer as she gets older?*

Chance...

by age 30	1 out of 2,525
by age 40	1 out of 217
by age 50	1 out of 50
by age 60	1 out of 24
by age 70	1 out of 14
by age 80	1 out of 10

Source: NCI Surveillance, Epidemiology and End Results Program & American Cancer Society, 1993

Who Is at Higher Than Average Risk for Breast Cancer?

One or more of the following conditions place a woman at higher than average risk for breast cancer:

- personal history of a prior breast cancer

- evidence of a specific genetic change that increases susceptibility to breast cancer (See Gene Testing for Breast Cancer Susceptibility)

- mother, sister, daughter, or two or more close relatives, such as cousins, with a history of breast cancer (especially if diagnosed at a young age)

- a diagnosis of a breast condition that may predispose a woman to breast cancer (i.e., atypical hyperplasia), or a history of two or more breast biopsies for benign breast disease (See Benign Breast Conditions and the Risk for Breast Cancer)

Also playing a role in a heightened risk for breast cancer is breast density. Women ages 45 or older who have at least 75 percent dense tissue on a mammogram are at elevated risk. And a slight increase in the risk of breast cancer is associated with having a first birth at age 30 or older.

In addition, women who receive chest irradiation for conditions such as Hodgkin's disease at age 30 or younger remain at higher risk for breast cancer throughout their lives. These women require meticulous surveillance for breast cancer.

These factors that increase cancer risk—risk factors—do not by themselves cause cancer. Having one or more does not mean that you are certain or even likely to develop breast cancer. Even among women with no other risk factors except a strong family history—for example, both a mother and a sister or two sisters with early onset breast cancer—three-fourths will not develop the disease.

On the other hand, not having any of the known risk factors does not mean that you are "safe." Most women who develop breast cancer do not have a strong family history of breast cancer or fall into any special higher risk category.

Clearly, there is much yet to be learned about what causes breast cancer.

What Are the Limitations of Screening Mammography?

Early detection by mammography does not guarantee that a woman's life will be saved. It may not help a woman who has a fast-growing cancer that has spread to other parts of her body before being detected. Also, about half of the women whose breast cancers are detected by mammography would not have died from cancer, even if they had waited until the lump could be felt, because their tumors are slow-growing and treatable.

False Negative Mammograms. Breasts of younger women contain many glands and ligaments. Because their breasts appear dense on mammograms, it is difficult to see tumors or to distinguish between normal and abnormal breast conditions. As a woman grows older, the glandular and fibrous tissues of her breasts gradually give way to less dense fatty tissues. Mammograms can then see into the breast tissue more easily to detect abnormal changes. About 25 percent of breast tumors are missed in women in their forties, compared to about 10 percent of women older than age 50. These are called false negatives. A normal mammogram in a woman with symptoms does not rule out breast cancer. Sometimes a clinical breast exam by a doctor or nurse can reveal a breast lump that is missed by a mammogram.

False Positive Mammograms. Between 5 and 10 percent of mammogram results are abnormal and require more testing (more mammograms, fine needle aspiration, ultrasound, or biopsy), and most of the followup tests confirm that no cancer was present. It is estimated that a woman who has yearly mammograms between ages 40 and 49 would have about a 30 percent chance of having a false positive mammogram at some point in that decade, and about a 7 to 8 percent chance of having a breast biopsy within the 10-year period. The estimate for false positive mammograms is about 25 percent for women ages 50 or older.

Increased Cases of Ductal Carcinoma *In Situ* (DCIS). The increased use of screening mammography has increased the detection of small abnormal tissue growths confined to the milk ducts in the breast, called ductal carcinoma *in situ* (DCIS). Doctors don't know which, if any, cases of DCIS may become life threatening. Usually, the growth is removed surgically, and radiation treatment is often given.

How Mammograms Are Made

Mammography is a simple procedure. It uses a "dedicated" x-ray machine specifically designed for x-raying the breast and used only for that purpose (in contrast to machines used to take x-rays of the bones or other parts of the body). The standard screening exam includes two views of each breast, one from above and one angled from the side. A registered technologist places the breast between two flat plastic plates. The two plates are then pressed together. The idea is to flatten the breast as much as possible; spreading the tissue out makes any abnormal details easier to spot with a minimum of radiation. The technologist takes the x-ray, then repeats the procedure for the next view.

The pressure from the plates may be uncomfortable, or even somewhat painful. It helps to remember that each x-ray takes less than one minute—and it could save your life. It also helps to schedule mammography just after your period, when your breasts are least likely to be tender, or at the same time each year, if you no longer have your period.

Although some women are concerned about radiation exposure, the risk of any harm is extremely small. The doses of radiation used for mammography are very low and considered safe. The exact amount of radiation needed for a specific mammogram will depend on several factors. For instance, breasts that are large or dense will require higher doses to get a clear image. Federal mammography guidelines limit the radiation used for each exposure of the breast to 0.3 rad. (A "rad" is a unit of measurement that stands for radiation absorbed dose.) In practice, most mammograms deliver just a small fraction of this amount.

Specialized mammography facilities have experienced personnel as well as modern equipment that is custom designed for mammograms. The combination of good technology and expertise makes it possible to obtain good-quality x-ray images with very low doses of radiation.

Reading a Mammogram

The mammogram is first checked by the technologist and then read by a diagnostic radiologist, a doctor who specializes in interpreting x-rays.

The radiologist looks for unusual shadows, masses, distortions, special patterns of tissue density, and differences between the two breasts. The shape of a mass can be important, too. A growth that is benign (noncancerous) such as a cyst, looks smooth and round and has a clearly defined edge. Breast cancer, in contrast, often has an irregular outline with finger-like extensions.

Many mammograms show nontransparent white specks. These are calcium deposits known as calcifications.

Macrocalcifications are coarse calcium deposits. They are often seen in both breasts. Macrocalcifications are most likely due to aging, old injuries, or inflammations. They usually are not signs of cancer.

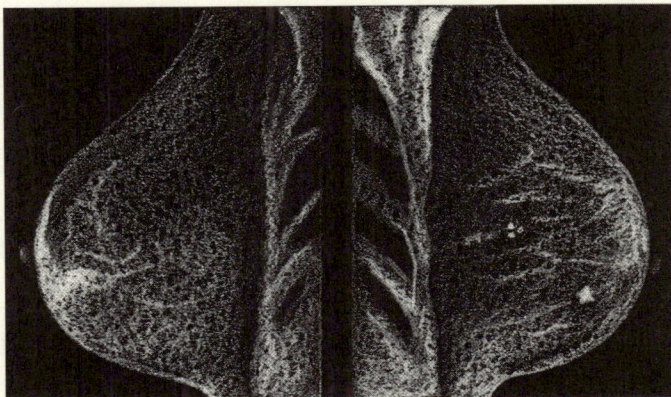

Figure 1.1. The radiologist looks for unusual shadows, masses, distortions, special patterns of tissue density, and differences between the two breasts.

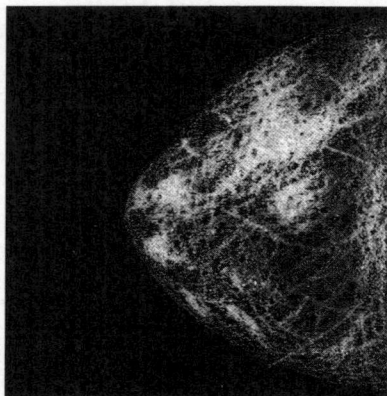

Figure 1.2. *Macrocalcifications are usually associated with benign breast conditions; many clusters of macrocalcifications in one area may be an early sign of breast cancer.*

Microcalcifications are tiny flecks of calcium found in an area of rapidly dividing cells. Clusters of numerous microcalcifications in one area can be a sign of ductal carcinoma *in situ*. (See DCIS) About half of the cancers found by mammography are detected as clusters of microcalcifications.

Reporting the Results

The radiologist will report the findings from your mammogram directly to you or to your doctor, who will contact you with the results. If you need further tests or exams, your doctor will let you know. If you don't get a report, you should call and ask for the results.

Don't simply assume that the mammogram is normal if you do not receive the results.

Your mammograms are an important part of your health history. Being able to compare earlier mammograms with new ones helps your doctor evaluate areas that look suspicious. If you move, ask your radiologist for your films and hand-carry them to your new physician, so they can be kept with your file. Always make sure that the radiologist who reads your mammogram has the old films to use for comparison.

Mammograms and Breast Implants

A woman who has had breast implants should continue to have mammograms. (A woman who has had an implant following breast cancer surgery should ask her doctor whether a mammogram is still necessary.) However, the woman should inform the technologist and radiologist beforehand and make sure they are experienced in x-raying patients with breast implants.

Because silicone implants are not transparent on x-ray, they can block a clear view of the tissues behind them. This is especially true if the implant has been placed in front of, rather than beneath, the chest muscles.

Experienced technologists and radiologists know how to carefully compress the breasts to avoid rupturing the implant. They can also use special techniques to detect abnormalities, sliding the implant backward against the chest wall, and pulling the breast tissue over and in front of it. Interpreting the mammogram can also be difficult, especially if scar tissue has formed around the implant or if silicone has leaked into nearby breast tissues.

Choose a Mammography Facility

Many places—breast clinics, radiology departments of hospitals, mobile vans, private radiology practices, doctors' offices—offer high-quality mammography. Your doctor can arrange for a mammogram for you, or you can schedule the appointment yourself. You can call NCI's Cancer Information Service (1-800-4-CANCER) to find a mammography facility in your community.

All facilities must be certified by the Food and Drug Administration (FDA). (See Assuring High-Quality Mammography) Staff of the facility are required to post the FDA certificate in a prominent place; if you don't see it, you should ask about certification. Without the FDA "seal of approval," it is now illegal for mammographic facilities to operate.

In addition to quality, another important consideration is cost. Most screening mammograms cost between $50 and $150. Most states now have laws requiring health insurance companies to reimburse all or part of the cost of screening mammograms; check with your insurance company. Medicare pays some of the cost for screening mammograms; check with your health care provider or call the Medicare Hotline (1-800-638-6833) for details.

Some health service agencies and some employers provide mammograms free or at low cost. Low cost does not mean low quality, however.

11

A large government survey found that some of the facilities charging the lowest fees (often because they serve large numbers of women) were among the best in terms of complying with high-quality standards.

Your doctor, local health department, clinic, or chapter of the American Cancer Society, as well as NCI's Cancer Information Service at 1-800-4-CANCER (1-800-422-6237), may be able to direct you to low-cost programs in your area.

Schedule a Regular Mammogram

Early detection of breast cancer is crucial for successful treatment, and regular screening mammography is currently the best tool for early detection. A 1993 survey by the National Center for Health Statistics found that 60 percent of all women ages 40 to 49 got a mammogram in the preceding 2 years, and 65 percent of women ages 50 to 64 had done so, but only 54 percent of women ages 65 and over had been screened during that time. It is clear that many women still do not get mammograms at regular intervals. Sadly, the women least likely to have regular exams include those at highest risk, women ages 60 and older.

The reason women most frequently give for having—or not having—a mammogram is whether or not the doctor suggested it. Although surveys show that more doctors routinely advise women about mammography, some fail to do so—because they forget, or because they assume that another doctor has done so. If your doctor doesn't suggest mammography, it will be up to you to raise the issue.

Assuring High-Quality Mammography

To make sure that all women have access to high-quality mammography, a federal law—the Mammography Quality Standards Act—now requires all mammography facilities to be certified by the FDA. Each facility must demonstrate that it meets federal standards for equipment, personnel, and practices.

Equipment must be capable of producing high-quality mammograms with the lowest possible amount of radiation exposure. Furthermore, it must be regularly checked by a radiological physicist and adjusted as necessary to be sure that its measurements and doses are correct.

Doctors and other staff members must be specially trained to perform and interpret breast x-rays. The technologists who take mammograms are certified by the American Registry of Radiological Technologists or licensed by the state; the doctors who read mammograms should be board-certified radiologists who have taken special courses in mammography.

The regulations also specify that mammography facilities must perform mammography regularly and frequently, maintain quality assurance programs, and ensure proper and timely reporting of test results.

Other Techniques for Detecting Breast Cancer

Clinical Breast Exam

Most professional medical organizations recommend that a woman have periodic breast exams by a doctor or nurse along with getting regular screening mammograms. You may find it convenient to schedule a breast exam during your routine physical.

The examiner will look at your breasts while you are sitting and while you are lying down. You may be asked to raise your arms over your head or let them hang by your sides, or to press your hands against your hips. The examiner checks your breasts carefully for changes in the skin such as dimpling, scaling, or puckering; any discharge from the nipples; or any difference in appearance between the two breasts, including differences in size or shape. The next step is palpation: Using the pads of the fingers to feel for lumps, the examiner will systematically inspect the entire breast, the underarm, and the collarbone area, first on one side, then on the other.

A lump is generally the size of a pea before a skilled examiner can detect it. Lumps that are soft, round, and smooth tend not to be cancerous. An irregular, hard lump that feels firmly anchored within the breast tissue is more likely to be a cancer. However, these are general observations, not hard and fast rules.

The only sure way to know if a solid lump is cancer is to have some tissue removed and examined under the microscope.

A breast exam by a doctor or nurse can find some cancers missed by mammography, even very small ones. In addition to the skill and carefulness of the examiner, the success of a physical exam can be influenced by your monthly cycle and by the size of your breast, as well as by the size and location of the lump itself. Lumps are harder to find in a large breast.

Currently, mammography and breast exams by the doctor or nurse are the most common and useful techniques for finding breast cancer early. Other methods such as ultrasound may be helpful in clarifying the diagnosis for women who have suspicious breast changes. However, no other procedure has yet proven to be more effective than mammography for screening women with no symptoms; thus, most alternative methods of breast cancer detection are used primarily in medical research programs.

Ultrasound

Ultrasound works by sending high-frequency sound waves into the breast. The pattern of echoes from these sound waves is converted into an image (sonogram) of the breast's interior. Ultrasound, which is painless and harmless, can distinguish between tumors that are solid and cysts, which are filled with fluid. Sonograms of the breast can also help radiologists to evaluate some lumps that can be felt but are hard to see on a mammogram, especially in the dense breasts of young women. Unlike mammography, ultrasound cannot detect the microcalcifications that sometimes indicate cancer, nor does it pick up small tumors.

CT Scanning

Computed tomography, or CT scanning, uses a computer to organize and stack the information from multiple x-ray, cross-sectional views of a body's organ or area. The scans are made by having the source of an x-ray beam rotate around the patient. X-rays passing through the body are detected by sensors that pass the information to computers. Once processed, the information is displayed as an image on a video screen. CT can separate overlapping structures precisely and is sometimes helpful in locating breast abnormalities that are difficult to pinpoint with mammography or ultrasound—for instance, a tumor that is so close to the chest wall that it shows up in only one mammographic view.

Research on New Techniques

Several new techniques for imaging the breast are in the research stage. These include the use of magnetic resonance imaging (MRI) and positron emission tomography (PET scanning) to identify tissues that are abnormally active. MRI uses a large magnet to surround the patient along with radio frequencies and a computer to produce its images. PET scanning uses signals from radioactive traces to construct images. Laser beam scanning shines a powerful laser beam through the breast, while a special camera on the far side of the breast records the image.

Researchers are also striving to improve the detection power and diagnostic accuracy of mammography. Digital mammography is a technique for recording x-ray images in computer code, improving the detection of breast abnormalities. Computer-aided diagnosis, or CAD, uses special computer programs to scan mammographic images and alert radiologists to areas that look suspicious.

Finally, medical researchers are exploring the use of biological tests to detect tumor markers for breast cancer in blood, urine, or nipple aspirates.

Gene Testing for Breast Cancer Susceptibility

A breast cell progresses from normal to cancerous through a series of several distinct changes, each one controlled by a different gene or set of genes. Researchers have precisely located the BRCA1 and BRCA2 genes, key regions within a woman's chromosomes that control cell growth in breast tissue. A woman can inherit a mutation, an alteration in these genes that are essential for normal growth of breast cells, and this inherited change may put her at greater risk for eventually developing breast cancer. The recent identification of genetic changes in BRCA1 and BRCA2 makes a gene test possible.

Scientists estimate that alterations in the BRCA1 and BRCA2 genes may be responsible for about 5 to 10 percent of all the cases of breast cancer and for about 25 percent of the cases in women under the age of 30. BRCA1 mutation testing is primarily done in certain families whose members are inclined to develop breast cancer at an early age because of an inherited change. Special counseling programs occur before and after the testing to inform women about the possible consequences of receiving test results. It is hoped that these genetic tests may one day enable scientists to delay or prevent breast cancer in high-risk families. Positive results may enable careful watchfulness when appropriate; negative results may reassure those women in high-risk families who are at no greater than average risk for breast cancer.

Scientists at NCI and elsewhere believe that tests for alterations in genes that control growth in breast tissue and in other genes throughout the body require careful study to establish their appropriate use. In addition to BRCA1 and BRCA2, other genes and the proteins they control may be involved in breast cancer, and much more needs to be learned about the risk associated with particular genetic alterations. NCI supports research on the development of new genetic tests offered within a research setting and accompanied by genetic counseling. Counseling is important because test results must be properly understood, and a counselor can help persons with a positive test to handle possible discrimination in health or life insurance or in the workplace.

About Breast Lumps and Other Changes

Over her lifetime, a woman can encounter a broad variety of breast conditions. These include normal changes that occur during the menstrual cycle as well as several types of benign lumps. What they have in common is that they are not cancer. Even for breast lumps that require a biopsy, some 80 percent prove to be benign.

Each breast has 15 to 20 sections, called lobes, each with many smaller lobules. The lobules end in dozens of tiny bulbs that can produce milk. Lobes, lobules, and bulbs are all linked by thin tubes called ducts. These ducts lead to the nipple, which is centered in a dark area of skin called the areola. The spaces between the lobules and ducts are filled with fat. There are no muscles in the breast, but muscles lie under each breast and cover the ribs.

These normal features can sometimes make the breasts feel lumpy, especially in women who are thin or who have small breasts.

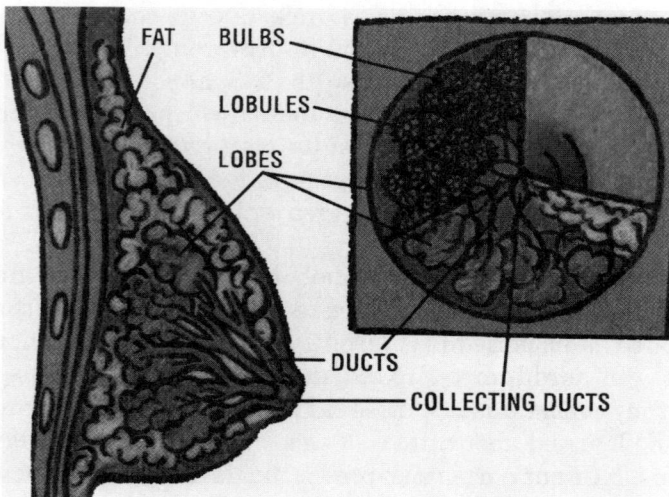

Figure 1.3. The breast's milk-producing system consists of lobes, lobules, and bulbs, all linked by thin tubes called ducts.

In addition, from the time a girl begins to menstruate, her breasts undergo regular changes each month. Many doctors believe that nearly all breasts develop some lasting changes, beginning when the woman is about 30 years old. Eventually, about half of all women will experience symptoms such as lumps, pain, or nipple discharge. Generally these disappear with menopause.

Some studies show that the chances of developing benign breast changes are higher for a woman who has never had children, has irregular menstrual cycles, or has a family history of breast cancer. Benign breast conditions are less common among women who take birth control pills or who are overweight. Because they generally involve the glandular tissues of the breast, benign breast conditions are more of a problem for women of child-bearing age, who have more glandular breasts.

Types of Benign Breast Changes

Common benign breast changes fall into several broad categories. These include generalized breast changes, solitary lumps, nipple discharge, and infection and/or inflammation.

Generalized Breast Changes

Generalized breast lumpiness is known by several names, including fibrocystic disease changes and benign breast disease. Such lumpiness, which is sometimes described as "ropy" or "granular," can often be felt in the area around the nipple and areola and in the upper-outer part of the breast. Such lumpiness may become more obvious as a woman approaches middle age and the milk-producing glandular tissue of her breasts increasingly gives way to soft, fatty tissue. Unless she is taking replacement hormones, this type of lumpiness generally disappears for good after menopause.

The menstrual cycle also brings cyclic breast changes. Many women experience swelling, tenderness, and pain before and sometimes during their periods. At the same time, one or more lumps or a feeling of increased lumpiness may develop because of extra fluid collecting in the breast tissue. These lumps normally go away by the end of the period.

During pregnancy, the milk-producing glands become swollen and the breasts may feel lumpier than usual. Although very uncommon, breast cancer has been diagnosed during pregnancy. If you have any questions about how your breasts feel or look, talk to your doctor.

17

Solitary Lumps

Benign breast conditions also include several types of distinct, solitary lumps. Such lumps, which can appear at any time, may be large or small, soft or rubbery, fluid-filled or solid.

Cysts are fluid-filled sacs. They occur most often in women ages 35 to 50, and they often enlarge and become tender and painful just before the menstrual period. They are usually found in both breasts. Some cysts are so small they cannot be felt; rarely, cysts may be several inches across. Cysts are usually treated by observation or by fine needle aspiration. They show up clearly on ultrasound. (See Aspirating a Cyst)

Fibroadenomas are solid and round benign tumors that are made up of both structural (fibro) and glandular (adenoma) tissues. Usually, these lumps are painless and found by the woman herself. They feel rubbery and can easily be moved around. Fibroadenomas are the most common type of tumors in women in their late teens and early twenties, and they occur twice as often in African-American women as in other American women.

Fibroadenomas have a typically benign appearance on mammography (smooth, round masses with a clearly defined edge), and they can sometimes be diagnosed with fine needle aspiration. Although fibroadenomas do not become malignant, they can enlarge with pregnancy and breast-feeding. Most surgeons believe that it is a good idea to remove fibroadenomas to make sure they are benign.

Fat necrosis is the name given to painless, round, and firm lumps formed by damaged and disintegrating fatty tissues. This condition typically occurs in obese women with very large breasts. It often develops in response to a bruise or blow to the breast, even though the woman may not remember the specific injury. Sometimes the skin around the lumps looks red or bruised. Fat necrosis can easily be mistaken for cancer, so such lumps are removed in a surgical biopsy. (See Biopsy)

Sclerosing adenosis is a benign condition involving the excessive growth of tissues in the breast's lobules. It frequently causes breast pain. Usually the changes are microscopic, but adenosis can produce lumps, and it can show up on a mammogram, often as calcifications. Short of biopsy, adenosis can be difficult to distinguish from cancer.

18

The usual approach is surgical biopsy, which furnishes both diagnosis and treatment.

Nipple Discharge

Nipple discharge accompanies some benign breast conditions. Since the breast is a gland, secretions from the nipple of a mature woman are not unusual, nor even necessarily a sign of disease. For example, small amounts of discharge commonly occur in women taking birth control pills or certain other medications, including sedatives and tranquilizers. If the discharge is being caused by a disease, the disease is more likely to be benign than cancerous.

Nipple discharges come in a variety of colors and textures. A milky discharge can be traced to many causes, including thyroid malfunction and oral contraceptives or other drugs. Women with generalized breast lumpiness may have a sticky discharge that is brown or green.

The doctor will take a sample of the discharge and send it to a laboratory to be analyzed. Benign sticky discharges are treated chiefly by keeping the nipple clean. A discharge caused by infection may require antibiotics.

One of the most common sources of a bloody or sticky discharge is an intraductal papilloma, a small, wartlike growth that projects into breast ducts near the nipple. Any slight bump or bruise in the area of the nipple can cause the papilloma to bleed. Single (solitary) intraductal papillomas usually affect women nearing menopause. If the discharge becomes bothersome, the diseased duct can be removed surgically without damaging the appearance of the breast. Multiple intraductal papillomas, in contrast, are more common in younger women. They often occur in both breasts and are more likely to be associated with a lump than with nipple discharge. Multiple intraductal papillomas, or any papillomas associated with a lump, need to be removed.

Infection and / or Inflammation

Infection and/or inflammation, including mastitis and mammary duct ectasia, are characteristic of some benign breast conditions.

Mastitis (sometimes called "postpartum mastitis") is an infection most often seen in women who are breast-feeding. A duct may become blocked, allowing milk to pool, causing inflammation, and setting the stage for infection by bacteria. The breast appears red and feels warm, tender, and lumpy.

19

In its earlier stages, mastitis can be cured by antibiotics. If a pus-containing abscess forms, it will need to be drained or surgically removed.

Mammary duct ectasia is a disease of women nearing menopause. Ducts beneath the nipple become inflamed and can become clogged. Mammary duct ectasia can become painful, and it can produce a thick and sticky discharge that is grey to green in color. Treatment consists of warm compresses, antibiotics, and, if necessary, surgery to remove the duct.

A word of caution: If you find a lump or other change in your breast, don't use this text to try to diagnose it yourself. There is no substitute for a doctor's evaluation.

Benign Breast Conditions and the Risk for Breast Cancer

Most benign breast changes do not increase a woman's risk for getting cancer. Recent studies show that only certain very specific types of microscopic changes put a woman at higher risk. These changes feature excessive cell growth, or hyperplasia.

About 70 percent of the women who have a biopsy showing a benign condition have no evidence of hyperplasia. These women are at no increased risk for breast cancer.

About 25 percent of benign breast biopsies show signs of hyperplasia, including conditions such as intraductal papilloma and sclerosing adenosis. Hyperplasia slightly increases the risk of developing breast cancer.

The remaining 5 percent of benign breast biopsies reveal both excessive cell growth—hyperplasia—and cells that are abnormal—atypia. A diagnosis of atypical hyperplasia, as it is called, moderately increases breast cancer risk.

If You Find a Lump

If you discover a lump in one breast, check the other breast. If both breasts feel the same, the lumpiness is probably normal. You should, however, mention it to your doctor at your next visit.

But if the lump is something new or unusual and does not go away after your next menstrual period, it is time to call your doctor. The same is true if you discover a discharge from the nipple or skin changes such as dimpling or puckering. If you do not have a doctor, your local medical society may be able to help you find one in your area.

You should not let fear delay you. It is natural to be concerned if you find a lump in your breast. But remember that four-fifths of all breast lumps are not cancer. The sooner any problem is diagnosed, the sooner you can have it treated.

Clinical Evaluation

No matter how your breast lump was discovered, the doctor will want to begin with your medical history. What symptoms do you have and how long have you had them? What is your age, menstrual status, general health? Are you pregnant? Are you taking any medications? How many children do you have? Do you have any relatives with benign breast conditions or breast cancer? Have you previously been diagnosed with benign breast changes?

The doctor will then carefully examine your breasts and will probably schedule you for a diagnostic mammogram, to obtain as much information as possible about the changes in your breast. This may be either a lump that can be felt or an abnormality discovered on a screening mammogram. Diagnostic mammography may include additional views or use special techniques to magnify a suspicious area or to eliminate shadows produced by overlapping layers of normal breast tissue. The doctor will want to compare the diagnostic mammograms with any previous mammograms. If the lump appears to be a cyst, your doctor may ask you to have a sonogram (ultrasound study).

Aspirating a Cyst

When a cyst is suspected, some doctors proceed directly with aspiration. This procedure, which uses a very thin needle and a syringe, takes only a few minutes and can be done in the doctor's office. The procedure is not usually very uncomfortable, since most of the nerves in the breast are in the skin.

Holding the lump steady, the doctor inserts the needle and attempts to draw out any fluid. If the lump is indeed a cyst, removing the fluid will cause the cyst to collapse and the lump to disappear. Unless the cyst reappears in the next week or two, no other treatment is needed. If the cyst reappears at a later date, it can simply be drained again.

If the lump turns out to be solid, it may be possible to use the needle to withdraw a clump of cells, which can then be sent to a laboratory for further testing. (Cysts are so rarely associated with cancer that the fluid removed from a cyst is not usually tested unless it is bloody or the woman is older than 55 years of age.)

Biopsy

The only certain way to learn whether a breast lump or mammographic abnormality is cancerous is by having a biopsy, a procedure in which tissue is removed by a surgeon or other specialist and examined under a microscope by a pathologist. A pathologist is a doctor who specializes in identifying tissue changes that are characteristic of disease, including cancer.

Tissue samples for biopsy can be obtained by either surgery or needle. The doctor's choice of biopsy technique depends on such things as the nature and location of the lump, as well as the woman's general health.

Surgical biopsies can be either excisional or incisional. An *excisional biopsy* removes the entire lump or suspicious area. Excisional biopsy is currently the standard procedure for lumps that are smaller than an inch or so in diameter. In effect, it is similar to a lumpectomy, surgery to remove the lump and a margin of surrounding tissue. Lumpectomy is usually used in combination with radiation therapy as the basic treatment for early breast cancer.

An excisional biopsy is typically performed in the outpatient department of a hospital. A local anesthetic is injected into the woman's breast. Sometimes she is given a tranquilizer before the procedure. The surgeon makes an incision along the contour of the breast and removes the lump along with a small margin of normal tissue. Because no skin is removed, the biopsy scar is usually small. The procedure typically takes less than an hour. After spending an hour or two in the recovery room, the woman goes home the same day.

An *incisional biopsy* removes only a portion of the tumor (by slicing into it) for the pathologist to examine. Incisional biopsies are generally reserved for tumors that are larger. They too are usually performed under local anesthesia, with the woman going home the same day.

Whether or not a surgical biopsy will change the shape of your breast depends partly on the size of the lump and where it is located in the breast, as well as how much of a margin of healthy tissue the surgeon decides to remove. You should talk with your doctor beforehand, so you understand just how extensive the surgery will be and what the cosmetic result will be.

Needle biopsies can be performed with either a very fine needle or a cutting needle large enough to remove a small nugget of tissue.

- *Fine needle aspiration* uses a very thin needle and syringe to remove either fluid from a cyst or clusters of cells from a solid mass. Accurate fine needle aspiration biopsy of a solid mass takes great skill, gained through experience with numerous cases.

- *Core needle biopsy* uses a somewhat larger needle with a special cutting edge. The needle is inserted, under local anesthesia, through a small incision in the skin, and a small core of tissue is removed. This technique may not work well for lumps that are very hard or very small. Core needle biopsy may cause some bruising, but rarely leaves an external scar, and the procedure is over in a matter of minutes.

At some institutions with extensive experience, aspiration biopsy is considered as reliable as surgical biopsy; it is trusted to confirm the malignancy of a clinically suspicious mass or to confirm a diagnosis that a lump is not cancerous. Should the needle biopsy results be uncertain, the diagnosis is pursued with a surgical biopsy. Some doctors prefer to verify all aspiration biopsy results with a surgical biopsy before proceeding with treatment.

Localization biopsy (also known as needle localization) is a procedure that uses mammography to locate and a needle to biopsy breast abnormalities that can be seen on a mammogram but cannot be felt (nonpalpable abnormalities). Localization can be used with surgical biopsy, fine needle aspiration, or core needle biopsy.

For a *surgical biopsy*, the radiologist locates the abnormality on a mammogram (or a sonogram) just prior to surgery. Using the mammogram as a guide, the radiologist inserts a fine needle or wire so the tip rests in the suspicious area—typically, an area of microcalcifications. The needle is anchored with a gauze bandage, and a second mammogram is taken to confirm that the needle is on target.

The woman, along with her mammograms, goes to the operating room, where the surgeon locates and cuts out the needle-targeted area. The more precisely the needle is placed, the less tissue needs to be removed.

Sometimes the surgeon will be able to feel the lump during surgery. In other cases, especially where the mammogram showed only microcalcifications, the abnormality can be neither seen nor felt. To make sure the surgical specimen in fact contains the abnormality, it is x-rayed on the spot. If this specimen x-ray fails to show the mass or the calcifications, the surgeon is able to remove additional tissue.

Stereotactic localization biopsy is a newer approach that relies on a three-dimensional x-ray to guide the needle biopsy of a nonpalpable mass. With one type of equipment, the patient lies face down on an examining table with a hole in it that allows the breast to hang through; the x-ray machine and the maneuverable needle "gun" are set up underneath. Alternatively, specialized stereotactic equipment can be attached to a standard mammography machine.

The breast is x-rayed from two different angles, and a computer plots the exact position of the suspicious area. (Because only a small area of the breast is exposed to the radiation, the doses are similar to those from standard mammography.) Once the target is clearly identified, the radiologist positions the gun and advances the biopsy needle into the lesion.

Tissue Studies

The cells or tissue removed through needle or surgical biopsy are promptly sent (along with the x-ray of the specimen, if one was made) to the pathology lab. If the excised lump is large enough, the pathologist can take a preliminary look by quick-freezing a small portion of the tissue sample. This makes the sample firm enough to slice into razor-thin sections that can be examined under the microscope. A "frozen section" provides an immediate, if provisional, diagnosis, and the surgeon may be able to give you the results before you go home.

The results of a frozen section are not 100 percent certain, however. A more thorough assessment takes several days, while the pathologist processes "permanent sections" of tissue that can be examined in greater detail.

When the biopsy specimen is small—as is often the case when the abnormality consists of mammographic calcifications only—many doctors prefer to bypass a frozen section so the tiny specimen can be analyzed in its entirety.

The pathologist looks for abnormal cell shapes and unusual growth patterns. In many cases the diagnosis will be clear-cut. However, the distinctions between benign and cancerous can be subtle, and even experts don't always agree. When in doubt, pathologists readily consult their colleagues. If there is any question about the results of your biopsy, you will want to make sure your biopsy slides have been reviewed by more than one pathologist.

Deciding to Biopsy

Not every lump or mammographic change merits a biopsy. Nearly all mammographic masses that look smooth and clearly outlined, for instance, are benign. Your doctor needs to thoughtfully weigh the findings from your physical exam and mammogram along with your background and your medical history when making a recommendation about a biopsy.

In general, doctors feel it is wise to biopsy any distinct and persistent lump.

Although benign lumps rarely, if ever, turn into cancer, cancerous lumps can develop near benign lumps and can be hidden on a mammogram. Even if you have had a benign lump removed in the past, you cannot be sure any new lump is also benign.

In some cases, the doctor may suggest watching the suspicious area for a month or two. Because many lumps are caused by normal hormonal changes, this waiting period may provide additional information.

Similarly, if the changes on your mammogram show all the signs of benign disease, your doctor may advise waiting several months and then taking another mammogram. This would be followed by more diagnostic mammograms over the next 3 years. If you choose this option, however, you must be strongly committed to regularly scheduled followups.

If you feel uncomfortable about waiting, express your concerns to your doctor. You may also want to get a second opinion, perhaps from a breast specialist or surgeon. Many cities have breast clinics where you can get a second opinion.

Biopsy: One Step or Two?

Not too many years ago, all women undergoing surgery for breast symptoms had a one-step procedure: If the surgical biopsy showed cancer, the surgeon performed a mastectomy immediately. The woman went into surgery not knowing if she had cancer or if her breast would be removed.

Today a woman facing biopsy has a broader range of options. In most cases, biopsy and diagnosis will be separated from any further treatment by an interval of several days or weeks. Such a two-step procedure does not harm the patient, and it has several benefits. It allows time for the tissue sample to be examined in detail and, if cancer is found, it gives the woman time to adjust to the diagnosis. She can review her treatment options, seek a second opinion, receive counseling, and arrange her schedule.

Some women, nonetheless, prefer a one-step procedure. They have decided beforehand that, if the surgical biopsy and frozen section show cancer, they want to go ahead with surgery, either mastectomy or lumpectomy and axillary dissection (removal of the underarm lymph nodes). If, on the other hand, the lump proves to be benign, the incision will be closed. The procedure will have taken less than an hour, and the woman may go home the same day or the next day.

A one-step procedure avoids the physical and psychological stress, as well as the costs in time and money, of two rounds of surgery and anesthesia—a particularly important consideration for women who are ill or frail. Women who have symptoms of breast cancer can find the wait between biopsy and surgery emotionally draining, and they may be relieved to have a one-step procedure to take care of the problem as quickly as possible.

No single solution is right for everyone. Each woman should consult with her doctors and her family, weigh the alternatives, and decide what approach is appropriate. Being involved in the decision-making process can give a woman a sense of control over her body and her life.

Prevention Research

Many of the factors that influence your chances of developing breast cancer—your age or inheritance of a breast cancer susceptibility gene—are beyond your control. Others present opportunities for change, and several large research studies are looking at possibilities for intervention—changing medication, diet, or behavior to prevent or delay onset of disease.

The Breast Cancer Prevention Trial is a randomized study of tamoxifen, a drug that has been widely used in the treatment of women with breast cancer. Because tamoxifen, when taken for 5 years, has been found to markedly reduce the occurrence of new cancers in the opposite breast of a woman who has already had breast cancer, it is now being tried as a prevention treatment in healthy women at increased risk for breast cancer either because they are age 60 or older, or because they are between the ages of 30 and 59 and have combinations of high-risk factors.

Nutrient chemoprevention is being tested in research studies in Italy, where women who have already been treated for breast cancer are taking 4-HPR, a synthetic form of vitamin A, in hopes of preventing cancer in the opposite breast. Other researchers are investigating the protective potential of several other vitamins, including C and E. Yet other scientists are checking out naturally occurring chemicals, called phytochemicals, found in common fruits, vegetables, and other edible plants, in hopes of finding cancer-fighting substances that can be extracted, purified, and added to our diets.

Diet itself is another target of prevention research. In the Women's Health Initiative, a project of the National Institutes of Health, 70,000 women over age 50 are enrolled in a series of clinical studies to measure the effectiveness of prevention strategies for coronary heart disease, cancer, and osteoporosis. Strategies under study include a low-fat diet (less than 20 percent of calories from fat) and calcium plus vitamin D supplements, along with hormone replacement therapy. Another large study evaluating a low-fat diet in high-risk women is under way in Canada.

A much more drastic approach to breast cancer prevention is surgery to remove both breasts. Such a procedure, known as prophylactic mastectomy, is sometimes chosen by women with a very high risk for breast cancer—for instance, carrying a genetic mutation in BRCA1 or BRCA2, having a mother and one or more sisters with premenopausal breast cancer, plus a diagnosis of atypical hyperplasia and a history of several breast biopsies.

Unless a woman finds that anxiety is undermining the quality of her life, she is usually counseled not to choose this physically and psychologically draining surgery. The vast majority of breasts removed prophylactically show no signs of cancer. Moreover, since even a total mastectomy can leave a small amount of breast tissue behind, it cannot guarantee the woman will remain cancer-free. The preferred approach for most high-risk women is careful watching with clinical breast exams and mammography once or twice a year.

If you are considering a prophylactic mastectomy, with or without subsequent breast reconstruction, you will want to get a second opinion, preferably from a breast specialist. There is seldom reason to rush your decision. Many doctors advise a woman to give herself several months to weigh the options.

If your risk for breast cancer is high, you might also consider talking with a genetic counselor about gene testing for breast cancer susceptibility. (See Gene Testing)

27

Steps to Take

Whether your risk of breast cancer is average or higher, there are some steps you can take:

- Follow early detection practices. Ask your doctor when you should begin mammograms at regular intervals. Get regular breast exams by a doctor or nurse.

- Consult your doctor about your personal situation and carefully weigh any potential risks against the benefits in making decisions about hormone-containing drugs. Stay informed as new research findings become available.

- Exercise and eat a balanced diet that provides a good variety of nutrients and plenty of fiber. Limit dietary fat and alcohol. These are good health measures that make sense for everyone.

Questions to Ask Your Doctor

We hope this information has answered many of your questions about breast changes and the early detection of breast cancer. However, no information in print or on the world wide web can take the place of talking with your doctor. Take any questions you have to your doctor. If you don't understand the answer, ask her or him to explain further.

Many women find it helpful to write down their questions ahead of time. Here is a list of some of the most common questions that women have. You may have others. Jot them down as you think of them, and take the list with you when you see your doctor.

- How often should I schedule appointments with you?

- How can I tell which lumps are not normal?

- What kind of lumps do I have?

- Do I need to have a mammogram? When? How often? Or if not, why not?

- Is there anything in my background that indicates I should have mammograms more often than your usual recommendations?

- Where should I have my mammogram?

- Did you receive the results of my mammogram? What does the report mean?

Chapter 2

Exercise Contributes to Breast Health

Exercise and the Risk of Breast Cancer

Exercise may be a way that women can lower their risk of breast cancer. Regular exercise is part of a healthy lifestyle and may help reduce the risk of several different diseases and improve the quality of life.

What evidence is there that exercise decreases a woman's risk of developing breast cancer?

There is encouraging evidence from both human and animal studies that exercise may reduce the risk of breast cancer. Among eleven human studies that took into account many of the established risk factors for breast cancer, eight reported a decrease in the risk of breast cancer in pre-menopausal, postmenopausal or all women with high levels of physical activity compared to women with low levels of activity. In the three studies in which exercise was not found to influence breast cancer risk, most of the women were younger and pre-menopausal. These results suggest that exercise may have a different influence on pre-menopausal versus postmenopausal breast cancer. The inconsistency of the results in these studies of exercise and breast cancer risk may also be due to

From "Exercise and the Risk of Breast Cancer," by Julie A. Napieralski, Ph.D. Research Associate, and Carol Devine, Ph.D., R.D. Division of Nutritional Sciences and Education Project Leader, Cornell University, Program on Breast Cancer and Environmental Risk Factors in New York State (BCERF), *FACT SHEET* #19, Institute for Comparative and Environmental Toxicology, Cornell Center for the Environment, January 1999; reprinted with permission.

differences in study design and how women reported their level of physical activity. Researchers are continuing to design studies to more specifically determine the relationship between exercise and breast cancer and to provide women with suggestions for incorporating appropriate levels of exercise in their daily routine.

In human studies, the relationship between exercise and breast cancer is complicated and difficult to study. Researchers must consider established risk factors for breast cancer, such as age at menarche (time of first menstrual cycle), age at first pregnancy, age at menopause, and family history, in their analysis. In addition, women who exercise may be different in other ways than women who do not exercise. For example, women who exercise may be less likely to smoke, may be leaner, and may eat differently than women who do not exercise. Researchers must consider all of these factors when trying to assess the influence of exercise on the risk of breast cancer.

In animal studies of exercise and breast cancer risk, the results depended on the kind of exercise program used. Animals that voluntarily exercised by using an exercise wheel placed in their cages had fewer mammary tumors compared to animals that did not have use of an exercise wheel. In other studies, a motorized treadmill was used to control the animal's level and frequency of exercise. Some researchers reported that this type of exercise, called involuntary exercise, reduced the incidence of mammary tumors while others reported that it either had no effect or increased the incidence of tumors. The stress of involuntary exercise may influence the growth of mammary tumors and account for the mixed results in these studies.

What is considered physical activity or exercise?

The words "physical activity" and "exercise" are used interchangeably in some studies and they are similar in some ways. Physical activity is a more general term to describe muscle movement that requires energy. For example, in the studies mentioned above, household chores, like vacuuming or cutting the grass, and work-related activities in occupations such as waitressing or nursing, were considered to be "physical activities". Exercise is a type of physical activity that a woman may plan to do specifically to improve her physical fitness. Exercise includes activities such as walking, dancing, playing tennis, or jogging. A complete assessment of all kinds of physical activity and exercise should include the frequency (times per week), duration (time spent in a particular activity), and intensity (how hard the body is working) of any kind of exercise or activity. Usually researchers measure work-related and leisure time activities separately to try to determine their effects on breast cancer risk independently.

Does occupational activity reduce the risk of breast cancer?

According to several large studies of occupational (work-related) activity, women who reported a high level of physical activity at work had an 18% to 52% reduction in their risk of developing breast cancer compared to women with low levels of activity at work. In these studies, some job titles that were considered to require high levels of physical activity were farmers, nurses and nurses' aides. Teachers, salespeople and waitresses were classified as having a moderate level of physical activity at work, and most office professionals as having very little activity. Job titles such as these are often used to study how work-related activity affected breast cancer risk. In other studies, women themselves were asked to rate how physically active they were at work. The difference in how researchers determined work-related activity may be one reason why these studies report such differences in risk reduction. It would be helpful if future studies consider the intensity, frequency, and duration of work-related activity and that women may have several different types of jobs or occupations during their lifetime.

Does recreational or leisure time activity reduce the risk of breast cancer?

In studies of recreational activity, women who exercised during their leisure time were reported to have a 12% to 60% reduction in their risk of developing breast cancer. This range in risk reduction may be due to differences in study design, such as how the researchers measured or defined different levels of physical activity and in how the researchers questioned women about their level of activity. Some of the researchers focused their attention on athletes, while others asked women to describe their level of activity based on a scale, or by selecting from a list of activities such as walking, jogging, aerobics, dancing or swimming. It may also be important for researchers to ask women about their lifetime participation in exercise activities, not just their recent levels of activity.

What kind of physical activity or exercise is the most beneficial?

It is not clear whether physical activity at work or exercise during leisure time is more effective at reducing the risk of breast cancer.

Also, studies that have attempted to combine occupational and recreational activities in one analysis have not shown any additional protective effects compared to studies that have analyzed one or the other separately. In most studies, women were asked if they participated in moderate or vigorous exercise that caused them to sweat. This could include specific kinds of activities, like participation in competitive sports, swimming, brisk walking or jogging. However, any activity that caused them to sweat and increased breathing and heart rate may have been called physical activity in these studies.

How much do I have to exercise to influence the risk of breast cancer?

Women need to consider their age, health, and overall fitness level and should consult with their physicians before starting any exercise program. In the report *Healthy People 2000*, the U.S. Department of Health and Human Services sets goals and provides suggestions regarding physical activity levels. *Americans should try to engage in light to moderate physical activity for at least 30 minutes, five or more times per week.* An example of this type of activity is a sustained walk. The report suggests that if this schedule is not possible, it is also acceptable to participate in physical activity intermittently, but at least three times per week. The goal is to make people aware of the importance of physical activity and to encourage them to make some daily life changes for their own health and well being.

Some studies have reported that athletes who exercised vigorously and participated in competitive sports had a lower risk of breast cancer than did non-athletes. However, others have reported that women who do not participate in competitive sports but who exercised regularly, such as three hours per week throughout their reproductive years, had a lower risk of breast cancer as compared to women who never exercised. Until researchers establish a more consistent and direct way of measuring exercise, it is not possible to specify the amount of exercise that is associated with reduced breast cancer risk.

When in a woman's life is exercise important?

The currently available information is contradictory as to whether exercise is more beneficial during adolescence, during adulthood or during a woman's entire life. It may be important to exercise early in life, such as during adolescence, because this may be a critical time period for the development of breast cancer. Also, establishing an exercise habit early may be important to maintain a good lifetime habit. One study demonstrated that women under age 40 who averaged 3.8 hours of exercise per week during their reproductive years had about a 60% decrease in the risk of breast cancer. Another study reported that women who were athletes in college remained more physically active than non-athletes later in life, and their risk of breast cancer was reduced by about 50%. Other researchers have not found that exercise during adolescence is any more helpful than current exercise habits.

Is exercise helpful for women who are undergoing treatment for breast cancer?

Several studies have reported that exercise benefits women diagnosed with breast cancer both during and after conventional treatments such as surgery, chemotherapy, and/or radiation. In particular, women with breast cancer who exercised reported having higher self-esteem, improved body image, less nausea during chemotherapy treatment, and less fatigue, depression and insomnia. Women who exercised also had improvements in physical performance and a higher quality of life. For example, in one study, women who walked at their own pace for 20 to 30 minutes 4-5 times per week, reported feeling less fatigued, less emotionally distressed, and had an improved physical performance level.

Also, weight gain is a troublesome and potentially serious problem for breast cancer patients undergoing chemotherapy. In one study, the patients who gained more weight during treatment were more likely to relapse and were more likely to die of their breast cancer than patients who gained less weight. Breast cancer patients who exercise while undergoing treatment may gain less weight compared to patients who do not exercise.

Women undergoing therapy for breast cancer may want to talk to their physicians about starting an exercise program.

How might exercise influence the risk of breast cancer?

There are several possible biological explanations for the influence of exercise on the development of breast cancer. Exercise may:

Influence age at menarche. An early age at menarche, the age at which a girl has her first menstrual period, is an established risk factor for breast cancer. Several studies have reported that girls who exercise regularly have a later age at menarche compared to inactive girls.

Alter the menstrual cycle. A few studies have reported that exercise may favorably alter the menstrual cycle. The alterations in the menstrual cycle caused by exercise may lead to a decrease in estrogen levels. Estrogen is a hormone necessary for reproductive development and health in women, but increased levels of estrogen over a lifetime have been associated with an increase in the risk of breast cancer. Activities that lower the level of estrogen in a woman's body may decrease her risk of developing breast cancer.

Decrease weight gain and overall weight. Some studies have reported that gaining weight during adulthood and being overweight as an adult are risk factors for postmenopausal breast cancer. Physical activity and exercise may help women to maintain a healthy weight and reduce their risk of breast cancer. Exercise may be particularly important to help postmenopausal women avoid weight gain.

Enhance the immune system. Several studies have reported that moderate exercise may enhance the immune system. A healthy immune system helps the body fight diseases such as cancer.

Should I exercise to reduce my risk of developing breast cancer?

While we wait for conclusive evidence regarding the influence of exercise on the risk of developing breast cancer, we already know that there are many other reasons for women to exercise. Regular physical activity in women reduces overall mortality, and the incidence of coronary heart disease, diabetes, stroke, osteoporosis, and obesity. Also, women who exercise report feeling better and have a better body image compared to women who don't exercise.

Below is a list of different kinds of physical activities and suggestions for how we can incorporate more activity into our daily lives:

- Walk briskly
- Clean the house
- Mow the lawn
- Golf: using a pull cart or carrying the clubs
- Dance
- Play table-tennis
- Use the stairs instead of the elevator
- Bike to work

- Park your car further from the entrance to the store or your workplace

People who are willing and physically able can also participate in other more vigorous activities such as running, swimming, aerobics, or competitive sports.

Cornell University Program on Breast Cancer and Environmental Risk Factors in New York State

An extensive bibliography on "Exercise and the Risk of Breast Cancer" is available on the BCERF web site http://www.cfe.cornell.edu/bcerf/

We hope you find this chapter informative. We welcome your comments. When reproducing this material, credit the Program on Breast Cancer and Environmental Risk Factors in New York State.

Funding for this fact sheet was made possible by the U.S. Department of Agriculture/Cooperative State Research, Education and Extension Service, and Cornell University.

Cornell University
Program on Breast Cancer and Environmental Risk Factors in New York State
112 Rice Hall
Ithaca, NY 14853-5601
Phone: (607) 254-2893
Fax: (607) 255-8207
email: breastcancer@cornell.edu
Internet: http://www.cfe.cornell.edu/bcerf/

—Julie A. Napieralski, Ph.D. Research Associate, BCERF and Carol Devine, Ph.D., R.D. Division of Nutritional Sciences and Education Project Leader, BCERF

Chapter 3

Breastfeeding and Its Role in Breast Health

Breastfeeding and the Risk of Breast Cancer

Breastfeeding may offer some modest protection against the development of breast cancer, particularly in young women. Considering the other health benefits of breastfeeding for both mothers and their babies, this information should encourage new mothers to try to arrange their schedules to accommodate breastfeeding.

Does breastfeeding influence the risk of breast cancer?

Breastfeeding may modestly reduce the risk of developing breast cancer. Out of 31 studies, more than half reported that women who breastfed had a decreased risk of developing breast cancer (ranging from 10%-64%) compared to women who never breastfed. The rest of the studies reported that breastfeeding had no influence on the risk of developing breast cancer.

The results of these studies may vary because of differences in the pattern of breastfeeding among women in different cultures, such as when solid foods are added, how often a child is fed, and the reasons for stopping breastfeeding. Another reason may be that some studies

From "Breast-feeding and the Risk of Breast Cancer," by Julie A. Napieralski, Ph.D. Research Associate, and Carol Devine, Ph.D., R.D. Division of Nutritional Sciences and Education Project Leader, Cornell University, Program on Breast Cancer and Environmental Risk Factors in New York State (BCERF), *FACT SHEET* #29, Institute for Comparative and Environmental Toxicology, Cornell Center for the Environment, May 1999; reprinted with permission.

used information on the average length of time of breastfeeding per child, while others asked for the total length of time of breastfeeding all children combined. In addition, other reproductive factors, such as number of children and a woman's age at first birth, are very closely related to breastfeeding and may also influence breast cancer risk. Other issues being studied include whether the age at which a woman first breastfeeds is important, and the effects of breastfeeding in women with a family history of breast cancer. Finally, it is also possible that breastfeeding has different effects on the risk of developing premenopausal breast cancer compared to postmenopausal breast cancer.

Does breastfeeding influence the risk of premenopausal and postmenopausal breast cancer differently?

Breastfeeding may be more protective against the development of premenopausal compared to postmenopausal breast cancer. In some studies where there was no overall reduction in breast cancer risk associated with breastfeeding, an analysis of the data by menopausal status revealed a slight protective effect of breastfeeding in younger premenopausal women. Many other studies that focused specifically on young women reported that the incidence of premenopausal breast cancer was lower among women who breastfed. Many researchers think that premenopausal breast cancer and postmenopausal breast cancer are different diseases. However, it is not clear why breastfeeding may be more protective against premenopausal breast cancer than postmenopausal breast cancer.

How long should women breastfeed?

Although there are a few studies that report a decrease in the risk of breast cancer after only three or more months of breastfeeding, the evidence for risk reduction becomes more consistent the longer women breastfeed. The most consistent evidence of a relationship between breastfeeding and the risk of breast cancer has been reported in studies of Chinese women who breastfed for long periods of time.

In these studies, women who breastfed for a total of six years or more (all children combined) over the course of their lives had as much as a 63% decrease in breast cancer incidence compared to women who never breastfed.

The American Academy of Pediatrics recommends that women begin breastfeeding within the first hour after birth if possible. For most women, exclusive breastfeeding is recommended for about the first six months and breastfeeding should continue for at least 12 months thereafter. In the report *Healthy People 2000*, the US Department of Health and Human Services set goals to: 1) increase to at least 75% the proportion of mothers who breastfeed their babies in the early postpartum period, and 2) increase to at least 50%, the proportion who continue breastfeeding until their babies are five to six months old.

Is there any evidence that drugs used to suppress lactation influence breast cancer risk?

Studies that examined the use of drugs to suppress lactation reported that these drugs do not have any influence on the risk of developing breast cancer.

Should breast cancer survivors breastfeed?

Since there are relatively few cases of breast cancer in premenopausal women, there are also very few studies that have looked at the effects of treatment for breast cancer on breastfeeding. The ability to breastfeed after treatment for breast cancer depends on the individual and on the treatment she received. Surgery and radiation may impair a woman's ability to breastfeed on the affected side. Radiation may cause skin damage during treatment similar to sunburn or chapped skin and, in order to avoid infection so treatment can continue, it is usually recommended that breastfeeding from the breast being treated be stopped. In some cases, women reported that there seemed to be less milk produced in the irradiated breast. However, they were able to breastfeed from the untreated breast. Other women have reported that they were able to breastfeed from both the treated and the untreated breast after radiation treatment.

Lumps are common in the breasts of women who are breastfeeding. Not all are cancer, but all should be evaluated seriously by a health care provider. Women should feel comfortable getting a second opinion about a persistent lump. Although physical changes in the breasts of women who are pregnant or breastfeeding may hide a lump, women who are breastfeeding should examine their breasts for changes or abnormalities. The best time to examine the breasts is immediately after a feeding. Women should talk to their health care providers about any unusual physical changes in their breasts while they are breastfeeding.

Women needing to undergo any kind of treatment for breast cancer, including surgery, chemotherapy, or radiation should talk with their health care providers if breastfeeding is a concern. It may be possible to breastfeed before and after surgery and through radiation, though probably not on the side being irradiated. Since many drugs may be passed to an infant through breast milk, breastfeeding women should always talk with their health care providers about any medications they are taking.

How might breastfeeding influence the risk of breast cancer?

There are several ways that breastfeeding may influence the risk of developing breast cancer. Breastfeeding may

- Cause hormonal changes, such as a decrease in the level of estrogen. Lower levels of estrogen may decrease a woman's risk of developing breast cancer.

- Suppress ovulation. According to some studies, women who have fewer ovulatory cycles over the course of their reproductive lives may have a decreased risk of developing breast cancer.

- Remove possible carcinogens that are stored in the adipose tissue of the breast (see below for more information).

- Cause physical changes in the cells that line the mammary ducts. These changes may make the cells more resistant to mutations that can lead to cancer.

Does breastfeeding influence the risk of breast cancer for the baby?

There is some preliminary evidence that there may be a slight decrease in the risk of developing breast cancer among women who were breastfed as infants. This protection may be due to the hormones and immune factors present in breast milk. It may also be due to the fact that babies who are breastfed take in fewer calories and gain weight more slowly than babies who are bottle fed. There are some studies that report that earlier maturation in childhood may increase the risk of developing breast cancer later in life.

In other preliminary studies, no association was found between being breastfed as an infant and the development of breast cancer later in life. In addition, one study reported that there was no difference in the risk of breast cancer among women who had been breastfed by a mother who eventually developed the disease.

Are there any health concerns associated with breast-feeding?

Breastmilk is considered to be the ideal nutrient source for infants. However, because certain chemicals persist in the environment, are stored in fat and secreted in breast milk, they have been studied by researchers at the National Institute of Environmental Health Sciences (NIEHS). These researchers concluded that in the *vast majority* of women the benefits of breastfeeding appear to outweigh possible risks.

In only a few cases, women should consult with their health care providers before breastfeeding. These cases include women with certain infectious diseases, women who have been taking prescription or street drugs, or women who may be exposed to high levels of certain environmental contaminants. There are only a few circumstances that may lead to some women having high levels of chemicals in their breast milk. These circumstances are 1) having a history of workplace exposure to environmental chemicals, 2) having a large accidental exposure and 3) regularly consuming fish that are caught in contaminated waters (this does not include fish bought in supermarkets).

Women can obtain information on the safety of consuming fish caught in different statewide bodies of water from the New York State Department of Health (DOH) by accessing their website at http://www.health.state.ny.us/nysdoh/environ/fish98.htm, by calling the Center for Environmental Health at 1-800-458-1158 to request a fish advisory, or by picking up a hunting and fishing guide at any store that sells hunting and fishing equipment. According to the 1998-1999 report on "Chemicals in Sportfish and Game", DOH recommends that women of childbearing age, infants, and children under the age of 15 do not eat any fish from the specific water bodies listed in the advisory. Information on the safety of consuming fish in bodies of water throughout the United States can be obtained by calling the Environmental Protection Agency at: 1-513-489-8190. Also, researchers at the Bureau of Toxic Substance Assessment in the DOH (led by Dr. Judith Schreiber) are continuing to assess the effects of various environmental chemicals on human health.

For more information, women can obtain a helpful review from the US Department of Health and Human Services by calling 1-703-356-1964 and requesting a copy of the "Maternal and Child Health Technical Information Bulletin: A review of the medical benefits and contraindications to breastfeeding in the United States" by Dr. Ruth Lawrence.

What are the other health benefits of breastfeeding?

There are many important health benefits associated with breastfeeding for both the mother and the baby. Babies who are breastfed have a lower incidence or severity of several childhood illnesses including diarrhea, lower respiratory infections, ear infections, and bacterial meningitis. Other possible protective effects have been reported against sudden infant death syndrome, allergic diseases, and chronic digestive diseases.

Women who breastfeed their infants have less postpartum bleeding and may have an earlier return to pre-pregnant weight. There is also some evidence that they have an improved bone remineralization after they stop breastfeeding, which may lead to a reduction in hip fractures during the postmenopausal years.

Cornell University Program on Breast Cancer and Environmental Risk Factors in New York State

An extensive bibliography on *Breastfeeding and the Risk of Breast Cancer* is available on the BCERF web site: http://www.cfe.cornell.edu/bcerf/

Funding for this project was made possible by Cornell University, the US Department of Agriculture/Cooperative State Research, Education and Extension Service and the New York State Department of Health.

We hope you find this text informative. We welcome your comments. When reproducing this material, credit the Program on Breast Cancer and Environmental Risk Factors in New York State.

Cornell University Program on Breast Cancer and Environmental Risk Factors in New York State
112 Rice Hall
Ithaca, NY 14853-5601
Phone: (607) 254-2893
Fax: (607) 255-8207
email: breastcancer@cornell.edu
Internet: http://www.cfe.cornell.edu/bcerf/

—Julie A. Napieralski, Ph.D. Research Associate, BCERF
and Carol Devine, Ph.D., R.D. Division of Nutritional Sciences
and Education Project Leader, BCERF

Chapter 4

Breast Self-Examination

One of the most important things you can do for your health is to get to know your breasts. Breast Self-Examination (BSE) is the way for you to notice any changes in your breasts—changes that could be signs of breast cancer. If you should notice an unusual lump, discharge or any other change during the month—whether or not you notice it during BSE—contact your doctor. The earlier the doctor can examine it, the better. Most lumps are not cancer but all changes that you find should be checked out. Do BSE every month, have an exam by a doctor each year and have regular mammograms. Doing these things can help save your life.

When to Do BSE

If you still menstruate (have your period), the best time is two or three days after your period ends. These are the days when your breasts are least likely to be tender or swollen. If you no longer menstruate, pick the same day of every month. It will be easy to remember.

If you take hormones, check with your doctor about the best time for your BSE.

"Keep in Touch: Do BSE," Document 0407, Department of Health, State of New York, March 2001; reprinted with permission.

How to Do BSE

Step 1: Stand in front of a mirror that lets you see your breasts clearly. Look at both breasts. You are looking for anything unusual. This includes puckered, dimpled or scaly skin, or any discharge (clear or colored fluid) from the nipples.

Step 2: Now, look carefully to see if there is any change in the shape of your breasts. First, clasp your hands behind your head and press your hands forward.

Step 3: Next, press your hands on your hips—firmly—and continue to look for changes in the shape of your breasts. Bend slightly toward the mirror as you hunch your shoulders and pull your elbows forward.

Step 4: Begin examining your breasts for lumps and thickness, using one of the different patterns shown in Figures 4.6 and 4.7. Raise one arm, putting your hand behind your head. With the opposite hand, use the pads of your fingers (the flat part) to check the breast, the area between the breast and underarm, the underarm itself and the area above the breast, up to the collarbone and over to your shoulder. Check each area firmly, carefully, and completely.

Some women prefer to do this in the shower. It's a good idea, because fingers glide easily over soapy skin, making it easier to feel for changes underneath.

Step 5: Repeat step 4 lying down. Lie flat on your back, with your right hand behind your head and a pillow or folded towel under your right shoulder. With your left hand, examine the right breast and area around it very carefully. Then switch hands and repeat the procedure for the left breast. You can use either of the patterns listed.

Choose Your Pattern

Use one of the following two patterns to examine your breasts. The one you choose is not important. What's important is that you don't miss any areas.

Lines

Begin in the underarm area and move your fingers down until they are below the breast. Move your fingers in toward the center and go slowly back up. Cover the whole area, going up and down.

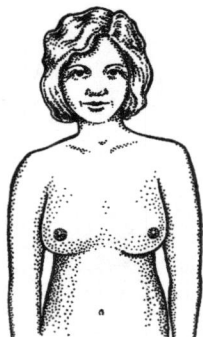

Figure 4.1. *Step 1. Check breasts in a mirror.*

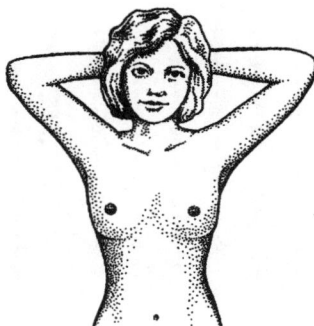

Figure 4.2. *Step 2. Check the shape of your breasts with hands behind head.*

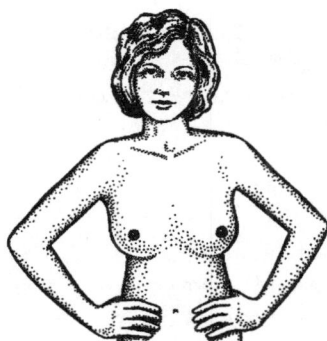

Figure 4.3. *Step 3. Check the shape of your breasts with hands on hips.*

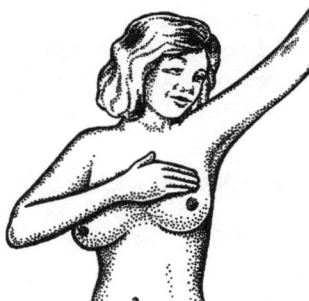

Figure 4.4. *Step 4. Use your fingers to examine your breasts for lumps and thickness.*

Figure 4.5. *Step 5. Repeat the examination while lying down.*

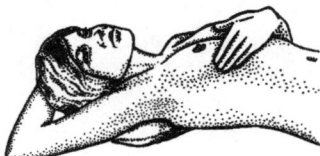

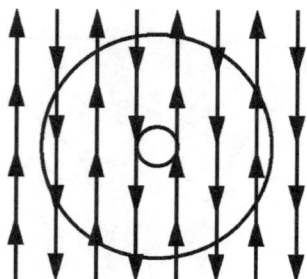

Lines

Figure 4.6. Line pattern for breast self-examination.

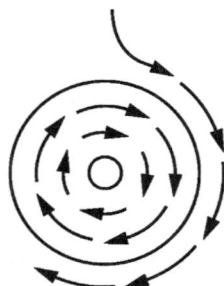

Circles

Figure 4.7. Circle pattern for breast self-examination.

Circles

Begin at the outer edge of your breast, moving your fingers slowly around the entire breast. When you come back to where you started, make a smaller circle and do it again. Continue, working toward the nipple. Check your underarm and upper chest areas, too.

Who Should Do BSE and Why?

Breast cancer is the number two cause of cancer-related deaths in women. Any woman can get breast cancer. Ninety-five percent of early breast cancer is curable. BSE can help you notice changes in your breasts. You can do BSE—and it only takes ten minutes a month.

Most (80%) lumps are not cancer (but all lumps and other changes in the breast should be checked out by a doctor). You should have a clinical breast exam every three years if you are between the ages of 20 and 40, and every year if you are over 40.

Have a mammogram. It can find breast cancer years before you can. The American Cancer Society recommends having a mammogram every year if you are 40 or older.

Women who do BSE and have regular exams and mammograms are keeping in touch with their breast health. Keep in touch for the rest of your life!

Chapter 5

Prevention of Breast Cancer

What Is Prevention?

Doctors can not always explain why one person gets cancer and another does not. However, scientists have studied general patterns of cancer in the population to learn what things around us and what things we do in our lives may increase our chance of developing cancer.

Anything that increases a person's chance of developing a disease is called a risk factor; anything that decreases a person's chance of developing a disease is called a protective factor. Some of the risk factors for cancer can be avoided, but many can not. For example, although you can choose to quit smoking, you can not choose which genes you have inherited from your parents. Both smoking and inheriting specific genes could be considered risk factors for certain kinds of cancer, but only smoking can be avoided. Prevention means avoiding the risk factors and increasing the protective factors that can be controlled so that the chance of developing cancer decreases.

Although many risk factors can be avoided, it is important to keep in mind that avoiding risk factors does not guarantee that you will not get cancer. Also, most people with a particular risk factor for cancer do not actually get the disease. Some people are more sensitive than others to factors that can cause cancer. Talk to your doctor about methods of preventing cancer that might be effective for you.

National Cancer Institute, PDQ®, August 2000.

The purposes of this summary on breast cancer prevention are to:

- give information on breast cancer and how often it occurs
- describe breast cancer prevention methods
- give current facts about which people or groups of people would most likely be helped by following breast cancer prevention methods

You can talk to your doctor or health care professional about cancer prevention methods and whether they would be likely to help you.

Breast Cancer Prevention

The breast consists of lobes, lobules, and bulbs that are connected by ducts. The breast also contains blood and lymph vessels. These lymph vessels lead to structures that are called lymph nodes. Clusters of lymph nodes are found under the arm, above the collarbone, in the chest, and in other parts of the body. Together, the lymph vessels and lymph nodes make up the lymphatic system, which circulates a fluid called lymph throughout the body. Lymph contains cells that help fight infection and disease.

When breast cancer spreads outside the breast, cancer cells are most often found under the arm in the lymph nodes. In many cases, if the cancer has reached the lymph nodes, cancer cells may have also spread to other parts of the body via the lymphatic system or through the bloodstream.

Breast cancer is second only to lung cancer as the leading cause of cancer death among women in the United States. Breast cancer occurs in men also, but the number of new cases is small. Early detection and effective treatment is expected to reduce the number of women who die from breast cancer, and development of new methods of prevention continue to be studied.

Breast cancer can sometimes be associated with known risk factors for the disease. Many risk factors are modifiable though not all can be avoided.

Tamoxifen for Prevention of Breast Cancer

Tamoxifen is a drug that blocks the effect of estrogen on breast cancer cells. A large study has shown that tamoxifen lowers the risk of getting breast cancer in women who are at elevated risk of getting breast cancer. However, tamoxifen may also increase the risk of getting some other serious diseases, including endometrial cancer, stroke, and blood clots in veins and in the lungs. Women who are concerned that they may be at an increased risk of developing breast cancer should talk with their doctor about whether to take tamoxifen to prevent breast cancer. It is important to consider both the benefits and risks of taking tamoxifen.

Hormonal Factors

Hormones produced by the ovaries appear to increase a woman's risk for developing breast cancer. The removal of one or both ovaries reduces the risk. The use of drugs that suppress the production of estrogen may inhibit tumor cell growth. The use of hormone replacement therapy may be associated with an increased risk of developing breast cancer, mostly in recent users. The use of oral contraceptives may also be associated with a slight increase in breast cancer risk.

Beginning to menstruate at an older age and having a full-term pregnancy reduces breast cancer risk. Also, a woman who has her first child before the age of 20 experiences a greater decrease in breast cancer risk than a woman who has never had children or who has her first child after the age of 35. Beginning menopause at a later age increases a woman's risk of developing breast cancer.

Radiation

Studies have shown that reducing the number of chest x-rays, especially at a young age, decreases the risk of breast cancer. Radiation treatment for childhood Hodgkin's disease may put women at a greater risk for breast cancer later in life. A small number of breast cancer cases can be linked to radiation exposure.

Diet and Lifestyle

Diet is being studied as a risk factor for breast cancer. Studies show that in populations that consume a high-fat diet, women are more likely to die of breast cancer than women in populations that consume a low-fat diet. It is not known if a diet low in fat will prevent breast cancer. Studies also show that certain vitamins may decrease a woman's risk of breast cancer, especially premenopausal women at high risk. Exercise, especially in young women, may decrease hormone levels and contribute to a decreased breast cancer risk. Breast feeding may also decrease a woman's risk of breast cancer. Studies suggest that the consumption of alcohol is associated with a slight increase in the risk of developing breast cancer. Postmenopausal weight gain, especially after natural menopause and/or after age 60, may increase breast cancer risk.

Prophylactic Mastectomy

Following cancer risk assessment and counseling, the removal of both breasts may reduce the risk of breast cancer in women with a family history of breast cancer.

Genetics

Women who inherit specific genes are at a greater risk for developing breast cancer. Research is underway to develop methods of identifying high-risk genes.

Drugs Being Studied

Fenretinide and raloxifene are two other drugs that are being studied for their usefulness as potential breast cancer prevention agents.

Part Two

Breast Cancer Fundamentals

Chapter 6

Lifetime Probability of Breast Cancer in American Women

A report from the National Cancer Institute (NCI) estimates that about 1 in 8 women in the United States (approximately 12.6 percent) will develop breast cancer during her lifetime.

This estimate is based on data from NCI's Surveillance, Epidemiology, and End Results Program (SEER) publication *SEER Cancer Statistics Review 1973-1996* and is based on cancer rates from 1994 through 1996. This figure includes all age groups in 5-year intervals up to an open-ended interval of 95 years and over. Each age interval is assigned a weight in the calculations based on the proportion of the population living to that age.

The 1 in 8 figure means that, if current rates stay constant, a female born today has a 1 in 8 chance of developing breast cancer sometime during her life. On the other hand, she has a 7 in 8 chance of never developing breast cancer. Because the SEER calculations are weighted, they take into account that not all women live to older ages, when breast cancer risk becomes the greatest. Table 6.1 provides details about a woman's chance of being diagnosed with breast cancer.

In evaluating cancer risk for a cancer-free individual at a specific point in time, age-specific (conditional) probabilities are more appropriate than lifetime probabilities. For example, at age 50, a cancer-free black woman has about a 2.4 percent chance of developing breast cancer by age 60, and a cancer-free white woman has about a 2.8 percent chance.

Cancer Facts, National Cancer Institute, March 2000.

Among the racial/ethnic groups studied by SEER, white, Hawaiian, and black women have the highest levels of breast cancer risk. Asian/Pacific Islander and Hispanic women have a lower level of risk; their chance of developing breast cancer is less than two-thirds of the risk of white women. The lowest levels of risk occur among Korean, Native American, and Vietnamese women.

These probabilities are based on population averages. An individual woman's breast cancer risk may be higher or lower, depending upon a variety of factors, including family history, reproductive history, and other factors that are not yet fully understood.

The NCI is directing special attention to women with disproportionately high rates of breast cancer and poor survival rates, including members of certain minority groups and the medically underserved. Efforts targeted at these groups are under way in all components of NCI's program: basic research, early detection, clinical trials, rehabilitation, education and information dissemination, and cancer centers.

Table 6.1. A Woman's Chance of Being Diagnosed with Breast Cancer

Age	Chance of Being Diagnosed with Breast Cancer
by age 30	1 out of 2,212
by age 40	1 out of 235
by age 50	1 out of 54
by age 60	1 out of 23
by age 70	1 out of 14
by age 80	1 out of 10
Ever	1 out of 8

Source: Feuer EJ, Wun LM. *DEVCAN: Probability of Developing or Dying of Cancer.* Version 4.0. Bethesda MD: National Cancer Institute. 1999.

Chapter 7

What You Need to Know about Breast Cancer

Introduction

Other than skin cancer, breast cancer is the most common type of cancer among women in the United States. More than 180,000 women are diagnosed with breast cancer each year. The National Cancer Institute (NCI) has written this text to help patients with breast cancer and their families and friends better understand this disease. We hope others will read it as well to learn more about breast cancer.

This chapter discusses screening and early detection, symptoms, diagnosis, treatment, and rehabilitation. It also has information to help patients cope with breast cancer.

Research has led to progress against breast cancer—better treatments, a lower chance of death from the disease, and improved quality of life. Through research, knowledge about breast cancer keeps increasing. Scientists are learning more about what causes breast cancer and are exploring new ways to prevent, detect, diagnose, and treat this disease.

Male Breast Cancer

Breast cancer affects more than 1,000 men in this country each year. Although this chapter was written mainly for women, much of the information on symptoms, diagnosis, treatment, and living with

National Cancer Institute (NCI), NIH Pub. No. 00-1556, updated December 2000.

the disease applies to men as well. However, the "Detecting Breast Cancer" section does not apply to men. Experts do not recommend routine screening for men.

The Breasts

Each breast has 15 to 20 sections called lobes. Within each lobe are many smaller lobules. Lobules end in dozens of tiny bulbs that can produce milk. The lobes, lobules, and bulbs are all linked by thin tubes called ducts. These ducts lead to the nipple in the center of a dark area of skin called the areola. Fat surrounds the lobules and ducts. There are no muscles in the breast, but muscles lie under each breast and cover the ribs.

Each breast also contains blood vessels and lymph vessels. The lymph vessels carry colorless fluid called lymph, and lead to small bean-shaped organs called lymph nodes. Clusters of lymph nodes are found near the breast in the axilla (under the arm), above the collarbone, and in the chest. Lymph nodes are also found in many other parts of the body.

Understanding the Cancer Process

Cancer is a group of many related diseases that begin in cells, the body's basic unit of life. To understand cancer, it is helpful to know what happens when normal cells become cancerous.

The body is made up of many types of cells. Normally, cells grow and divide to produce more cells only when the body needs them. This orderly process helps keep the body healthy. Sometimes, however, cells keep dividing when new cells are not needed. These extra cells form a mass of tissue, called a growth or tumor. Tumors can be benign or malignant.

- **Benign tumors** are not cancer. They can usually be removed, and in most cases, they do not come back. Cells from benign tumors do not spread to other parts of the body. Most important, benign breast tumors are not a threat to life.

- **Malignant tumors** are cancer. Cells in these tumors are abnormal. They divide without control or order, and they can invade and damage nearby tissues and organs. Also, cancer cells can break away from a malignant tumor and enter the bloodstream or the lymphatic system. That is how cancer spreads from the original (primary) cancer site to form new tumors in other organs. The spread of cancer is called metastasis.

56

When cancer arises in breast tissue and spreads (metastasizes) outside the breast, cancer cells are often found in the lymph nodes under the arm (axillary lymph nodes). If the cancer has reached these nodes, it means that cancer cells may have spread to other parts of the body—other lymph nodes and other organs, such as the bones, liver, or lungs. When cancer spreads from its original location to another part of the body, the new tumor has the same kind of abnormal cells and the same name as the primary tumor. For example, if breast cancer spreads to the brain, the cancer cells in the brain are actually breast cancer cells. The disease is called metastatic breast cancer. (It is not brain cancer.) Doctors sometimes call this "distant" disease.

This chapter deals with breast cancer. For information about benign breast lumps and other benign breast changes, read NCI's booklet, *Understanding Breast Changes: A Health Guide for All Women*.

Breast Cancer: Who's at Risk?

The exact causes of breast cancer are not known. However, studies show that the risk of breast cancer increases as a woman gets older. This disease is very uncommon in women under the age of 35. Most breast cancers occur in women over the age of 50, and the risk is especially high for women over age 60. Also, breast cancer occurs more often in white women than African American or Asian women.

Research has shown that the following conditions increase a woman's chances of getting breast cancer:

- **Personal history of breast cancer.** Women who have had breast cancer face an increased risk of getting breast cancer in their other breast.

- **Family history.** A woman's risk for developing breast cancer increases if her mother, sister, or daughter had breast cancer, especially at a young age.

- **Certain breast changes.** Having a diagnosis of atypical hyperplasia or lobular carcinoma *in situ* (LCIS) may increase a woman's risk for developing cancer.

- **Genetic alterations.** Changes in certain genes (BRCA1, BRCA2, and others) increase the risk of breast cancer. In families in which many women have had the disease, gene testing can sometimes show the presence of specific genetic changes that increase the risk of breast cancer. Doctors may suggest ways to try to delay or prevent breast cancer, or to improve the detection of this disease in women who have these changes in their genes. For more information about gene testing, read the "Causes and Prevention" section under "The Promise of Cancer Research."

Other factors associated with an increased risk for breast cancer include:

- **Estrogen.** Evidence suggests that the longer a woman is exposed to estrogen (estrogen made by the body, taken as a drug, or delivered by a patch), the more likely she is to develop breast cancer. For example, the risk is somewhat increased among women who began menstruation at an early age (before age 12), experienced menopause late (after age 55), never had children, or took hormone replacement therapy for long periods of time. Each of these factors increases the amount of time a woman's body is exposed to estrogen.

  DES (diethylstilbestrol) is a synthetic form of estrogen that was used between the early 1940s and 1971. Women who took DES during pregnancy to prevent certain complications are at a slightly higher risk for breast cancer. This does not appear to be the case for their daughters who were exposed to DES before birth. However, more studies are needed as these daughters enter the age range when breast cancer is more common.

- **Late childbearing.** Women who have their first child late (after about age 30) have a greater chance of developing breast cancer than women who have a child at a younger age.

- **Breast density.** Breasts that have a high proportion of lobular and ductal tissue appear dense on mammograms. Breast cancers nearly always develop in lobular or ductal tissue (not fatty tissue). That's why cancer is more likely to occur in breasts that have a lot of lobular and ductal tissue (that is, dense tissue) than in breasts with a lot of fatty tissue. In addition, when breasts are dense, it is more difficult for doctors to see abnormal areas on a mammogram.

- **Radiation therapy.** Women whose breasts were exposed to radiation during radiation therapy before age 30, especially those who were treated with radiation for Hodgkin's disease, are at an increased risk for developing breast cancer. Studies show that the younger a woman was when she received her treatment, the higher her risk for developing breast cancer later in life.

- **Alcohol.** Some studies suggest a slightly higher risk of breast cancer among women who drink alcohol.

Most women who develop breast cancer have none of the risk factors listed above, other than the risk that comes with growing older. Scientists are conducting research into the causes of breast cancer to learn more about risk factors and ways of preventing this disease.

Detecting Breast Cancer

Women should talk with their doctor about factors that can increase their chance of getting breast cancer. Women of any age who are at higher risk for developing this disease should ask their doctor when to start and how often to be checked for breast cancer. Breast cancer screening has been shown to decrease the risk of dying from breast cancer.

Women can take an active part in the early detection of breast cancer by having regularly scheduled screening mammograms and clinical breast exams (breast exams performed by health professionals). Some women also perform breast self-exams.

A screening mammogram is the best tool available for finding breast cancer early, before symptoms appear. A mammogram is a special kind of x-ray. Screening mammograms are used to look for breast changes in women who have no signs of breast cancer.

Mammograms can often detect a breast lump before it can be felt. Also, a mammogram can show small deposits of calcium in the breast. Although most calcium deposits are benign, a cluster of very tiny specks of calcium (called microcalcifications) may be an early sign of cancer.

If an area of the breast looks suspicious on the screening mammogram, additional (diagnostic) mammograms may be needed. Depending on the results, the doctor may advise the woman to have a biopsy.

Although mammograms are the best way to find breast abnormalities early, they do have some limitations. A mammogram may miss some cancers that are present (false negative) or may find things that turn out not to be cancer (false positive). And detecting a tumor early does not guarantee that a woman's life will be saved. Some fast-growing breast cancers may already have spread to other parts of the body before being detected.

Nevertheless, studies show that mammograms reduce the risk of dying from breast cancer. Most doctors recommend that women in their forties and older have mammograms regularly, every 1 to 2 years.

59

Some women perform monthly breast self-exams to check for any changes in their breasts. When doing a breast self-exam, it's important to remember that each woman's breasts are different, and that changes can occur because of aging, the menstrual cycle, pregnancy, menopause, or taking birth control pills or other hormones. It is normal for the breasts to feel a little lumpy and uneven. Also, it is common for a woman's breasts to be swollen and tender right before or during her menstrual period. Women in their forties and older should be aware that a monthly breast self-exam is not a substitute for regularly scheduled screening mammograms and clinical breast exams by a health professional.

Recognizing Symptoms

Early breast cancer usually does not cause pain. In fact, when breast cancer first develops, there may be no symptoms at all. But as the cancer grows, it can cause changes that women should watch for:

- A lump or thickening in or near the breast or in the underarm area;
- A change in the size or shape of the breast;
- Nipple discharge or tenderness, or the nipple pulled back (inverted) into the breast;
- Ridges or pitting of the breast (the skin looks like the skin of an orange); or
- A change in the way the skin of the breast, areola, or nipple looks or feels (for example, warm, swollen, red, or scaly).

A woman should see her doctor about any symptoms like these. Most often, they are not cancer, but it's important to check with the doctor so that any problems can be diagnosed and treated as early as possible.

Diagnosing Breast Cancer

To help find the cause of any sign or symptom, a doctor does a careful physical exam and asks about personal and family medical history. In addition, the doctor may do one or more breast exams:

- **Clinical breast exam.** The doctor can tell a lot about a lump by carefully feeling it and the tissue around it. Benign lumps often feel different from cancerous ones. The doctor can examine the size and texture of the lump and determine whether the lump moves easily.

- **Mammography.** X-rays of the breast can give the doctor important information about a breast lump.

- **Ultrasonography.** Using high-frequency sound waves, ultrasonography can often show whether a lump is a fluid-filled cyst (not cancer) or a solid mass (which may or may not be cancer). This exam may be used along with mammography.

Based on these exams, the doctor may decide that no further tests are needed and no treatment is necessary. In such cases, the doctor may need to check the woman regularly to watch for any changes.

Biopsy

Often, fluid or tissue must be removed from the breast so the doctor can make a diagnosis. A woman's doctor may refer her for further evaluation to a surgeon or other health care professional who has experience with breast diseases. These doctors may perform:

- **Fine-needle aspiration.** A thin needle is used to remove fluid and/or cells from a breast lump. If the fluid is clear, it may not need to be checked by a lab.

- **Needle biopsy.** Using special techniques, tissue can be removed with a needle from an area that looks suspicious on a mammogram but cannot be felt. Tissue removed in a needle biopsy goes to a lab to be checked by a pathologist for cancer cells.

- **Surgical biopsy.** In an incisional biopsy, the surgeon cuts out a sample of a lump or suspicious area. In an excisional biopsy, the surgeon removes all of a lump or suspicious area and an area of healthy tissue around the edges. A pathologist then examines the tissue under a microscope to check for cancer cells.

When a woman needs a biopsy, these are some questions she may want to ask her doctor:

- What type of biopsy will I have? Why?

- How long will it take? Will I be awake? Will it hurt?

- How soon will I know the results?

- If I do have cancer, who will talk with me about treatment? When?

When Cancer Is Found

The most common type of breast cancer is ductal carcinoma. It begins in the lining of the ducts. Another type, called lobular carcinoma, arises in the lobules. When cancer is found, the pathologist can tell what kind of cancer it is (whether it began in a duct or a lobule) and whether it is invasive (has invaded nearby tissues in the breast).

Special lab tests of the tissue help the doctor learn more about the cancer. For example, hormone receptor tests (estrogen and progesterone receptor tests) can help determine whether hormones help the cancer to grow. If test results show that hormones do affect the cancer's growth (a positive test result), the cancer is likely to respond to hormonal therapy. This therapy deprives the cancer cells of estrogen. More information about hormonal therapy can be found in the "Planning Treatment" section.

Other tests are sometimes done to help the doctor predict whether the cancer is likely to progress. For example, the doctor may order x-rays and lab tests. Sometimes a sample of breast tissue is checked for a gene (the human epidermal growth factor receptor-2 or HER-2 gene) that is associated with a higher risk that the breast cancer will come back. The doctor may also order special exams of the bones, liver, or lungs because breast cancer may spread to these areas.

If the diagnosis is breast cancer, a woman may want to ask these questions:

- What kind of breast cancer do I have?

- What did the hormone receptor test show? What other lab tests were done on the tumor tissue, and what did they show?

- How will you determine whether the disease has spread?

- How will this information help in deciding what type of treatment or further tests will be best for me?

Planning Treatment

Many women with breast cancer want to take an active part in decisions about their medical care. They want to learn all they can about their disease and their treatment choices. However, the shock and stress that people often feel after a diagnosis of cancer can make it hard for them to think of everything they want to ask the doctor. Often it is helpful to prepare a list of questions in advance. To help remember what the doctor says, patients may take notes or ask whether they may use a tape recorder. Some people also want to have a family member or friend with them when they talk to the doctor—to take part in the discussion, to take notes, or just to listen.

The patient's doctor may refer her to doctors who specialize in treating cancer, or she may ask for a referral. Treatment generally begins within a few weeks after the diagnosis. There will be time for the woman to talk with the doctor about her treatment choices, to get a second opinion, and to prepare herself and her loved ones.

Second Opinion

Before starting treatment, the patient might want a second opinion about the diagnosis and the treatment plan. Some insurance companies require a second opinion; others may cover a second opinion if the woman requests it. It may take a little while to arrange to see another doctor. In most cases, a brief delay (up to 3 or 4 weeks) between biopsy and treatment does not make breast cancer treatment less effective. There are a number of ways to find a doctor for a second opinion:

- The patient's doctor may refer her to one or more specialists. Specialists who treat women with breast cancer include surgeons, medical oncologists, plastic surgeons, and radiation oncologists. At cancer centers or special centers for breast diseases, these doctors often work together as a team.

- The Cancer Information Service, at 1-800-4-CANCER, can tell callers about treatment facilities, including cancer centers and other NCI-supported programs, in their area.

- Patients can get the names of specialists from their local medical society, a nearby hospital, or a medical school.

- The Official ABMS Directory of Board Certified Medical Specialists lists doctors' names along with their specialty and their educational background. This resource, produced by the American Board of Medical Specialties (ABMS), is available in most public libraries. The ABMS also provides an online service to help people locate doctors (http://www.certifieddoctor.org/).

Methods of Treating Breast Cancer

Breast cancer may be treated with local or systemic therapy. Some patients have both kinds of treatment.

Local therapy is used to remove or destroy breast cancer in a specific area. Surgery and radiation therapy are local treatments. They are used to treat the disease in the breast. When breast cancer has spread to other parts of the body, local therapy may be used to control cancer in those specific areas, such as in the lung or bone.

Systemic treatments are used to destroy or control cancer throughout the body. Chemotherapy, hormonal therapy, and biological therapy are systemic treatments. Some patients have systemic therapy to shrink the tumor before local therapy. Others have systemic therapy to prevent the cancer from coming back, or to treat cancer that has spread.

Surgery is the most common treatment for breast cancer, and there are several types of surgery. The doctor can explain each type, discuss and compare their benefits and risks, and describe how each will affect the patient's appearance.

- An operation to remove the cancer but not the breast is called breast-sparing surgery or breast-conserving surgery. Lumpectomy and segmental mastectomy (also called partial mastectomy) are types of breast-sparing surgery. After breast-sparing surgery, most women receive radiation therapy to destroy cancer cells that remain in the area.

- An operation to remove the breast (or as much of the breast as possible) is a mastectomy. Breast reconstruction is often an option at the same time as the mastectomy, or later on.

- In most cases, the surgeon also removes lymph nodes under the arm to help determine whether cancer cells have entered the lymphatic system. This is called an axillary lymph node dissection.

Breast reconstruction (surgery to rebuild the shape of a breast) is often an option after mastectomy. Women considering reconstruction should discuss this with a plastic surgeon before having a mastectomy.

Here are some questions a woman may want to ask her doctor before having surgery:

- What kinds of surgery can I consider? Is breast-sparing surgery an option for me? Which operation do you recommend for me? What are the risks of surgery?

- Should I store some of my own blood in case I need a transfusion?

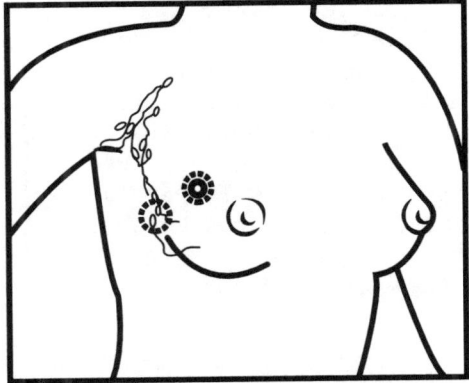

Figure 7.1. In **lumpectomy**, the surgeon removes the breast cancer and some normal tissue around it. (Sometimes an excisional biopsy serves as a lumpectomy.) Often, some of the lymph nodes under the arm are removed.

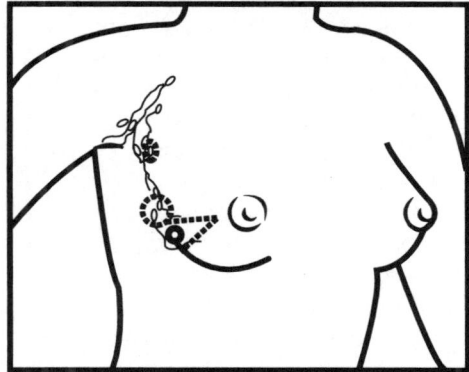

Figure 7.2. In **segmental mastectomy**, the surgeon removes the cancer and a larger area of normal breast tissue around it. Occasionally, some of the lining over the chest muscles below the tumor is removed as well. Some lymph nodes under the arm may also be removed.

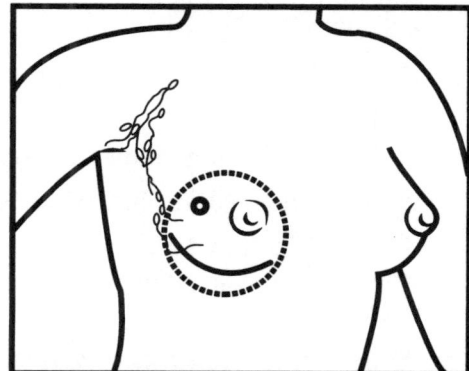

Figure 7.3. In **total (simple) mastectomy**, the surgeon removes the whole breast. Some lymph nodes under the arm may also be removed.

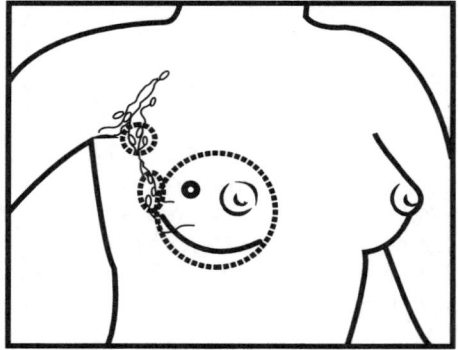

*Figure 7.4. In **modified radical mastectomy**, the surgeon removes the whole breast, most of the lymph nodes under the arm, and, often, the lining over the chest muscles. The smaller of the two chest muscles also may be taken out to help in removing the lymph nodes.*

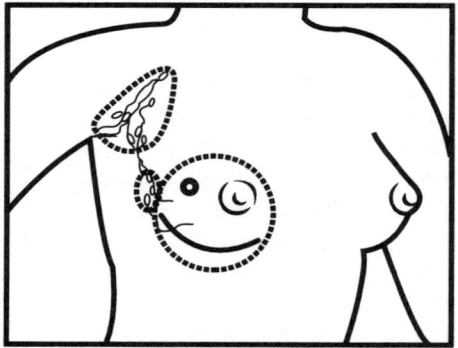

*Figure 7.5. In **radical mastectomy** (also called Halsted radical mastectomy), the surgeon removes the breast, both chest muscles, all of the lymph nodes under the arm, and some additional fat and skin. For many years, this operation was considered the standard one for women with breast cancer, but it is almost never used today. In rare cases, radical mastectomy may be suggested if the cancer has spread to the chest muscles.*

- Do I need my lymph nodes removed? How many? Why? What special precautions will I need to take if lymph nodes are removed?

- How will I feel after the operation?

- Will I need to learn how to do special things to take care of myself or my incision when I get home?

- Where will the scars be? What will they look like?

- If I decide to have plastic surgery to rebuild my breast, how and when can that be done? Can you suggest a plastic surgeon for me to contact?

- Will I have to do special exercises?

66

- When can I get back to my normal activities?
- Is there someone I can talk with who has had the same treatment I'll be having?

Radiation therapy (also called radiotherapy) is the use of high-energy rays to kill cancer cells. The radiation may be directed at the breast by a machine (external radiation). The radiation can also come from radioactive material placed in thin plastic tubes that are placed directly in the breast (implant radiation). Some women have both kinds of radiation therapy.

For external radiation therapy, the patient goes to the hospital or clinic, generally 5 days a week for several weeks. For implant radiation, a patient stays in the hospital. The implants remain in place for several days. They are removed before the woman goes home.

Sometimes, depending on the size of the tumor and other factors, radiation therapy is used after surgery, especially after breast-sparing surgery. The radiation destroys any breast cancer cells that may remain in the area.

Before surgery, radiation therapy, alone or with chemotherapy or hormonal therapy, is sometimes used to destroy cancer cells and shrink tumors. This approach is most often used in cases in which the breast tumor is large or not easily removed by surgery.

Before having radiation therapy, a patient may want to ask her doctor these questions:

- Why do I need this treatment?
- What are the risks and side effects of this treatment?
- Are there any long-term effects?
- When will the treatments begin? When will they end?
- How will I feel during therapy?
- What can I do to take care of myself during therapy?
- Can I continue my normal activities?
- How will my breast look afterward?
- What are the chances that the tumor will come back in my breast?

Chemotherapy is the use of drugs to kill cancer cells. Chemotherapy for breast cancer is usually a combination of drugs. The drugs may be given in a pill or by injection. Either way, the drugs enter the bloodstream and travel throughout the body.

Most patients have chemotherapy in an outpatient part of the hospital, at the doctor's office, or at home. Depending on which drugs are given and her general health, however, a woman may need to stay in the hospital during her treatment.

Hormonal therapy keeps cancer cells from getting the hormones they need to grow. This treatment may include the use of drugs that change the way hormones work, or surgery to remove the ovaries, which make female hormones. Like chemotherapy, hormonal therapy can affect cancer cells throughout the body.

Biological therapy is a treatment designed to enhance the body's natural defenses against cancer. For example, Herceptin® (trastuzumab) is a monoclonal antibody that targets breast cancer cells that have too much of a protein known as human epidermal growth factor receptor-2 (HER-2). By blocking HER-2, Herceptin slows or stops the growth of these cells. Herceptin may be given by itself or along with chemotherapy.

Patients may want to ask these questions about systemic therapy (chemotherapy, hormonal therapy, or biological therapy):

- Why do I need this treatment?
- If I need hormonal treatment, which would be better for me, drugs or an operation?
- What drugs will I be taking? What will they do?
- Will I have side effects? What can I do about them?
- How long will I be on this treatment?

Treatment Choices

Women with breast cancer now have many treatment options. Many women want to learn all they can about the disease and their treatment choices so that they can take an active part in decisions about their medical care. They are likely to have many questions and concerns about their treatment options.

The doctor is the best person to answer questions about treatment for a particular patient: what her treatment choices are and how successful her treatment is expected to be. Most patients also want to know how they will look after treatment and whether they will have to change their normal activities. A woman should not feel that she needs to ask all her questions or understand all the answers at once. She will have many chances to ask the doctor to explain things that are not clear and to ask for more information.

A woman may want to talk with her doctor about taking part in a clinical trial, a research study of new treatment methods. Clinical trials are an important option for women with all stages of breast cancer. The Promise of Cancer Research section has more information.

A woman's treatment options depend on a number of factors. These factors include her age and menopausal status; her general health; the size and location of the tumor and the stage of the cancer; the results of lab tests; and the size of her breast. Certain features of the tumor cells (such as whether they depend on hormones to grow) are also considered. In most cases, the most important factor is the stage of the disease. The stage is based on the size of the tumor and whether the cancer has spread. The following are brief descriptions of the stages of breast cancer and the treatments most often used for each stage. (Other treatments may sometimes be appropriate.)

- **Stage 0** is sometimes called noninvasive carcinoma or carcinoma *in situ*.

  Lobular carcinoma *in situ* (LCIS) refers to abnormal cells in the lining of a lobule. These abnormal cells seldom become invasive cancer. However, their presence is a sign that a woman has an increased risk of developing breast cancer. This risk of cancer is increased for both breasts. Some women with LCIS may take a drug called tamoxifen, which can reduce the risk of developing breast cancer. Others may take part in studies of other promising new preventive treatments. Some women may choose not to have treatment, but to return to the doctor regularly for checkups. And, occasionally, women with LCIS may decide to have surgery to remove both breasts to try to prevent cancer from developing. (In most cases, removal of underarm lymph nodes is not necessary.)

  Ductal carcinoma *in situ* (DCIS) refers to abnormal cells in the lining of a duct. DCIS is also called intraductal carcinoma. The abnormal cells have not spread beyond the duct to invade the surrounding breast tissue. However, women with DCIS are at an increased risk of getting invasive breast cancer. Some women with DCIS have breast-sparing surgery followed by radiation therapy. Or they may choose to have a mastectomy, with or without breast reconstruction (plastic surgery) to rebuild the breast. Underarm lymph nodes are not usually removed. Also, women with DCIS may want to talk with their doctor about tamoxifen to reduce the risk of developing invasive breast cancer.

- **Stage I** and **stage II** are early stages of breast cancer in which the cancer has spread beyond the lobe or duct and invaded nearby tissue. Stage I means that the tumor is no more than about an inch across and cancer cells have not spread beyond the breast. Stage II means one of the following: the tumor in the breast is less than 1 inch across and the cancer has spread to the lymph nodes under the arm; or the tumor is between 1 and 2 inches (with or without spread to the lymph nodes under the arm); or the tumor is larger than 2 inches but has not spread to the lymph nodes under the arm.

  Women with early stage breast cancer may have breast-sparing surgery followed by radiation therapy to the breast, or they may have a mastectomy, with or without breast reconstruction to rebuild the breast. These approaches are equally effective in treating early stage breast cancer. (Sometimes radiation therapy is also given after mastectomy.)

  The choice of breast-sparing surgery or mastectomy depends mostly on the size and location of the tumor, the size of the woman's breast, certain features of the cancer, and how the woman feels about preserving her breast. With either approach, lymph nodes under the arm usually are removed.

  Many women with stage I and most with stage II breast cancer have chemotherapy and/or hormonal therapy after primary treatment with surgery or surgery and radiation therapy. This added treatment is called adjuvant therapy. If the systemic therapy is given to shrink the tumor before surgery, this is called neoadjuvant therapy. Systemic treatment is given to try to destroy any remaining cancer cells and prevent the cancer from recurring, or coming back, in the breast or elsewhere.

- **Stage III** is also called locally advanced cancer. In this stage, the tumor in the breast is large (more than 2 inches across) and the cancer has spread to the underarm lymph nodes; or the cancer is extensive in the underarm lymph nodes; or the cancer has spread to lymph nodes near the breastbone or to other tissues near the breast.

Inflammatory breast cancer is a type of locally advanced breast cancer. In this type of cancer the breast looks red and swollen (or inflamed) because cancer cells block the lymph vessels in the skin of the breast.

Patients with stage III breast cancer usually have both local treatment to remove or destroy the cancer in the breast and systemic treatment to stop the disease from spreading. The local treatment may be surgery and/or radiation therapy to the breast and underarm. The systemic treatment may be chemotherapy, hormonal therapy, or both. Systemic therapy may be given before local therapy to shrink the tumor or afterward to prevent the disease from recurring in the breast or elsewhere.

- **Stage IV** is metastatic cancer. The cancer has spread beyond the breast and underarm lymph nodes to other parts of the body.

Women who have stage IV breast cancer receive chemotherapy and/or hormonal therapy to destroy cancer cells and control the disease. They may have surgery or radiation therapy to control the cancer in the breast. Radiation may also be useful to control tumors in other parts of the body.

- **Recurrent cancer** means the disease has come back in spite of the initial treatment. Even when a tumor in the breast seems to have been completely removed or destroyed, the disease sometimes returns because undetected cancer cells remained somewhere in the body after treatment.

Most recurrences appear within the first 2 or 3 years after treatment, but breast cancer can recur many years later. Cancer that returns only in the area of the surgery is called a local recurrence. If the disease returns in another part of the body, the distant recurrence is called metastatic breast cancer. The patient may have one type of treatment or a combination of treatments for recurrent cancer.

Side Effects of Treatment

It is hard to protect healthy cells from the harmful effects of breast cancer treatment. Because treatment does damage healthy cells and tissues, it causes side effects. The side effects of cancer treatment depend mainly on the type and extent of the treatment. Also, the effects may not be the same for each person, and they may be different from one treatment to the next. An important part of the treatment plan is the management of side effects.

A patient's reaction to treatment is closely monitored by physical exams, blood tests, and other tests. Doctors and nurses will explain the possible side effects of treatment, and they can suggest ways to deal with problems that may occur during and after treatment. The NCI provides helpful, informative booklets about cancer treatments and coping with side effects. Patients may want to read *Understanding Breast Cancer Treatment: A Guide for Patients*, as well as *Radiation Therapy and You*, *Chemotherapy and You*, and *Eating Hints for Cancer Patients*.

Surgery

Surgery causes short-term pain and tenderness in the area of the operation, so women may need to talk with their doctor about pain management. Any kind of surgery also carries a risk of infection, poor wound healing, bleeding, or a reaction to the anesthesia used during surgery. Women who experience any of these problems should tell their doctor or nurse right away.

Removal of a breast can cause a woman's weight to be out of balance—especially if she has large breasts. This imbalance can cause discomfort in her neck and back. Also, the skin in the area where the breast was removed may be tight, and the muscles of the arm and shoulder may feel stiff. After a mastectomy, some women have some permanent loss of strength in these muscles, but for most women, reduced strength and limited movement are temporary. The doctor, nurse, or physical therapist can recommend exercises to help a woman regain movement and strength in her arm and shoulder.

Because nerves may be injured or cut during surgery, a woman may have numbness and tingling in the chest, underarm, shoulder, and upper arm. These feelings usually go away within a few weeks or months, but some women have permanent numbness.

Removing the lymph nodes under the arm slows the flow of lymph. In some women, this fluid builds up in the arm and hand and causes swelling (lymphedema). Women need to protect the arm and hand on the treated side from injury or pressure, even long after surgery. They should ask the doctor how to handle any cuts, scratches, insect bites, or other injuries to the arm or hand. Also, they should contact the doctor if an infection develops in that arm or hand.

Radiation Therapy

During radiation therapy, patients may become extremely tired, especially after several treatments. This feeling may continue for a while after treatment is over. Resting is important, but doctors usually advise their patients to try to stay reasonably active, matching their activities to their energy level. It is also common for the skin in the treated area to become red, dry, tender, and itchy. The breast may feel heavy and hard, but these conditions will clear up with time. Toward the end of treatment, the skin may become moist and "weepy." Exposing this area to air as much as possible will help the skin heal. Because bras and some types of clothing may rub the skin and cause irritation, patients may want to wear loose-fitting cotton clothes. Gentle skin care is important at this time, and patients should check with their doctor before using any deodorants, lotions, or creams on the treated area. These effects of radiation therapy on the skin are temporary, and the area gradually heals once treatment is over. However, there may be a permanent change in the color of the skin.

Chemotherapy

As with radiation, chemotherapy affects normal as well as cancer cells. The side effects of chemotherapy depend mainly on the specific drugs and the dose. In general, anticancer drugs affect rapidly dividing cells. These include blood cells, which fight infection, help the blood to clot, and carry oxygen to all parts of the body. When blood cells are affected, patients are more likely to get infections, may bruise or bleed easily, and may feel unusually weak and very tired. Rapidly dividing cells in hair roots and cells that line the digestive tract may also be affected. As a result, side effects may include loss of hair, poor appetite, nausea and vomiting, diarrhea, or mouth and lip sores. Many of these side effects can now be controlled, thanks to new or improved drugs. Side effects generally are short-term and gradually go away. Hair grows back, but it may be different in color and texture.

Some anticancer drugs can damage the ovaries. If the ovaries fail to produce hormones, the woman may have symptoms of menopause, such as hot flashes and vaginal dryness. Her periods may become irregular or may stop, and she may not be able to become pregnant. Other long-term side effects are quite rare, but there have been cases in which the heart is weakened, and second cancers such as leukemia (cancer of the blood cells) have occurred.

73

Women who are still menstruating may still be able to get pregnant during treatment. Because the effects of chemotherapy on an unborn child are not known, it is important for a woman to talk with her doctor about birth control before treatment begins. After treatment, some women regain their ability to become pregnant, but in women over the age of 35, infertility is likely to be permanent.

Hormonal Therapy

The side effects of hormonal therapy depend largely on the specific drug or type of treatment. Tamoxifen is the most common hormonal treatment. This drug blocks the cancer cells' use of estrogen but does not stop estrogen production. Tamoxifen may cause hot flashes, vaginal discharge or irritation, nausea, and irregular periods. Women who are still menstruating and having irregular periods may become pregnant more easily when taking tamoxifen. They should discuss birth control methods with their doctor.

Serious side effects of tamoxifen are rare. It can cause blood clots in the veins, especially in the legs and in the lungs, and in a small number of women, it can slightly increase the risk of stroke. Also, tamoxifen can cause cancer of the lining of the uterus. Any unusual vaginal bleeding should be reported to the doctor. The doctor may do a pelvic exam, as well as a biopsy of the lining of the uterus, or other tests. (This does not apply to women who have had a hysterectomy, surgery to remove the uterus.)

Young women whose ovaries are removed to deprive the cancer cells of estrogen experience menopause immediately. Their symptoms are likely to be more severe than symptoms associated with natural menopause.

Biological Therapy

The side effects of biological therapy differ with the types of substances used, and from patient to patient. Rashes or swelling where the biological therapy is injected are common. Flu-like symptoms also may occur.

Herceptin may cause these and other side effects, but these effects generally become less severe after the first treatment. Less commonly, Herceptin can also cause damage to the heart that can lead to heart failure. It can also affect the lungs, causing breathing problems that require immediate medical attention. For these reasons, women are checked carefully for heart and lung problems before taking Herceptin. Patients who do take it are watched carefully during treatment.

Breast Reconstruction

After a mastectomy, some women decide to wear a breast form (prosthesis). Others prefer to have breast reconstruction, either at the same time as the mastectomy or later on. Each option has its pros and cons, and what is right for one woman may not be right for another. What is important is that nearly every woman treated for breast cancer has choices. It is best to consult with a plastic surgeon before the mastectomy, even if reconstruction will be considered later on.

Various procedures are used to reconstruct the breast. Some use implants (either saline or silicone); others use tissue moved from another part of the woman's body. The safety of silicone breast implants has been under review by the Food and Drug Administration (FDA) for several years. Women interested in having silicone implants should talk with their doctor about the FDA's findings and the availability of silicone implants. Which type of reconstruction is best depends on a woman's age, body type, and the type of surgery she had. A woman should ask the plastic surgeon to explain the risks and benefits of each type of reconstruction. The National Cancer Institute booklet *Understanding Breast Cancer Treatment: A Guide for Patients* contains more information about breast reconstruction. The Cancer Information Service at 1-800-4-CANCER can suggest other sources of information about breast reconstruction and can talk with callers about breast cancer support groups.

Rehabilitation

Rehabilitation is a very important part of breast cancer treatment. The health care team makes every effort to help women return to their normal activities as soon as possible. Recovery will be different for each woman, depending on the extent of the disease, the type of treatment, and other factors.

Exercising the arm and shoulder after surgery can help a woman regain motion and strength in these areas. It can also reduce pain and stiffness in her neck and back. Carefully planned exercises should be started as soon as the doctor says the woman is ready, often within a day or so after surgery. Exercising begins slowly and gently and can even be done in bed. Gradually, exercising can be more active, and regular exercise becomes part of a woman's normal routine. (Women who have a mastectomy and immediate breast reconstruction need special exercises, which the doctor or nurse will explain.)

Often, lymphedema after surgery can be prevented or reduced with certain exercises and by resting with the arm propped up on a pillow. If lymphedema occurs, the doctor may suggest exercises and other ways to deal with this problem. For example, some women with lymphedema wear an elastic sleeve or use an elastic cuff to improve lymph circulation. The doctor also may suggest other approaches, such as medication, manual lymph drainage (massage), or use of a machine that gently compresses the arm. The woman may be referred to a physical therapist or another specialist.

Followup Care

Regular followup exams are important after breast cancer treatment. Regular checkups ensure that changes in health are noticed. Followup exams usually include examination of the breasts, chest, neck, and underarm areas, as well as periodic mammograms. If a woman has a breast implant, special mammogram techniques can be used. Sometimes the doctor may order other imaging procedures or lab tests.

A woman who has had cancer in one breast should report any changes in the treated area or in the other breast to her doctor right away. Because a woman who has had breast cancer is at risk of getting cancer in the other breast, mammograms are an important part of followup care.

Also, a woman who has had breast cancer should tell her doctor about other physical problems, such as pain, loss of appetite or weight, changes in menstrual cycles, unusual vaginal bleeding, or blurred vision. She should also report headaches, dizziness, shortness of breath, coughing or hoarseness, backaches, or digestive problems that seem unusual or that don't go away. These symptoms may be a sign that the cancer has returned, but they can also be signs of various other problems. It's important to share these concerns with a doctor.

Support for Women with Breast Cancer

The diagnosis of breast cancer can change a woman's life and the lives of those close to her. These changes can be hard to handle. It is common for the woman and her family and friends to have many different and sometimes confusing emotions. Having helpful information and support services can make it easier to cope with these problems.

People living with cancer may worry about caring for their families, keeping their jobs, or continuing daily activities. Concerns about

76

tests, treatments, hospital stays, and medical bills are also common. Doctors, nurses, and other members of the health care team can answer questions about treatment, working, or other activities. Meeting with a social worker, counselor, or member of the clergy can be helpful to people who want to talk about their feelings or discuss their concerns. Often, a social worker can suggest resources for help with rehabilitation, emotional support, financial aid, transportation, or home care.

Friends and relatives can be very supportive. Also, it helps many patients to discuss their concerns with others who have cancer. Women with breast cancer often get together in support groups, where they can share what they have learned about coping with their disease and the effects of their treatment. It is important to keep in mind, however, that each person is different. Treatments and ways of dealing with cancer that work for one person may not be right for another— even if they both have the same kind of cancer. It is always a good idea to discuss the advice of friends and family members with the doctor.

Several organizations offer special programs for patients with breast cancer. Trained volunteers, who have had breast cancer themselves, may talk with or visit patients, provide information, and lend emotional support before and after treatment. They often share their experiences with breast cancer treatment, rehabilitation, and breast reconstruction.

Sometimes women who have had breast cancer are afraid that changes to their body will affect not only how they look but how other people feel about them. They may be concerned that breast cancer and its treatment will affect their sexual relationships. Many couples find that talking about these concerns helps them find ways to express their love during and after treatment. Some seek counseling or a couples' support group.

The Promise of Cancer Research

Doctors all over the country are conducting many types of clinical trials (research studies in which people take part voluntarily). These include studies of ways to prevent, detect, diagnose, and treat breast cancer; studies of the psychological effects of the disease; and studies of ways to improve comfort and quality of life. Research already has led to significant advances in these areas, and researchers continue to search for more effective approaches.

People who take part in clinical trials have the first chance to benefit from new approaches. They also make important contributions to medical science. Although clinical trials may pose some risks, researchers take very careful steps to protect people who take part.

Women who are interested in being part of a clinical trial should talk with their doctor. They may want to read the National Cancer Institute booklets *Taking Part in Clinical Trials: What Cancer Patients Need To Know* or *Taking Part in Clinical Trials: Cancer Prevention Studies*, which describe how research studies are carried out and explain their possible benefits and risks. NCI's cancerTrials™ Web site at http://cancertrials.nci.nih.gov/ provides general information about clinical trials. It also offers detailed information about specific ongoing studies of breast cancer by linking to PDQ®, a cancer information database developed by the NCI.

Causes and Prevention

Doctors can seldom explain why one woman gets breast cancer and another doesn't. It is clear, however, that breast cancer is not caused by bumping, bruising, or touching the breast. And this disease is not contagious; no one can "catch" breast cancer from another person.

Scientists are trying to learn more about factors that increase the risk of developing this disease. For example, they are looking at whether the risk of breast cancer might be affected by environmental factors. So far, scientists do not have enough information to know whether any factors in the environment increase the risk of this disease. (The main known risk factors are listed in the "Breast Cancer: Who's at Risk?" section.)

Some aspects of a woman's lifestyle may affect her chances of developing breast cancer. For example, recent studies suggest that regular exercise may decrease the risk in younger women. Also, some evidence suggests a link between diet and breast cancer. Ongoing studies are looking at ways to prevent breast cancer through changes in diet or with dietary supplements. However, it is not yet known whether specific dietary changes will actually prevent breast cancer. These are active areas of research.

Scientists are trying to learn whether having a miscarriage or an abortion increases the risk of breast cancer. Thus far, studies have produced conflicting results, and this question is still unresolved.

Research has led to the identification of changes (mutations) in certain genes that increase the risk of developing breast cancer. Women with a strong family history of breast cancer may choose to have a blood test to see if they have inherited a change in the BRCA1 or BRCA2 gene. Women who are concerned about an inherited risk for breast cancer should talk to their doctor. The doctor may suggest seeing a health professional trained in genetics. Genetic counseling can help a woman decide whether testing would be appropriate for her. Also, counseling before and after testing helps women understand and deal with the possible results of a genetic test. Counseling can also help with concerns about employment or about health, life, and disability insurance. The Cancer Information Service can supply additional material on genetic testing.

Scientists are looking for drugs that may prevent the development of breast cancer. In one large study, the drug tamoxifen reduced the number of new cases of breast cancer among women at an increased risk for the disease. Doctors are now studying how another drug called raloxifene compares to tamoxifen. This study is called STAR (Study of Tamoxifen and Raloxifene). For more information about prevention clinical trials, call the Cancer Information Service.

Detection and Diagnosis

At present, mammograms are the most effective tool we have to detect breast cancer. Researchers are looking for ways to make mammography more accurate, such as using computers to read mammograms (digital mammography). They are also exploring other techniques, such as magnetic resonance imaging (MRI), breast ultrasonography, and positron emission tomography (PET), to produce detailed pictures of the tissues in the breast.

In addition, researchers are studying tumor markers. These are substances that may be present in abnormal amounts in people with cancer. Tumor markers may be found in blood or urine, or in fluid from the breast (nipple aspirate). Some of these markers may be used to check women who have already been diagnosed with breast cancer. At this time, however, no tumor marker test is reliable enough to be used routinely to detect breast cancer.

Treatment

Through research, doctors try to find new, more effective ways to treat cancer. Many studies of new approaches for patients with breast cancer are under way. When laboratory research shows that a new treatment method has promise, cancer patients receive the new approach in treatment clinical trials. These studies are designed to answer important questions and to find out whether the new approach is safe and effective. Often, clinical trials compare a new treatment with a standard approach.

Researchers are testing new anticancer drugs, doses, and treatment schedules. They are working with various drugs and drug combinations, as well as with several types of hormonal therapy. They also are looking at the effectiveness of using chemotherapy before surgery (called neoadjuvant chemotherapy) and at new ways of combining treatments, such as adding hormonal therapy or radiation therapy to chemotherapy.

New biological approaches also are under study. For example, several cancer vaccines have been designed to stimulate the immune system to mount a response against breast cancer cells. Combinations of biological treatments with other agents are also undergoing clinical study.

Researchers are exploring ways to reduce the side effects of treatment (such as lymphedema from surgery), improve the quality of patients' lives, and reduce pain. One procedure under study is called sentinel lymph node biopsy. Researchers are trying to learn whether this procedure may reduce the number of lymph nodes that must be removed during breast cancer surgery. Before surgery, the doctor injects a radioactive substance near the tumor. The substance flows through the lymphatic system to the first lymph node or nodes where cancer cells are likely to have spread (the "sentinel" node or nodes). The doctor uses a scanner to locate the radioactive substance in the sentinel nodes. Sometimes the doctor also injects a blue dye near the tumor. The dye travels through the lymphatic system to collect in the sentinel nodes. The surgeon makes a small incision and removes only the nodes with radioactive substance or blue dye. A pathologist checks the sentinel lymph nodes for cancer cells. If no cancer cells are detected, it may not be necessary to remove additional nodes. If sentinel lymph node biopsy proves to be as effective as the standard axillary lymph node dissection, the new procedure could prevent lymphedema.

Chemotherapy can reduce the ability of bone marrow to make blood cells. That is why researchers are studying ways to help the blood cells recover so that high doses of chemotherapy can be given. These studies use biological therapies (known as colony-stimulating factors), autologous bone marrow transplants, or peripheral stem cell transplants.

Chapter 8

The Biology of Breast Cancer

To reduce cancer risk, we first need to understand how cancer develops in the body. Understanding how cancer develops can help us find ways to slow down its progress or perhaps stop it from occurring in the first place. For example, understanding that breast tissue of girls and young women is especially sensitive to cancer causing agents can help direct risk reduction efforts to these groups. Making sense of cancer means taking a step toward more informed decisions about our bodies, our selves, and our environment.

How Does Breast Cancer Develop?

Cancer develops through a multistep process in which normal, healthy cells in the body go through stages that eventually change them to abnormal cells that multiply out of control. In most cases, cancer takes many years to develop.

Normal cells in the body communicate with each other and regulate each other's proliferation (division). Cells proliferate to replace worn-out cells. When cancer occurs, cells escape the normal controls

From "The Biology of Breast Cancer," prepared by Rachel Ann Clark, M.S. Science Writer, Cornell University; Roy Levine, Ph.D. Department of Pathology College of Veterinary Medicine, Cornell University; and Suzanne Snedeker, Ph.D., Research Project leader, Cornell University, Program on Breast Cancer and Environmental Risk Factors in New York State (BCERF), *FACT SHEET* #5, Institute for Comparative and Environmental Toxicology, Cornell Center for the Environment, October 1997; reprinted with permission.

on their growth and proliferation. This escape from control can happen through a variety of pathways.

Part of the multistep process to cancer includes acquiring damage (mutations) to genes that normally regulate cell proliferation. A series of permanent mutations in tumor suppressor genes and proto-oncogenes are needed before cancer develops. Buildup of damage in these genes can result in uncontrolled cell proliferation. In some cases, further damage can lead to cells that can break away from the primary tumor and form cancers at other sites in the body (metastasis).

Breast tissue is particularly sensitive to developing cancer for several reasons. The female hormone estrogen stimulates breast cell division. This division can increase the risk of making damage to DNA permanent. Furthermore, breast cells are not fully matured in girls and young women who have not had their first full-term pregnancy. Breast cells that are not fully mature bind carcinogens (cancer causing agents) more strongly and are not as efficient at repairing DNA damage as mature breast cells.

How Do Things Go Wrong?

When cancer develops it is because things go wrong in the cells of the body. In the breast tissue of young women and girls, cells are especially sensitive to DNA damage from cancer causing agents.

Mutations in DNA

In every one of the trillions of cells in the body, there is an "operations manual" made up of DNA molecules. The information in the manual is separated into chapters, called genes which are made up of small units of DNA. Genes are written in a DNA code that must be transcribed and translated in order for the cell to make the protein signals specified in each gene. These proteins are signals which tell the cell how to function.

A change in the genetic code is a mutation. Mutations can happen by subtracting from, adding to, or rearranging the original code. Mutations can happen randomly within the cell's DNA, but they can also be induced. A substance that causes mutations in DNA is called a mutagen. Mutations in a gene may interfere with its ability to make a functional signal, or cause it to code for a protein that sends an incorrect signal to the cell.

Most mutations are repaired by the cell, but in rare cases mutations do not get repaired. If a mutation is not repaired before a cell copies its DNA and divides into two cells, then the mutation is passed on to the two new daughter cells and becomes permanent. Rare genetic disorders (e.g., Ataxia Telangiectasia) are one way that cells are deprived of the ability to repair DNA, and may experience buildup of mutations in cells.

Mutations in most of a cell's DNA have no effect on whether the cell will become cancerous. However, the protein signals coded by a very small proportion of the total genes in each cell regulate cell growth and division. These regulatory genes include the two groups of genes called proto-oncogenes and tumor suppressor genes. A series of mutations in the DNA of either and/or both groups of these growth controlling genes can eventually lead to cancer. Buildup of these mutations may take years to develop.

Breast Biology and Susceptibility to Cancer

Cells that divide are at a higher risk of acquiring mutations than cells that don't divide. Cancer is generally rare in tissues in which cells don't divide, like nerve tissue. Alternatively, cancer is more common in tissues in which cells divide frequently such as with breast, skin, colon, and uterine tissues.

Young women and girls have breast tissue that is especially sensitive to cancer causing agents (carcinogens). Unlike other tissues in the body like the liver and heart that are formed at birth, breast tissue in newborns consists only of a tiny duct. At puberty, in response to hormones (like estrogen that is secreted by the ovary), the breast duct grows rapidly into a tree-like structure composed of many ducts. Most breast development occurs between puberty and a woman's first pregnancy. The immature breast cells, called "stem cells", divide rapidly during puberty. The cells in the immature, developing breast are not very efficient at repairing mutations, and they are more likely to bind carcinogens.

Therefore it is important to reduce the exposure of young women and girls to carcinogens that might damage DNA during this phase of rapid breast development. For example, Japanese infants and young women exposed to ionizing radiation from atomic bombing during WWII have high rates of breast cancer as adults. It is also important to reduce exposure to environmental estrogens during these critical times. Environmental estrogens (estrogen 'mimics') are synthetic chemicals that can act like human estrogen in a woman's body, and may stimulate cell division in the breast.

After a woman's first full-term pregnancy, hormonal influences transform a high proportion of her breast cells into mature, differentiated cells which make milk. Milk producing cells are fully mature and less sensitive to DNA damage than immature undifferentiated cells. Therefore, susceptibility to mutations declines in the breast cells of women who have had an early full-term pregnancy. Some evidence also suggests that breast feeding further reduces the breast cells' sensitivity to mutations.

Though much of what we know about the biology of breast tissue susceptibility to cancer is based on research in animals, it is believed most of this knowledge can be applied to human biology.

The Stages of Tumor Development

Cancer develops through different stages. These stages may or may not eventually lead to invasive and metastatic cancer. In most cases

Table 8.1. Susceptibility to Breast Cancer

Critical Periods of Susceptibility
    Birth to 4 years
    Puberty
    End of Puberty to 1st full-term pregnancy

    Biological Characteristics of Critical Periods
        Rapid cell division
        Breast cells have higher proportion of "stem cells"
        Mutations can be passed on if not repaired
        Stem cells are more susceptible to carcinogens.

After 1st Full-Term Pregnancy
    Biological Characteristics AFTER Critical Periods
        Fewer stem cells
        Less cell division
        More cells are differentiated
        Differentiated cells repair DNA more efficiently
        Differentiated cells bind carcinogens more weakly than stem cells

Original hypothesis and animal modeling done by Drs. Irma and Jose Russo it takes many years for cancer to develop. Early detection of any tumor is important because it increases the chances of removing the cancer before it becomes life-threatening.

Normal: There are trillions of cells in the healthy human body. Even though adults stop growing, the body constantly replaces worn-out cells with new ones to stay healthy. Cells must communicate and respond to each other's checks and balances to maintain the correct number of healthy cells.

Genetically altered cell(s): Tumor development begins when at least one cell has a genetic mutation (mistake in DNA) which causes it to divide and proliferate when it normally would not. This leads to more cells with the same mistake.

Hyperplasia: Cells look normal but grow too much. Further damage can lead to "dysplasia."

Dysplasia: Cells proliferate too much *and* look abnormal in shape and orientation. Cells are less responsive to surrounding cells and the body's signals to stop proliferating. Further damage and/or cell changes can lead to *"in situ"* (pronounced "in-SIGH-two") cancer.

Atypia: Cells look abnormal. Atypia is a general term describing how cells look. For example, one cell can appear atypical, but a group of cells display "dysplasia."

Benign tumor (not life-threatening): Although cells are not normal, they do not have the ability to travel to other parts of the body. Cells in benign tumors are typically more differentiated (mature) and organized than cells in cancerous tumors. In some cases a benign tumor may eventually become an invasive or metastatic tumor.

In situ **carcinoma (cancer):** Cells become even more abnormal in growth and appearance but the tumor cells have not broken through the boundary around the tumor that separates it from surrounding tissues. This boundary is like a capsule that contains the tumor. Cells may acquire additional damage and/or changes which can lead to invasive cancer.

Invasive cancer (can be life-threatening—primary tumor): The uncontrolled growth of cells in the tumor allow some cells to break through the capsule-like boundary and invade nearby tissues. Generally, invasive tumors are life-threatening if the cancer cells are present within a vital organ like the kidneys, lungs, or liver. Invasive tumors in non-vital organs like the breasts are not necessarily life-threatening unless they become malignant and migrate to a vital organ. Therefore, early detection of any tumor is important because it increases the chances of removing the cancer before it becomes life-threatening.

- **Malignant:** Cells from the invasive (primary) tumor gain the ability to enter the blood stream or lymphatic system and to travel to distant areas in the body (metastasize).

Metastatic cancer (life-threatening—secondary tumors that come from the primary invasive tumor). Cells from the malignant primary tumor gain the ability to re-establish somewhere else in the body where they form new cancerous tumors. The secondary tumors are called metastases. Metastatic tumors can become fatal because they may disrupt the function of vital organs.

Where Can Things Go Wrong?

Cells in the body are regulated through the cell cycle. Damaged cells may eventually become deaf to normal regulation and multiply out of control.

Cell Cycle

Even though adults are no longer growing, many cells in an adult's body continue to divide to replace worn out cells. To divide, a cell must enter a "highway" called the cell cycle. There are specific signals that tell a cell when to enter the cell cycle and how long to stay there and divide. For example, cyclins are molecules that help control the cell cycle. There are also signals which tell the cell when to exit the cell cycle. When a cell divides, it copies its DNA and produces two new daughter cells. If any of the signals controlling the cell cycle fail, cell division may go unchecked.

The female hormone estrogen is one signal that tells certain kinds of breast cells to enter the cell cycle. This leads to increased cell division. In addition, researchers suspect an interaction between estrogen and certain cyclins (e.g. cyclin-D1) which stimulates the cell cycle.

Factors that are locally produced by breast cells can also affect cell division. One example is the growth factor TGF-alpha (transforming growth factor alpha). Researchers have shown that over-expression of TGF-alpha is associated with increased cell division in breast cells, and hence may be associated with breast tumor progression (see Stages of Tumor Development). Over-expression of growth factors may be related to damage in proto-oncogenes.

Proto-Oncogenes and Oncogenes: "Go" Genes

Proto-oncogenes are normal genes that code for the "go" signals controlling the cell cycle. These signals tell a cell to enter the cell cycle and code for how long it should stay there and divide. If a proto-oncogene loses the ability to regulate the cell cycle, the cell may reproduce uncontrollably because it stays in the cell cycle and continues to divide. A mutated proto-oncogene that has lost control of its "go" signal is called an oncogene.

Oncogenes code for protein signals that stimulate the cell to enter or continue in the cell cycle. This leads to inappropriate cell division and growth of a developing tumor. For example, a mutation in a proto-oncogene may cause the over expression of certain growth factors, and lead to inappropriate division of cells. That is why some growth factors are seen at higher levels in many breast tumors.

Another example is the erb-B2 receptor gene, an oncogene which codes for a receptor protein. The receptor in normal cells must be bound to a certain growth factor before it can stimulate the cell to enter the cell cycle and divide. But in faulty versions of the erb-B2 receptor gene, the receptors specified by this gene can release a flood of signals to stimulate increased cell division without being bound to the growth factor. Researchers have shown that up to 30% of primary breast cancers have too many copies of the erb-B2 gene.

Other oncogenes that researchers have found to be related to breast cancer include the tyrosine kinase family of growth factor receptors, the c-myc oncogene, cyclin D-1, and the cyclin regulator, CDK-1.

Tumor Suppressor Genes: "Stop" Genes

Just as the cell has "go" signals that tell it when to enter the cell cycle, it also has genes which control the "brakes." Cells with tumor suppressor genes that are mutated or inactivated lose control over their brakes. Brakes are important in the cell cycle. Putting on brakes at certain "check points," allows the cell to check for any damage in its DNA. Repairs must be made before the cell is allowed to go on in the cycle. Without these brakes, cells with damaged DNA would copy

87

the mutations, divide, and pass on the damage to daughter cells. The damage is then established as a permanent mutation in subsequent generations of new cells. Therefore, an important function of tumor suppressor genes is to maintain the integrity of the DNA in cells.

An example of a vital tumor suppressor ("stop") gene is the p53 gene. A mutation in the p53 gene is the most common genetic change found in breast cancer. One function of this gene is to keep cells with damaged DNA from entering the cell cycle. The p53 gene can tell a normal cell with DNA damage to stop proliferating and repair the damage. In cancer cells, p53 recognizes damaged DNA and tells the cell to "commit suicide" (apoptosis). If the p53 gene is damaged and loses its function, cells with damaged DNA continue to reproduce when normally they would have been removed through apoptosis. This is why the p53 gene has been termed "The Guardian of the Genome."

A small proportion of breast cancer cases (5%) are related to the inheritance of susceptibility genes. Alterations of the recently discovered "breast cancer susceptibility genes," BRCA 1 & 2, are involved in some inherited cases of breast cancer. If inactivated, these tumor suppressor genes can act indirectly in the cell by disrupting DNA repair. This allows the cell to accumulate DNA damage, including mutations that can encourage cancer development.

Other tumor suppressor genes that researchers have found may be related to breast cancer include the Retino blastoma, Brush-1, Maspin, nm23, and the TSG101 genes.

Cell Adhesion Proteins

Healthy cells in the body are contained in a very orderly arrangement, like cobblestones in a street. Cobblestones are cemented in position and are contained by a curb. Like cobblestones, cells are cemented in position by cell adhesion proteins and are contained in their proper location by a curb called the basement membrane. In order for cells that have become cancerous to metastasize, the cells have to "break through" the basement membrane and enter the blood stream or lymphatic system.

Certain genes code for molecules which signal the cell to make cell adhesion proteins. If these genes are damaged by mutations the resulting adhesion protein may no longer function properly. Without the cell adhesion proteins, cells do not stick as strongly to each other and to the basement membrane. The cells themselves may no longer stay in their orderly arrangement and may escape the boundaries of the basement membrane. Researchers have shown that expression of normally functioning adhesion molecules is progressively reduced in more advanced tumors. Two types of cell adhesion protein that researchers have found to be related to breast cancer are the cadherins and integrins.

Early detection of tumors is vitally important because damage to the genes governing cell adhesion molecules can be one of the life-threatening stages of tumor progression. Removing a tumor when it is still contained and before cells have escaped the confines of the original tumor reduces the chance that cells may have metastasized and generated new tumors in other areas of the body.

Summary

- Cancer is a multistep process in which normal, healthy cells in the body go through stages that eventually change them to abnormal cells that multiply out of control. In most cases, cancer takes many years to develop.

- Breast tissue can be sensitive to developing cancer. The female hormone estrogen stimulates breast cell division, which can increase the risk of breast cancer. Furthermore, breast cells are not fully mature in girls and young women who have not had their first full-term pregnancy. Breast cells which are not fully mature bind carcinogens more strongly than and are not as efficient at repairing DNA damage as mature breast cells. Therefore, it is very important to reduce exposure to cancer causing agents during the critical periods in a woman's life.

- Part of the multistep process to cancer includes buildup of mutations to genes that normally regulate cell division. Damage to tumor suppressor genes and/or proto-oncogenes can eventually cause cancer. Damage to genes that code for cell adhesion proteins can lead to cells that can break away from the primary tumor and form cancers at other sites in the body.

- Development of invasive and metastatic cancer is a multi-step process. Early detection of tumors is vitally important. Removing a tumor before cells can escape the confines of the original tumor reduces the chance that cells will metastasize and generate new tumors in other areas of the body.

- Taking steps to reduce risk includes understanding cancer and making more informed decisions about our bodies, our selves, and our environment.

Breast Cancer Sourcebook, First Edition

This text benefited from the suggestions of numerous reviewers including the BCERF Educational Advisory Committee, Dr. Cora Foster, Dr. Renu Gandhi, and Dr. Andrew Yen who generously provided insight and comment.

Key References

Breast Cancer Dictionary, 1996. American Cancer Society, Inc.

Dairkee, S.H., and H.S. Smith, 1996. The Genetic Analysis of Breast Cancer Progression. *Journal of Mammary Gland Biology and Neoplasia*. Vol. 1, No. 2. pp. 139-149.

Cavenee, W. K., and R.L. White, March 1995. The Genetic Basis of Cancer. *Scientific American*. pp. 72-79.

Putta, M., (in prep). Tumor Suppressor Genes: Guardians of Our Cells. BCERF *Fact Sheet #6*.

Russo, J., and I.H. Russo, 1987. Biology of Disease: Biological and Molecular Bases of Mammary Carcinogenesis. *Laboratory Investigation*. Vol. 57, No. 2. pp. 112-137.

Weinberg, R.A., September 1996. How Cancer Arises. *Scientific American*. pp. 62-70.

A complete bibliography is also available at http://www.cfe.cornell.edu/bcerf/

Cornell University Program on Breast Cancer and Environmental Risk Factors in New York State (BCERF)

This text is a publication of the Cornell University Program on Breast Cancer and Environmental Risk Factors in New York State (BCERF). The Program is housed within the university-wide Institute for Comparative and Environmental Toxicology (ICET) in the Cornell Center for the Environment. BCERF strives to better understand the relationship between breast cancer and other hormonally-related cancers to environmental risk factors and to make this information available on an on-going basis to the citizens of New York State.

The program involves faculty and staff from the Cornell Ithaca campus (College of Agriculture and Life Sciences, College of Arts and Sciences, the College of Human Ecology, the College of Veterinary Medicine, the Division of Biological Sciences and the Division of

90

Nutritional Sciences), Cornell Cooperative Extension, and the Cornell Medical College and Strang Cancer Prevention Center.

If you would like to be added to our mailing list to receive future copies of our newsletter, *THE RIBBON*, please contact the Administrative/Outreach Coordinator at the address below. Also included in the newsletter is a tear-off sheet listing other fact sheets.

We hope you find this text informative. We welcome your comments. When reproducing this material, credit the Program on Breast Cancer and Environmental Risk Factors in New York State.

Funding for this project was made possible by the U.S. Department of Agriculture Cooperative State Research, Education and Extension Service, the New York State Department of Environmental Conservation, and Cornell University.

Cornell University
Program on Breast Cancer and
Environmental Risk Factors in New York State
110 Rice Hall
Ithaca, NY 14853-5601
Phone: (607) 254-2893
FAX: (607) 255-8207
email: breastcancer@cornell.edu
Internet: http://www.cfe.cornell.edu/bcerf/

—Prepared by Rachel Ann Clark, M.S. Science Writer BCERF Cornell University; Roy Levine, Ph.D. Department of Pathology College of Veterinary Medicine Cornell University; Suzanne Snedeker, Ph.D. Research Project leader BCERF Cornell University

Chapter 9

Inflammatory Breast Cancer

Inflammatory breast cancer is an uncommon type of breast cancer in which cancer cells block the lymph vessels in the skin of the breast. This blockage causes the breast to become red, swollen, and warm. The skin of the breast may have ridges or appear pitted, like the skin of an orange (called peau d'orange). This type of breast cancer may also cause a discharge from the nipple, and the nipple may be pulled back. Another possible sign of inflammatory breast cancer is the presence of swollen lymph nodes under the arm or above the collarbone. Often, a tumor cannot be felt, even though one may appear on a mammogram. A biopsy is done to confirm the diagnosis of inflammatory breast cancer.

Inflammatory breast cancer generally grows rapidly, and the cancer cells often spread to other parts of the body. Treatment for inflammatory breast cancer usually involves local treatment to remove or destroy the cancer in the breast and systemic treatment to stop the disease from spreading to other parts of the body. Local treatment affects only cells in the tumor and the area close to it; systemic treatment affects cells throughout the body. The local treatment may be surgery and/or radiation therapy to the breast and underarm. The systemic treatment may be chemotherapy (anticancer drugs), hormonal therapy (drugs that interfere with the effects of the female hormone estrogen), or both. Systemic treatment is generally given before the surgery and/or radiation therapy.

Cancer Facts, National Cancer Institute, January 1999.

Researchers are studying the effectiveness of high-dose chemo-therapy with bone marrow or peripheral blood stem cell transplantation (replacing blood-forming cells destroyed by treatment) in improving the outcome of patients with inflammatory breast cancer. They are also studying biological therapy (stimulating the immune system to fight the cancer), new chemotherapy and hormonal drugs, and new combinations of chemotherapy and hormonal drugs. Information about ongoing clinical trials (research studies) is available from the Cancer Information Service or from the National Cancer Institute's cancerTrials web site at http://cancertrials.nci.nih.gov on the internet.

Cancer Information Service (CIS) provides accurate, up-to-date infor-mation on cancer to patients and their families, health professionals, and the general public. Information specialists translate the latest scientific information into understandable language and respond in English, Spanish, or on TTY equipment.

Telephone 1-800-4-CANCER (1-800-422-6237)
TTY: 1-800-332-8615 (for deaf and hard of hearing callers)

Chapter 10

Male Breast Cancer

What Is Male Breast Cancer?

Male breast cancer is rare, accounting for less than 1% of all cases of breast cancer. The average age of men who are found to have breast cancer is between 60 and 70 years of age, although men of all ages can develop breast cancer.

Risk factors for male breast cancer appear to include exposure to radiation, the administration of estrogen (a hormone), and diseases associated with hyperestrogenism (producing too much estrogen), such as cirrhosis (liver disease) or Klinefelter's syndrome (a genetic disorder). Male breast cancer tends to run in families, with the risk of breast cancer increasing in men who have multiple female relatives who have had breast cancer. Men who have the BRCA2 genetic alteration appear to have a higher risk of developing breast cancer.

The types of breast cancer found in men are similar to those seen in women. The most common type of breast cancer is infiltrating ductal cancer (cancer that has spread beyond the cells lining ducts in the breast). Intraductal cancer (abnormal cells found in the lining of a duct; also called ductal carcinoma *in situ*), inflammatory cancer (a rare cancer in which the breast looks as if it is inflamed because of its red appearance and warmth), and Paget's disease of the nipple (the tumor has grown from ducts beneath the nipple onto the surface of the nipple) have also been seen in men. Lobular cancer *in situ* (abnormal

CancerNet, National Cancer Institute, PDQ®, updated November 2000.

cells found in the one of the lobes or sections of the breast) has not been seen in men. Breast cancer in men is staged (tests done to find out if the cancer has spread from the breast to other parts of the body) the same as it is in women.

Overall survival for men who have breast cancer is similar to that of women with breast cancer. Breast cancer in men, however, is frequently diagnosed at a later stage, affecting the likelihood of survival.

Types of Treatment

There are treatments for men with breast cancer. Four types of treatment are used:

- surgery (taking out the cancer in an operation)
- radiation therapy (using high-dose x-rays to kill cancer cells)
- chemotherapy (using drugs to kill cancer cells)
- hormone therapy (using drugs that change the way hormones work or taking out organs that make hormones, such as the testicles)

Surgery for men with breast cancer is usually a modified radical mastectomy (removal of the breast, the lining over the chest muscles, and sometimes part of the chest wall muscles). In addition, some of the lymph nodes (small organs that fight infection and disease) under the arm may also be removed and sent to a laboratory to be examined under a microscope by a doctor of pathology to see if the lymph nodes contain any microscopic cancer cells.

Radiation therapy is the use of high-energy x-rays to kill cancer cells and shrink tumors. Radiation will usually be given by a machine outside the body (external radiation therapy).

Chemotherapy is the use of drugs to kill cancer cells. Chemotherapy may be taken by mouth or it may be put into the body by inserting a needle into a vein or muscle. Chemotherapy is called a systemic treatment because the drugs enter the bloodstream, travel through the body, and can kill cancer cells outside the breast area.

Hormone therapy may be given if tests show that the breast cancer cells have estrogen receptors or progesterone receptors (certain proteins in cancer tissue). Hormone therapy is used to change the way hormones in the body help cancers grow. This may be done by using drugs that change the way hormones work or by surgery to take out organs that make hormones, such as the testicles. Hormone therapy with tamoxifen is often given to patients with early stages of breast cancer.

Initial Surgical Management

Most men diagnosed with breast cancer will receive a modified radical mastectomy followed by removal of some of the lymph nodes located under the arm.

Adjuvant Therapy

Even if the doctor removes all the cancer that can be seen at the time of the operation, the patient may be given radiation therapy, chemotherapy, and/or hormone therapy after surgery to try to kill any cancer cells that may be left. Therapy given after an operation when there are no cancer cells that can be seen is called adjuvant therapy.

If cancer is found in the lymph nodes, treatment consisting of chemotherapy plus tamoxifen (to block the effect of estrogen) and other hormone therapy appears to increase survival in men as it does in women. The patient's response to hormone therapy depends on the presence of hormone receptors in the tumor. The majority of breast cancers in men have these receptors. Hormone therapy is usually recommended for male breast cancer patients, but it can have many side effects, such as hot flashes and impotence (the inability to have an erection adequate for sexual intercourse).

Locally Recurrent Disease

For locally recurrent disease (cancer that has come back in a limited area after treatment), treatment is usually surgery and radiation therapy combined with chemotherapy.

Distant Metastases

For distant metastases (cancer that has spread to other parts of the body), hormone therapy, chemotherapy, or a combination of both have shown some success. Hormone therapy may include:

- Orchiectomy (removal of the testicles to decrease hormone production)
- Luteinizing hormone-releasing hormone with or without total androgen blockade (to decrease the production of sex hormones)

- Tamoxifen for cancer that is estrogen-receptor positive
- Progesterone (a female hormone)
- Aminoglutethimide (reduces the production of estrogen)

Hormone therapies may be used in sequence (one after the other). Standard chemotherapy regimens may be used if hormone therapy does not work. Men usually respond to therapy no differently than women who have breast cancer.

For More Information

For more information, call the National Cancer Institute's Cancer Information Service at 1-800-4-CANCER (1-800-422-6237); TTY at 1-800-332-8615. The call is free and a trained information specialist is available to answer your questions.

The National Cancer Institute has booklets and other materials for patients, health professionals, and the public. These publications discuss types of cancer, methods of cancer treatment, coping with cancer, and clinical trials. Some publications provide information on tests for cancer, cancer causes and prevention, cancer statistics, and NCI research activities. NCI materials on these and other topics may be ordered online from the NCI Publications Locator Service at http://publications.nci.nih.gov/ or by telephone from the Cancer Information Service toll free at 1-800-4-CANCER.

There are many other places where people can get materials and information about cancer treatment and services. Local hospitals may have information on local and regional agencies that offer information about finances, getting to and from treatment, receiving care at home, and dealing with problems associated with cancer treatment. A list of organizations and websites that offer information and services for cancer patients and their families is available on CancerNet at http://cancernet.nci.nih.gov/cancerlinks.html.

For more information from the National Cancer Institute, please write to this address:

National Cancer Institute
Office of Cancer Communications
31 Center Drive, MSC 2580
Bethesda, MD 20892-2580

Chapter 11

Metastatic Cancer

Questions and Answers about Metastatic Cancer

What is cancer?

Cancer is a group of many related diseases that begin in cells, the body's basic unit of life. The body is made up of many types of cells. Normally, cells grow and divide to produce more cells only when the body needs them. This orderly process helps keep the body healthy. Sometimes cells keep dividing when new cells are not needed. These extra cells may form a mass of tissue, called a growth or tumor. Tumors can be either benign (not cancerous) or malignant (cancerous).

Cancer can begin in any organ or tissue of the body. The original tumor is called the primary cancer or primary tumor and is usually named for the part of the body in which it begins.

What is metastasis?

Metastasis means the spread of cancer. Cancer cells can break away from a primary tumor and travel through the bloodstream or lymphatic system to other parts of the body.

Cancer cells may spread to lymph nodes near the primary tumor (regional lymph nodes). This is called nodal involvement, positive nodes, or regional disease. Cancer cells can also spread to other parts of the body, distant from the primary tumor. Doctors use the term

Cancer Facts, National Cancer Institute, August 2000.

99

metastatic disease or distant disease to describe cancer that spreads to other organs or to lymph nodes other than those near the primary tumor.

When cancer cells spread and form a new tumor, the new tumor is called a secondary, or metastatic, tumor. The cancer cells that form the secondary tumor are like those in the original tumor. That means, for example, that if breast cancer spreads (metastasizes) to the lung, the secondary tumor is made up of abnormal breast cells (not abnormal lung cells). The disease in the lung is metastatic breast cancer (not lung cancer).

Is it possible to have a metastasis without having a primary cancer?

No. A metastasis is a tumor that started from a cancer cell or cells in another part of the body. Sometimes, however, a primary cancer is discovered only after a metastasis causes symptoms. For example, a man whose prostate cancer has spread to the bones in the pelvis may have lower back pain (caused by the cancer in his bones) before experiencing any symptoms from the prostate tumor itself.

How does a doctor know whether a cancer is a primary or a secondary tumor?

The cells in a metastatic tumor resemble those in the primary tumor. Once the cancerous tissue is examined under a microscope to determine the cell type, a doctor can usually tell whether that type of cell is normally found in the part of the body from which the tissue sample was taken.

For instance, breast cancer cells look the same whether they are found in the breast or have spread to another part of the body. So, if a tissue sample taken from a tumor in the lung contains cells that look like breast cells, the doctor determines that the lung tumor is a secondary tumor.

Metastatic cancers may be found at the same time as the primary tumor, or months or years later. When a second tumor is found in a patient who has been treated for cancer in the past, it is more often a metastasis than another primary tumor.

In a small number of cancer patients, a secondary tumor is diagnosed, but no primary cancer can be found, in spite of extensive tests. Doctors refer to the primary tumor as unknown or occult, and the patient is said to have cancer of unknown primary origin (CUP).

What treatments are used for metastatic cancer?

When cancer has metastasized, it may be treated with chemotherapy, radiation therapy, biological therapy, hormone therapy, surgery, or a combination of these. The choice of treatment generally depends on the type of primary cancer, the size and location of the metastasis, the patient's age and general health, and the types of treatments used previously. In patients diagnosed with CUP, it is still possible to treat the disease even when the primary tumor cannot be located.

New cancer treatments are currently under study. To develop new treatments, the National Cancer Institute (NCI) sponsors clinical trials (research studies) with cancer patients in many hospitals, universities, medical schools, and cancer centers around the country. Clinical trials are a critical step in the improvement of treatment. Before any new treatment can be recommended for general use, doctors conduct studies to find out whether the treatment is both safe for patients and effective against the disease. The results of such studies have led to progress not only in the treatment of cancer, but in the detection, diagnosis, and prevention of the disease as well. Patients interested in participating in research should ask their doctor to find out whether they are eligible for a clinical trial.

Part Three

Evaluating Breast Cancer Risk Factors

Chapter 12

Genetic Testing for Breast Cancer Risk

For American women, breast cancer is the second most common form of cancer and the second leading cause of cancer deaths. Each year, more than 180,000 women in the United States learn that they have breast cancer.

Some kinds of cancer, such as breast cancer, seem to run in families. There is a test that may tell some people if they are at risk for this kind of breast cancer. Before getting tested, however, there are many factors to consider.

This chapter provides a general overview on testing for breast and ovarian cancer risk. It describes the pros and cons of this kind of testing and explains terms like "family history," "genes," and "genetic testing." For more information about cancer and genetic testing, you should talk to a doctor or other health care professionals trained in genetics or call the National Cancer Institute's Cancer Information Service at 1-800-4-CANCER.

Who Is at Increased Risk for Breast and Ovarian Cancer?

A woman with a significant family history of breast and/or ovarian cancer has an increased risk of getting these cancers. You have a significant family history if:

National Action Plan on Breast Cancer, National Cancer Institute, NIH Pub. No. 00-4252, revised August 1999.

- you have two or more close family members who have had breast and/or ovarian cancer and
- the breast cancer in the family members has been found before the age of 50.

A close family member can be your:

- mother
- sister
- grandparent (on either your mother's or father's side)
- mother's sister
- father's sister

A close family member can also be your father, brother, or uncle, but breast cancer is very rare in men. Your family history of cancer can be assessed by a doctor or other health care professional trained in genetics who will determine if you have a significant family history of breast and/or ovarian cancer. Having this information may help you learn about your cancer risk and help you decide if genetic testing is right for you.

It is important to know that a family history of cancer does not mean you are going to get cancer. Many things such as family history and age may increase a person's chance (or risk) of getting cancer, but family history alone is not the only reason people get cancer. Scientists do not know all the reasons why people get cancer.

What Is a Gene?

Genes are nature's blueprints for every living thing. Genes come in pairs: one set of genes is passed down (or inherited) from your mother and the other set from your father. Genes determine how your body will function and grow, as well as the color of your hair and eyes.

How Might Genes Affect Breast Cancer Risk?

Some genes do not function properly because there is a mistake in them. If a gene has a mistake, it is said to be mutated or altered. In fact, all people have altered forms of some genes. Some alterations can increase your risk for certain illnesses such as cancer. In recent years, gene alterations have been found in some families with a history of breast cancer. Some women in these families also have had ovarian cancer.

These alterations are most often found in genes named BRCA1 and BRCA2 (BReast CAncer Gene 1 and BReast CAncer Gene 2). Both men and women have BRCA1 and BRCA2 genes, so alterations in these genes can be passed down from either the mother or the father. It is likely that more genes like these will be discovered in the future.

Does Every Woman with an Altered Breast Cancer Gene Get Cancer?

A woman with a BRCA1 or BRCA2 alteration is more likely to develop breast or ovarian cancer than is a woman without an alteration. However, not every woman who has an altered BRCA1 or BRCA2 gene will get breast or ovarian cancer, because genes are not the only factor that affect cancer risk. Therefore, an altered gene is not sufficient to cause cancer.

Most cases of breast cancer do not involve an altered BRCA1 or BRCA2 gene. At most, 1 in 10 breast cancer cases involves an inherited altered gene, and not all inherited breast cancer involves BRCA1 or BRCA2.

Do Men with an Altered BRCA1 or BRCA2 Gene Have an Increased Cancer Risk?

Although breast cancer is rare even in men with an altered gene, men with an altered BRCA2 gene have higher rates of breast cancer than men without an altered gene. Men with an altered BRCA1 or BRCA2 gene may also have a slightly increased risk of prostate cancer. Even if a man never develops cancer, he can pass the altered gene to his sons and daughters.

What Is Genetic Testing for Cancer Risk?

Genetic testing is a process in which it is possible to look for genetic alterations that may be associated with an increased risk of particular cancers. Genetic testing may reveal whether the cancer risk in a family is passed through their genes.

Although the lab test itself is quite complex, only a blood sample is needed. Genetic testing for breast and ovarian cancer risk involves looking for altered genes such as BRCA1 and BRCA2.

Because finding an altered gene can take several weeks or months, test results may not be readily available. The price of testing also varies. The price can be quite high and may not be covered by health insurance, or you may not want your insurance company to know you were tested. Ask your doctor or other health professionals for more information on genetic testing and health insurance coverage.

What Should I Think about Before Getting Tested?

- limitations of the test
- coping with cancer risk
- advantages of testing
- disadvantages of testing

What Are the Limitations of the Test?

Testing for breast cancer risk will not give you a simple "yes" or "no" answer. Finding a gene alteration in BRCA1 or BRCA2 indicates an increased risk of getting cancer, but it will not indicate if or when cancer will develop.

Currently, altered genes cannot be "fixed," but some day research may make it possible to prevent the disease in people who carry an altered gene.

What Can I Do If I Have an Altered Gene?

If you are at increased risk for breast or ovarian cancer, you can make choices that may help reduce your risk of getting cancer or help find cancer early. Of course, you can take these steps with or without getting tested for a BRCA1 or BRCA2 alteration.

Increased surveillance: You may choose to be monitored more closely for any sign of cancer. This may include more frequent mammograms, breast exams by your doctor, breast self-exams, and an ultrasound exam of the ovaries.

Prophylactic surgery: You may choose to have your healthy breasts and/or ovaries removed. This surgery may reduce the risk of cancer, but doctors do not know by how much. Because the surgery cannot remove all of the breast or ovarian tissue, some women who have chosen this surgery have later developed breast or ovarian cancer in the tissue that was left behind.

Join a research study: Because it is not yet possible to prevent cancer, you may choose to join a research study that is looking at ways to reduce cancer risk. This may entail changing your diet, reducing the amount of alcohol you drink, or trying new drugs to reduce the risk of cancer.

What we know now about cancer is due in large part to research. By taking part in a study, you could help researchers find better ways of preventing and treating cancer.

What Are the Advantages and Disadvantages of Testing?

Genetic testing may help you to:

- Make medical and lifestyle choices.
- Find out you do not have an altered gene.
- Cope with your cancer risk.
- Decide whether or not to have prophylactic surgery.
- Give other family members useful information (if you choose to share your test results).
- Contribute to research.

There are also disadvantages to testing:

- There is no proven way to reduce cancer risk.
- There is no guarantee that test results will remain private.
- You may face discrimination for health insurance, life insurance, or employment.
- You may find it harder to cope with your cancer risk when you know your test results.
- Negative test results may provide a false sense of security because you think you have no chance of getting cancer, which is not true. You would still have the same risk as women in the general population.

Lastly, genetic testing can affect relationships with family members. You should think about who in your family might want to know your test results, and whom you might want to tell.

If you are thinking about being tested, you should decide what the advantages and disadvantages of testing are *for you*. What is right for one person is not always right for another.

What Is Informed Consent?

If you are thinking about genetic testing, you should be informed, verbally and in writing, about the risks of getting tested as well as what the test can and cannot tell you. You should also sign a form to show that you have been given this information and want to be tested.

After reading the consent form, you can decide if testing is or is not right for you. You may also choose to delay the decision, if perhaps this is not the best time for you to be tested.

Questions You May Want to Ask Your Doctor or Other Health Professional

If you are thinking about genetic testing, be sure to talk with your doctor, genetic counselor, or other health professionals and take some time to answer these questions. You may want to get more than one opinion.

- What are the chances that a gene alteration is involved in the cancer in my family?

- What are my chances of having an altered gene?

- Besides altered BRCA1 or BRCA2 genes, what are other risk factors for breast and ovarian cancer?

- Are all genetic tests the same? How much does the test cost? How long will it take to get my results?

- What are the possible results of the test?

- What would a positive result mean for me?

- What would a negative result mean for me?

- How might a positive test result affect my health insurance? life insurance? employment?

- Do I want to submit my test results to an insurance company? If yes, will they pay for the testing?

- Where will my test results be placed/recorded? How might this affect me? Who will have access to them?

- Will having the test do anything to make me change my current health practices?

- What are my reasons for wanting to be tested?

- What type of cancer screening would be recommended if I don't get tested?

Other questions to think about and discuss with your family:

- What effect will the test results have on me and on my relationships with my family members if I have an altered gene? If I don't have an altered gene?

- Should I share my test results with my partner? parents? children? friends? others? How will they react to the news, which also affects them?

- Are my children ready to learn new information that may one day affect their own health?

Who Can I Call?

A person who is considering genetic testing should speak with a professional trained in genetics before deciding whether to be tested. For more information on genetic testing or for a referral to centers that have health care professionals trained in genetics, call the National Cancer Institute's Cancer Information Service at 1-800-4-CAN-CER. The Cancer Information Service can also provide information about clinical trials and research studies.

The National Action Plan on Breast Cancer (NAPBC) is a unique public-private partnership whose mission is to stimulate rapid progress in the fight against breast cancer. The NAPBC has identified genetic testing concerns as a high priority issue. Breast cancer survivors, researchers, and health care professionals from many fields worked together to produce educational materials to explain the risks and benefits of genetic testing. The NAPBC is coordinated by the U.S. Public Health Service's Office on Women's Health within the U.S. Department of Health and Human Services.

National Action Plan on Breast Cancer
U.S. Public Health Service's Office on Women's Health
U.S. Department of Health and Human Services
200 Independence Ave., S.W., Room 718F
Washington, D.C. 20201
http://www.4woman.gov/napbc

The National Cancer Institute (NCI) is the lead federal agency for cancer research. Since Congress passed the National Cancer Act in 1971, NCI has collaborated with top researchers and medical facilities throughout the country to conduct innovative research leading to progress in cancer prevention, detection, diagnosis, and treatment. These efforts have resulted in a recent decrease in the overall cancer death rate, and have helped improve and extend the lives of millions of Americans.

National Cancer Institute
31 Center Drive, MSC 2580
Bethesda, MD 20892-2580

Chapter 13

Hormone Replacement Therapy and Breast Cancer Risk

Menopause

Menopause is the time in a woman's life when hormonal changes cause menstruation to stop permanently. For most women, menopause is the last stage of a gradual biological process that actually begins during their mid-thirties.

Menopause is considered complete when a woman has stopped menstruating, or having her period, for 1 year. This usually occurs between ages 45 and 55, with variations in timing from woman to woman. By the time natural menopause is complete, hormone output has decreased significantly, but does not completely stop. Women who have surgery to remove both of their ovaries (an operation called bilateral oophorectomy) experience "surgical menopause," the immediate cessation of ovarian hormone production and menstruation. Doctors may recommend hormone replacement therapy (HRT), using either estrogen alone or estrogen in combination with progestin (a form of progesterone) to counter some of the possible effects of natural or surgical menopause on a woman's health and quality of life.

Because of advances in medical care and fewer deaths during childbirth, the average life expectancy for women in the United States increased from 51 years in 1900 to 79 years in 1990. A 50-year-old

This chapter includes text from "Menopausal Hormone Replacement Therapy," CancerNet, National Cancer Institute, April 2000; and "Adding Progestin to Hormone Replacement Therapy Increases Risk of Breast Cancer," Cancer Facts, National Cancer Institute, March 2000.

113

woman today can expect to live at least one-third of her life after menopause. An estimated 40 million women will go through menopause in the next 20 years. Thus, an increasing number of women will need to weigh the benefits and risks of HRT.

Although menopause is defined by many people as simply the end of a woman's menstrual cycles and her ability to bear children, it is also the beginning of a new and distinct phase of her life, with its own special health issues.

Symptoms of Menopause

Each woman experiences menopause differently. Some women have minimal discomfort, while others have moderate or even severe problems. Hot flashes, the most common symptom, occur in more than 60 percent of menopausal women. Hot flashes often begin several years before other symptoms of menopause occur.

Other changes involve the vagina and urinary tract. Declining estrogen levels can make vaginal tissue drier, thinner, and less elastic, which can make sexual intercourse painful. Urinary tract tissue also becomes less elastic, sometimes leading to involuntary loss of urine upon coughing, laughing, sneezing, exercising, or sudden exertion (stress incontinence). Urinary tract infections tend to occur more frequently. Other possible effects of menopause include sleep disturbances, mood swings, depression, and anxiety.

Health Effects of Menopause

In addition to producing some potentially uncomfortable symptoms, menopause can have more serious, long-term effects on a woman's overall health and potential years of life. For example, the drop in estrogen that occurs at menopause is thought to cause adverse changes in levels of cholesterol and other blood lipids (fats), and in levels of fibrinogen (a substance that affects blood clotting). These changes may increase the risk of heart disease (the leading cause of death among American women) and stroke. More than 370,000 women in this country die each year from heart disease, and about 93,000 die from stroke.

Osteoporosis (thinning of the bones), another serious concern during later life, is aggravated by menopause. Menopause speeds up the bone depletion that occurs during normal aging processes. About 20 percent of women over age 50 have or are at risk for bone fragility and fractures as their estrogen levels decline. Fractures, which often require a long recovery period, are a common injury in women with osteoporosis. Fractures of the vertebrae can cause curvature of the spine (also called kyphosis), loss of height, and pain.

Hormone Replacement Therapy

Most women will eventually need to make decisions about whether to take HRT and, if so, for how long. Hormone replacement therapy can have beneficial effects, but there are also some concerns associated with it. Each woman should consider both risks and benefits when making her decisions.

Benefits of HRT

It has been well documented for several decades that HRT is the most effective remedy for the hot flashes and sleep disturbances that often accompany menopause. Hormone replacement therapy has also consistently been shown to decrease vaginal discomfort by increasing the thickness, elasticity, and lubricating ability of vaginal tissue. Urinary tract tissue also becomes thicker and more elastic, reducing the incidence of stress incontinence and urinary tract infections.

Some women and their doctors report that HRT can be helpful in relieving the depression and mood swings that may occur during menopause and can produce a general sense of well being and increased energy. Also, some find that HRT increases skin thickness and elasticity, decreasing the appearance of wrinkles.

Although HRT was used initially to reduce the discomfort from short-term menopausal symptoms, studies have provided evidence that it may prevent or reduce some of the negative long-term health effects of menopause. Scientists continue to gather information to define the potential benefits from HRT and to identify the women for whom it may be most useful. Further research is also needed to determine when HRT should be started and how long it should be continued to achieve the greatest benefits.

Hormone replacement therapy plays a significant role in building and maintaining bone, thus helping to prevent osteoporosis. HRT is also sometimes used to treat bone loss that has already begun. HRT can prevent the decline of bone density and may reduce the incidence of fractures. It has been shown, however, that bone loss resumes upon discontinuation of HRT.

Research shows that HRT improves blood lipids and lowers fibrinogen levels. Some studies suggest that HRT may reduce the risk of heart disease and stroke. However, scientists are concerned that some of the apparent benefits of HRT in these studies may be due to the fact that healthier or more health-conscious women may be more likely to take replacement hormones. In one study of postmenopausal women with heart disease, the use of HRT did not prevent further heart attacks or death from heart disease. Additional research is in progress to clarify this issue.

Some studies suggest that taking estrogen may reduce the risk of developing Alzheimer's disease. However, scientists caution that additional research is needed to explore this possibility.

Concerns about HRT

Although HRT has potential benefits for many menopausal and postmenopausal women, it can also have drawbacks. Concerns about HRT center on the risk of endometrial cancer and breast cancer, especially after long-term use (more than 10 years).

Endometrial Cancer (Cancer of the Uterus)

When estrogen replacement became available for menopausal women in the 1940s, it was administered in high doses without progestin. As it became more popular in the 1960s, it was given to increasing numbers of women. In the 1970s, however, it became clear that women who received estrogen alone had a six- to eightfold increased risk of developing cancer of the endometrium (lining of the uterus).

Now, most doctors prescribe HRT that includes progestin, along with much lower doses of estrogen, for women who have not had a hysterectomy (surgery to remove the uterus). Progestin counteracts estrogen's negative effect on the uterus by preventing the overgrowth of the endometrial lining. Adding progestin to HRT substantially reduces the increased risk of endometrial cancer associated with taking estrogen alone. (A woman who has had a hysterectomy does not need progestin and can receive HRT with estrogen alone.)

Because reports have shown that estrogen increases the risk of developing endometrial cancer, many women and their doctors are also concerned that HRT may increase the risk of recurrence in women with a history of endometrial cancer. At present, however, there is no scientific evidence that taking estrogen increases this risk. To help resolve this issue, the National Cancer Institute is sponsoring a clinical trial to determine the effects of estrogen in women treated for early stage endometrial cancer. The study will compare recurrence rates between women who are given estrogen and those who are not given estrogen.

Breast Cancer

The relationship between HRT and breast cancer is not clear. The possible increased risk of developing breast cancer is consistently cited by menopausal and postmenopausal women as the main reason they are reluctant to use HRT. Many women and their doctors have particular concerns about the effects of long-term HRT use on breast cancer risk.

One of the most important risk factors for developing breast cancer is a woman's lifelong exposure to naturally occurring hormones; the longer her body produces hormones, the more likely she is to develop breast cancer. Factors such as early menstruation (before age 12) and late menopause (after age 55) contribute to prolonged hormone exposure. Because of this relationship between prolonged hormone exposure and breast cancer risk, scientists have been concerned that increasing a woman's lifelong exposure to hormones with HRT would result in increased breast cancer risk.

Over the last 25 years, numerous observational studies have examined the possible relationship between HRT and breast cancer. These studies have varied widely in terms of study design; size of populations studied; and doses, timing, and types of hormones used. Results of these studies have been inconsistent. Some of the early studies that followed women who used high doses of estrogen alone showed increased breast cancer risk. Other studies have looked at the experience of women who took estrogen combined with progestin. Some have shown an increased risk, while others have not.

Two studies compared the risk of breast cancer for women who had taken estrogen-only HRT with the risk for women who had taken HRT using estrogen combined with progestin. The first study analyzed data on 46,000 women. The researchers found that the risk for breast cancer among women who had used HRT during the past 4 years was higher than the risk for women who did not use HRT. For women who had taken the combination HRT, the risk of breast cancer increased by 8 percent per year; the risk was increased by 1 percent per year for women who had taken the estrogen-only therapy. There was no increase in risk among women who had stopped using either type of HRT for 4 years or more.

The second study focused on nearly 1,900 postmenopausal women diagnosed with breast cancer and more than 1,600 controls matched for age, race, and neighborhood. The researchers found that, for combined HRT, the risk of developing breast cancer increased by 24 percent for every 5 years of use; for estrogen-only therapy, the risk increased by 6 percent every 5 years. Both studies reported that the increased risk of breast cancer associated with either type of HRT was more pronounced in thin women.

In addition, data from the Postmenopausal Estrogen/Progestin Interventions (PEPI) trial indicate that about 25 percent of women who use HRT that includes a combination of progestin and estrogen have an increase in breast density on their mammograms. In the PEPI study, about 8 percent of women taking estrogen-only HRT also had increased breast density. Increased density is a concern because other studies have shown that women age 45 and older whose mammograms show at least 75 percent dense tissue are at increased risk for breast cancer. However, researchers do not know if increased breast density due to HRT carries the same risk for breast cancer as having naturally dense breasts.

Increased breast density from HRT makes it more difficult for a radiologist to read some mammograms, sometimes leading to the need for followup mammograms and breast biopsies. One study showed that stopping HRT for about 2 weeks before having a mammogram improved the readability of the mammogram. However, further research is needed to confirm the usefulness of this approach.

There is also considerable uncertainty about the relationship between a woman's risk of developing breast cancer and the length of time she receives HRT. Some women take HRT for only a few years, until the worst of their menopausal symptoms have passed, while others take it for a decade or more. Some researchers believe that there is little or no increased risk of breast cancer associated with short-term use (3 years or less) of either HRT with estrogen alone or estrogen combined with progestin, while long-term use is linked to an increased risk.

Still another area of controversy centers on whether women who have had breast cancer can take HRT, especially since treatments for breast cancer can often lead to early menopause in younger women. Use of HRT in breast cancer survivors is widely discouraged because of the concern that exposure to the estrogen in HRT would increase their risk for recurrence. Some scientists question the validity of this concern, since the prognosis of women who took HRT before developing breast cancer seems to be better than that of women who did not do so. However, this finding may be a result of increased doctor visits leading to earlier detection and may not be due to the HRT. Women with a history of breast cancer should talk with their doctor about HRT so that they can make an informed decision.

Phytoestrogens

Some women who are concerned about conventional HRT have turned to nonprescription remedies, such as foods containing phytoestrogens, to relieve their menopausal symptoms. Phytoestrogens are weak estrogen-like substances that are found in foods such as soy products, whole-grain cereals, seeds, and certain fruits and vegetables. Phytoestrogens can also be obtained in the form of soy tablets.

Researchers are studying the use of phytoestrogens as an alternative to conventional HRT, particularly in women with a history of breast cancer. However, studies conducted with breast cancer survivors have not shown a significant improvement in menopausal symptoms with increased intake of phytoestrogens. Researchers continue to study whether phytoestrogens affect a woman's risk of cancer. To make an informed decision about the use of phytoestrogens and HRT, women should talk with their doctor.

The Future of HRT

Many women decide against using HRT because they are concerned about the risk of developing cancer. Often, they prefer to take other steps (such as exercise and a well-balanced diet along with calcium supplementation) to reduce their risk of osteoporosis and heart disease.

In an effort to find definitive answers, the Women's Health Initiative (WHI) and other carefully designed studies are evaluating the effects of long-term use of HRT in postmenopausal women. Sponsored by the National Institutes of Health, the WHI is a 15-year nationwide clinical trial that is investigating heart disease, osteoporosis, and breast and colon cancers in 63,000 women ages 50 to 79. Long-term, well-designed studies such as the WHI should be able to answer many of the lingering questions about the true effects of HRT.

Weighing benefits and risks is part of all medical decisions. Some women and their doctors feel that HRT's potential beneficial effects on cardiovascular disease, osteoporosis, and general quality of life outweigh the risk of developing cancer. Others are concerned about the possible negative effects of long-term HRT use. Many women choose to reduce the risks of osteoporosis and heart disease by exercising regularly, avoiding tobacco products, eating a balanced diet, and/or taking dietary supplements or other medications.

Ultimately, physicians emphasize that each woman's decision about whether to take HRT and, if so, for how long, must be an individual one made in cooperation with her physician. This decision should be based on the woman's individual risk profile—her personal and family medical history, not only of cancer, but also of heart disease, stroke, and osteoporosis.

Adding Progestin to Hormone Replacement Therapy Increases Risk of Breast Cancer

Postmenopausal women taking the hormone estrogen in combination with progestin have an increased risk of breast cancer.

Dr. Ronald Ross, M.D., and colleagues at the University of Southern California Norris Comprehensive Cancer Center, present their results on this topic in the February 16 issue of the *Journal of the National Cancer Institute*.

Estrogen given to postmenopausal women may decrease the incidence of cardiovascular disease. However, the use of estrogen is associated with a substantially increased risk of endometrial cancer and slightly increased risk of breast cancer. Use of both estrogen and progestin, which is termed combined therapy, was introduced to reduce the increased risk of endometrial cancer, but the impact of combined therapy on breast cancer risk was not clear.

In response, the authors conducted a study of 1,897 postmenopausal women in Los Angeles County, California, who were diagnosed with breast cancer in the late 1980s and 1990s. These case patients were matched with 1637 postmenopausal women control subjects on the basis of age, race, and neighborhood of residence. Each participant was interviewed at home to collect information on a number of topics related to breast cancer, including a detailed history of the use of hormone replacement therapy and oral contraceptives.

Basic hormone replacement therapy, meaning the use of estrogen alone, was associated with a 6% increase in the risk of breast cancer for each 5 years of use, but this association was not statistically significant. However, combined therapy resulted in a 24% increase in risk of breast cancer for every 5 years of use. When estrogen use was followed in the monthly cycle by progestin, termed sequential combined therapy, the risk increased to 38% for each 5 years of use.

The authors conclude that even with the increases in endometrial and breast cancer risk associated with estrogen use, there is an overall benefit due to the marked reduction in risk from cardiovascular disease. They calculate, assuming the associations reflect causal relationships, that for every case of breast cancer due to estrogen use, more than six deaths from heart disease are prevented. However, their data suggest that the overall benefit from combined therapy (estrogen and progestin) could be considerably less favorable than that from estrogen alone, as the adverse effect on the breast may outweigh the beneficial effect on the endometrium. They conclude that women should be provided this information, and should be told where uncertainty still lies in the risk-benefit equation.

Resources

The following Federal Government agencies can provide information related to hormone replacement therapy:

National Institute on Aging (NIA)
Public Information Office
Building 31, Room 5C27
31 Center Drive, MSC 2292
Bethesda, MD 20892
Telephone 301-496-1752 or 1-800-222-2225
TTY: 1-800-222-4225 (for deaf and hard of hearing callers)
Internet Web site: http://www.nih.gov/nia/

The NIA Public Information Office offers printed material about menopause, osteoporosis, heart disease, and stroke.

National Institutes of Health (NIH)
Osteoporosis and Related Bone Diseases
National Resource Center
1232 22nd Street, NW.
Washington, DC 20037-1292
Telephone: 1-800-624-BONE (1-800-624-2663)
TTY: 202-466-4315 (for deaf and hard of hearing callers)
Fax: 202-293-2356
Internet Web site: http://www.osteo.org

The Osteoporosis and Related Bone Diseases National Resource Center distributes printed material about osteoporosis prevention and treatment.

National Heart, Lung, and Blood Institute (NHLBI)
Information Center
Post Office Box 30105
Bethesda, MD 20824-0105 *(continued on next page)*

National Heart, Lung, and Blood Institute (NHLBI) *(continued)*
Telephone: 301-592-8573
Fax: 301-592-8563
Internet Web site: http://www.nhlbi.nih.gov/index.htm

The NHLBI Information Center provides printed material about heart disease and its risk factors.

National Institute of Neurological Disorders and Stroke (NINDS)
Office of Communications and Public Liaison
Post Office Box 5801
Bethesda, MD 20824
Internet Web site: http://www.ninds.nih.gov

The NINDS Office of Communications and Public Liaison distributes printed material about stroke and other neurological disorders.

Women's Health Initiative (WHI)
Program Office
Suite 300 MS 7966
One Rockledge Centre
6705 Rockledge Drive
Bethesda, MD 20892-7966
Telephone: (301) 402-2900
Fax: (301) 480-5158
Internet Web site: http://www.nhlbi.nih.gov/whi/

The WHI Program Office provides information about the WHI.

National Cancer Institute Information Resources

You may want more information for yourself, your family, and your doctor. The following National Cancer Institute (NCI) services are available to help you.

Telephone: Cancer Information Service (CIS) provides accurate, up-to-date information on cancer to patients and their families, health professionals, and the general public. Information specialists translate the latest scientific information into understandable language and respond in English, Spanish, or on TTY equipment.
Telephone 1-800-4-CANCER (1-800-422-6237)
TTY: 1-800-332-8615 (for deaf and hard of hearing callers)

Internet: These web sites may be useful:

NCI's primary web site; contains information about the Institute and its programs. http://www.nci.nih.gov/

CancerNet; contains material for health professionals, patients, and the public, including information from PDQ about cancer treatment, screening, prevention, genetics, supportive care, and clinical trials, and CANCERLIT, a bibliographic database. http://cancernet.nci.nih.gov/

cancerTrials; NCI's comprehensive clinical trials information center for patients, health professionals, and the public. Includes information on understanding trials, deciding whether to participate in trials, finding specific trials, plus research news and other resources. http://cancertrials.nci.nih.gov/

E-mail: CancerMail includes NCI information about cancer treatment, screening, prevention, genetics, and supportive care. To obtain a contents list, send e-mail to cancermail@icicc.nci.nih.gov with the word "help" in the body of the message.

Fax: CancerFax includes NCI information about cancer treatment, screening, prevention, genetics, and supportive care. To obtain a contents list, dial 301-402-5874 or 1-800-624-2511 from a touch-tone telephone or fax machine hand set and follow the recorded instructions.

References

Andrews WC. The transitional years and beyond. *Obstetrics & Gynecology* 1995; 85(1):1-5.

Bonnier P, Romain S, Giacalone PL, et al. Clinical and biologic prognostic factors in breast cancer diagnosed during postmenopausal hormone replacement therapy. *Obstetrics & Gynecology* 1995; 85(1):11-17.

Brinton LA, Schairer C. Postmenopausal hormone-replacement therapy: time for a reappraisal? *New England Journal of Medicine* 1997; 336(25):1821-1822.

Bush TL. Feminine forever revisited: menopausal hormone therapy in the 1990s. *Journal of Women's Health* 1992; 1(1):1-4.

Bush TL, Whiteman MK. Hormone replacement therapy and risk of breast cancer. Editorial. *Journal of the American Medical Association* 1999; 281(22):2140-2141.

Davidson NE. Is hormone replacement therapy a risk? *Scientific American* 1996; 275(3):101.

Gapstur SM, Morrow M, Sellers TA. Hormone replacement therapy and risk of breast cancer with a favorable histology: results of the Iowa Women's Health Study. *Journal of the American Medical Association* 1999; 281(22):2091-2097.

Gottlieb, N. "Soybean" in a haystack? Pinpointing an anti-cancer effect. *Journal of the National Cancer Institute* 1999; 91(19):1610-1612.

Greendale GA, Reboussin BA, Sie A, et al. Effects of estrogen and estrogen-progestin on mammographic parenchymal density. Postmenopausal estrogen/progestin interventions (PEPI) investigators. *Annals of Internal Medicine* 1999; 130(4 Part 1):262-269.

Grodstein F, Stampfer MJ, Colditz GA, et al. Postmenopausal hormone therapy and mortality. *New England Journal of Medicine* 1997; 336(25):1769-1775.

Harvey JA, Pinkerton JV, Herman CR. Short-term cessation of hormone replacement therapy and improvement of mammographic specificity. *Journal of the National Cancer Institute* 1997; 89(21):1623-1625.

Hulley S, Grady D, Bush T, et al. Randomized trial of estrogen plus progestin for secondary prevention of coronary heart disease in postmenopausal women. *Journal of the American Medical Association* 1998; 280(7):605-613.

Keller C, Fullerton J, Mobley C. Supplemental and complementary alternatives to hormone replacement therapy. *Journal of the American Academy of Nurse Practitioners* 1999; 11(5):187-198.

Mayeaux EJ Jr., Johnson C. Current concepts in postmenopausal hormone replacement therapy. *The Journal of Family Practice* 1996; 43(1):69-75.

Quella SK, Loprinzi CL, Barton DL, et al. Evaluation of soy phytoestrogens for the treatment of hot flashes in breast cancer survivors: a North Central Cancer Treatment Group trial. *Journal of Clinical Oncology* 2000; 18(5):1068-1074.

Ross RK, Paganini-Hill A, Wan PC, Pike MC. Effect of hormone replacement therapy on breast cancer risk: estrogen versus estrogen plus progestin. *Journal of the National Cancer Institute* 2000; 92(4):328-332.

Schairer C, Lubin J, Troisi R, et al. Menopausal estrogen and estrogen-progestin replacement therapy and breast cancer risk. *Journal of the American Medical Association* 2000; 283(4): 485-491.

Willett W, Colditz G, Stampfer M. Postmenopausal estrogens opposed, unopposed, or none of the above. *Journal of the American Medical Association* 2000; 283(4):534-535.

Women's Health Initiative Study Group. Design of the women's health initiative clinical trial and observational study. *Controlled Clinical Trials* 1998; 19:61-109.

Writing Group for the PEPI Trial. Effects of estrogen or estrogen/progestin regimens on heart disease risk factors in postmenopausal women. The postmenopausal estrogen/progestin interventions (PEPI) trial. *Journal of the American Medical Association* 1995; 273(3):199-208.

Writing Group for the PEPI Trial. Effects of hormone therapy on bone mineral density: results from the postmenopausal estrogen/progestin interventions (PEPI) trial. *Journal of the American Medical Association* 1996; 276(17):1389-1396.

Wysowski DK, Golden L, Burke L. Use of menopausal estrogens and medroxyprogesterone in the United States, 1982-1992. *Obstetrics & Gynecology* 1995; 85(1):6-10.

Chapter 14

Alcohol and the Risk of Breast Cancer

The relationship between alcohol consumption and the risk of breast cancer is currently the focus of much research. Since alcohol consumption is a modifiable behavior, information regarding its association with breast cancer may offer women a practical way to decrease their risk of developing this disease.

Does the consumption of alcohol increase the risk of breast cancer?

The results of most studies indicate that there is a weak association between drinking alcoholic beverages and the incidence of breast cancer at low levels of consumption, and that the risk of breast cancer increases as the amount of alcohol consumed increases. In a recent summary of 63 published studies, 65% reported that consuming alcohol was associated with an increased risk of breast cancer. These studies involved different populations of women in several countries.

Women who drink alcohol may be different in many ways from those who do not drink alcohol. In order to determine if the consumption of alcohol is associated with breast cancer, researchers must take

From "Alcohol and the Risk of Breast Cancer," by Julie A. Napieralski, Ph.D. Research Associate, and Carol Devine, Ph.D., R.D. Division of Nutritional Sciences and Education Project Leader, Cornell University, Program on Breast Cancer and Environmental Risk Factors in New York State (BCERF), *FACT SHEET* #13, Institute for Comparative and Environmental Toxicology, Cornell Center for the Environment, March 1998; reprinted with permission.

into account other factors that have been previously shown to influence breast cancer risk. For example, getting older, having a family history of breast cancer, and an earlier age at menarche (the age when a girl has her first menstrual period) are established risk factors for breast cancer. When assessing the influence of alcohol consumption on breast cancer risk, it is important for researchers to account for these as well as other potential risk factors such as diet and smoking. These factors may be more common among women who drink alcoholic beverages and may actually be contributing to the reported association between alcohol and breast cancer.

Many of the studies of alcohol consumption and breast cancer risk have taken established breast cancer risk factors into account and some have also included other types of habits and behavioral differences, such as diet and smoking. The results of most of these studies suggest that the consumption of alcohol may have an independent and direct effect on a woman's risk of developing breast cancer. However, other researchers are not convinced that alcohol is acting independently and they are continuing to analyze the relationship between alcohol and other lifestyle and personal characteristics.

How much alcohol is thought to increase the risk of breast cancer?

Researchers have reported that there is a weak association between alcohol consumption and breast cancer in women who drink one alcoholic beverage a day. Drinking more, about 2 to 5 drinks per day, may be associated with a rate of breast cancer that is about 40% higher than the rate for non-drinkers. This level of risk is similar in proportion to that of other well-established risk factors. For example, breast cancer risk is reported to be about 25% higher in women whose age at menarche was 12 years or younger versus 15 years or older. Also, the risk of breast cancer among women whose mother or sister had breast cancer is increased about 50% or more as compared to women who do not have a family history of the disease.

Is there an age at which the consumption of alcohol has the greatest effect?

If alcohol is associated with breast cancer risk, it is important to understand whether the age at which a woman starts to drink alcohol is an important factor in this relationship. Some studies have reported that drinking before the age of 30 is more closely tied to breast cancer risk than recent or current drinking habits. Others have reported that current or recent drinking habits have a greater influence on breast cancer rates than drinking at an early age. Lifetime consumption of alcohol has also been suggested as an important factor when determining breast cancer risk. In other words, it may be the total amount of alcohol consumed during a lifetime regardless of the age at which the habit starts that is most important. Although researchers have not been able to establish the age at which consumption of alcohol has the greatest effect, drinking at any age may contribute to the risk.

Does the pattern of drinking affect the risk of breast cancer?

There are no studies that compare the effects of drinking every day to the effects of drinking only occasionally. In other words, it is not known whether drinking one drink every day, such as drinking wine with a meal, has the same relationship to breast cancer risk as binge drinking, such as having 7 drinks on a Saturday night.

What kinds of alcoholic beverages have been associated with breast cancer risk?

Some researchers reported that the consumption of beer and hard liquor, such as vodka and gin, had a greater association with breast cancer risk than the consumption of wine. Others have reported no difference in the type of alcoholic beverage consumed. Studies in European countries, such as Italy, where wine is consumed regularly at dinner, have also reported that the consumption of alcohol is associated with increased breast cancer risk. Therefore, the current evidence suggests that it is probably the alcohol in wine, beer and liquor and not some other component of these beverages that is associated with the risk of breast cancer.

How might alcohol increase the risk of breast cancer?

Several possible biological pathways by which alcohol might be acting to influence the risk of breast cancer have been suggested. Many researchers are analyzing the influence of alcohol on the levels of hormones in the body, particularly estrogen. Estrogen is important for normal development of the reproductive system, and lifetime estrogen exposure is thought to influence the development of breast cancer. In some studies, the consumption of alcohol has been observed to lead to increases in the level of estrogen in a woman's body. This overall increase in body estrogen levels may be due to an increase in the production of estrogen or a decrease in the breakdown of estrogen.

Since the studies on alcohol and estrogen are not yet conclusive, researchers are also studying other ways that alcohol may influence biological systems that affect breast cancer risk. For example, alcohol has a strong effect on the liver, an organ that helps rid the body of potentially harmful material. If the liver is not able to function properly, it may not be able to get rid of potential cancer-causing agents (carcinogens). There is also evidence that alcohol may be acting as a co-carcinogen.

More research is needed to discover the mechanism by which alcohol may influence the risk of breast cancer. This information will help researchers determine if alcohol works alone or along with some other breast cancer risk factors.

What about the positive health effects of alcohol consumption?

Researchers have reported that women who consume light to moderate amounts of alcohol have a decreased risk of developing and dying from cardiovascular disease. Since more women are affected by and may die from cardiovascular diseases than breast cancer, the recommendations regarding alcohol and breast cancer may seem to contradict the reports regarding cardiovascular disease. The *1996 Guidelines on Diet, Nutrition and Cancer Prevention* from the American Cancer Society suggest that most adults can drink, but they should limit their intake. Given the complex relationship between alcohol consumption and different diseases, any recommendations should be based on information about all health risks and benefits.

What kinds of research are needed to fully explain the relationship between alcohol and breast cancer?

- More research is needed to determine whether or not the age at which a woman starts to drink is important in determining breast cancer risk.

- Studies are needed to determine whether regular drinking during the week or binge drinking on the weekends has a greater influence on breast cancer risk.

- More research is needed to discover the mechanism(s) by which alcohol may be acting to influence the risk of breast cancer.

- More studies are needed which analyze the relationship of alcohol to other risk factors for breast cancer, such as menopausal status and hormone replacement therapy.

- Research is needed on the relationship of alcohol to other factors such as diet, body fat distribution, and genetics.

Should women drink alcoholic beverages?

The decision whether or not to drink alcoholic beverages needs to be made by a woman herself with the help of her physician. Women who have other well-established risk factors for breast cancer, such as a family history of the disease, may want to seriously consider limiting their alcohol consumption.

Cornell University Program on Breast Cancer and Environmental Risk Factors in New York State (BCERF)

Acknowledgment: BCERF would like to acknowledge the members of the Educational Advisory Board and the Technical Advisory Reviewers for their critical review of this information.

This text is a publication of the Cornell University Program on Breast Cancer and Environmental Risk Factors in New York State (BCERF). The Program is housed within the university-wide Institute for Comparative and Environmental Toxicology (ICET) in the Cornell Center for the Environment. BCERF strives to better understand the relationship between breast cancer and other hormonally-related cancers to environmental risk factors and to make this information available on an on-going basis to the citizens of New York State.

The program involves faculty and staff from the Cornell Ithaca campus (College of Agriculture and Life Sciences, College of Arts and Sciences, the College of Human Ecology, the College of Veterinary Medicine, the Division of Biological Sciences and the Division of Nutritional Sciences), Cornell Cooperative Extension, and the Cornell Medical College and Strang Cancer Prevention Center.

If you would like to be added to our mailing list to receive future copies of our newsletter, *THE RIBBON*, please contact the Administrative/Outreach Coordinator at the address below. Also included in the newsletter is a tear-off sheet listing other fact sheets.

We hope you find this text informative. We welcome your comments. When reproducing this material, credit the Program on Breast Cancer and Environmental Risk Factors in New York State.

Funding for this project was made possible by the New York State Department of Health.

An extensive bibliography on *Alcohol and the Risk of Breast Cancer* is available on the BCERF web site http://www.cfe.cornell.edu/bcerf/

Cornell University
Program on Breast Cancer and Environmental
Risk Factors in New York State
112 Rice Hall
Ithaca, NY 14853-5601
Phone: 607 254-2893
FAX: 607-255-8027
email: breastcancer@cornell.edu
Internet: http://www.cfe.cornell.edu/bcerf/

—*Julie A. Napieralski, Ph.D Research Associate, BCERF; and Carol Devine, Ph.D., R.D. Division of Nutritional Sciences and Education Project Leader, BCERF*

Chapter 15

Oral Contraceptives and Cancer Risk

Oral contraceptives (OCs) first became available to American women in the early 1960s. The convenience, effectiveness, and reversibility of action of birth control pills (which are popularly known as "the pill") has made them the most popular form of birth control in the United States. However, a correlation between estrogen and increased risk of breast cancer has led to continuing controversy about a possible link between OCs and cancer.

This chapter addresses only what is known about OC use and the risk of developing cancer. It does not deal with the most serious side effect of OC use—the increased risk of cardiovascular disease for certain groups of women.

Oral Contraceptives

Currently, two types of OCs are available in the United States. The most commonly prescribed OC contains two synthetic versions of natural female hormones (estrogen and progesterone) that are similar to the hormones the ovaries normally produce. Estrogen stimulates the growth and development of the uterus at puberty, thickens the endometrium (the inner lining of the uterus) during the first half of the menstrual cycle, and stimulates changes in breast tissue at puberty and childbirth. Two types of synthetic estrogens are used in OCs, ethinyl estradiol and mestranol.

Cancer Facts, National Cancer Institute, February 2000.

Progesterone, which is produced during the last half of the menstrual cycle, prepares the endometrium to receive the egg. If the egg is fertilized, progesterone secretion continues, preventing release of additional eggs from the ovaries. For this reason, progesterone is called the "pregnancy-supporting" hormone, and scientists believe it to have valuable contraceptive effects. The synthetic progesterone used in OCs is called progestogen or progestin. Norethindrone and levonorgestrel are examples of synthetic progesterones used in OCs.

The second type of OC available in the United States is called the minipill and contains only a progestogen. The minipill is less effective in preventing pregnancy than the combination pill, so it is prescribed less often.

Because medical research suggests that cancers of the female reproductive organs sometimes depend on naturally occurring sex hormones for their development and growth, scientists have been investigating a possible link between OC use and cancer risk. Medical researchers have focused a great deal of attention on OC users over the past 30 years. This scrutiny has produced a wealth of data on OC use and the development of certain cancers, although results of these studies have not always been consistent.

Breast Cancer

A woman's risk of developing breast cancer depends on several factors, some of which are related to her natural hormones. Hormonal factors that increase the risk of breast cancer include conditions that allow high levels of estrogen to persist for long periods of time, such as early age at first menstruation (before age 12), late age at menopause (after age 55), having children after age 30, and not having children at all. A woman's risk of breast cancer increases with the amount of time she is exposed to estrogen.

Because many of the risk factors for breast cancer are related to natural hormones, and because OCs work by manipulating these hormones, there has been some concern about the possible effects of medicines such as OCs on breast cancer risk, especially if women take them for many years. Sufficient time has elapsed since the introduction of OCs to allow investigators to study large numbers of women who took birth control pills for many years beginning at a young age and to follow them as they became older.

However, studies examining the use of OCs as a risk factor for breast cancer have produced inconsistent results. Most studies have not found an overall increased risk for breast cancer associated with

OC use. In June 1995, however, investigators at the National Cancer Institute (NCI) reported an increased risk of developing breast cancer among women under age 35 who had used birth control pills for at least 6 months, compared with those who had never used OCs. They also saw a slightly lower, but still elevated, risk among women ages 35 to 44. In addition, their research showed a higher risk among long-term OC users, especially those who had started to take the pill before age 18.

A 1996 analysis of worldwide epidemiologic data, which included information from the 1995 study, found that women who were current or recent users of birth control pills had a slightly elevated risk of developing breast cancer. However, 10 years or more after they stopped using OCs, their risk of developing breast cancer returned to the same level as if they had never used birth control pills.

To conduct this analysis, the researchers examined the results of 54 studies conducted in 25 countries that involved 53,297 women with breast cancer and 100,239 women without breast cancer. More than 200 researchers participated in this combined exhaustive analysis of their original studies, which represented about 90 percent of the epidemiological studies throughout the world that had investigated the possible relationship between OCs and breast cancer.

The return of risk to normal levels after 10 years or more of not taking OCs was consistent regardless of family history of breast cancer, reproductive history, geographic area of residence, ethnic background, differences in study designs, dose and type of hormone, and duration of use. The change in risk also generally held true for age at first use; however, for reasons that were not fully understood, there was a continued elevated risk among women who had started to use OCs before age 20.

One encouraging aspect of the study is that the slightly elevated risk seen in both current OC users and those who had stopped use less than 10 years previously may not be due to the contraceptive itself. The slightly elevated risk may result from the potential of estrogen to promote the growth of breast cancer cells that are already present, rather than its potential to initiate changes in normal cells leading to the development of cancer.

Furthermore, the observation that the slightly elevated risk of developing breast cancer that was seen in this study peaked during use, declined gradually after OC use had stopped, then returned to normal risk levels 10 years or more after stopping, is not consistent with the usual process of carcinogenesis. It is more typical for cancer risk to peak decades after exposure, not immediately afterward. Cancer usually is more likely to occur with increased duration and/or degree of exposure to a carcinogen. In this analytical study, neither the dose and type of hormone nor the duration of use affected the risk of developing breast cancer.

Ovarian and Endometrial Cancers

Many studies have found that using OCs reduces a woman's risk of ovarian cancer by 40 to 50 percent compared with women who have not used OCs. The Centers for Disease Control and Prevention's (CDC) Cancer and Steroid Hormone Study (CASH), along with other research conducted over the past 20 years, shows that the longer a woman uses OCs, the lower her risk of ovarian cancer. Moreover, this lowered risk persists long after OC use ceases. The CASH study found that the reduced risk of ovarian cancer is seen in women who have used OCs for as little as 3 to 6 months, and that it continues for 15 years after use ends. Other studies have confirmed that the reduced risk of ovarian cancer continues for at least 10 to 15 years after a woman has stopped taking OCs. Several hypotheses have been offered to explain how oral contraceptives might protect against ovarian cancer, such as a reduction in the number of ovulations a woman has during her lifetime, but the exact mechanism is still not known.

Researchers have also found that OC use may reduce the risk of endometrial cancer. Findings from the CASH study and other reports show that combination OC use can protect against the development of endometrial cancer. The CASH study found that using combination OCs for at least 1 year reduced the risk of developing endometrial cancer to that of women who never took birth control pills. In addition, the beneficial effect of OC use persisted for at least 15 years after OC users stopped taking birth control pills. Some researchers have found that the protective effect of OCs against endometrial cancer increases with the length of time combination OCs are used, but results have not been consistent.

The reduction in risk of ovarian and endometrial cancers from OC use does not apply to the sequential type of pill, in which each monthly cycle contains 16 estrogen pills followed by 5 estrogen-plus-progesterone pills. (Sequential OCs were taken off the market in 1976, so few women have been exposed to them.) Researchers believe OCs reduce cancer risk only when the estrogen content of birth control pills is balanced by progestogen in the same pill.

Cancer of the Cervix

There is some evidence that long-term use of OCs may increase the risk of cancer of the cervix (the narrow, lower portion of the uterus).

The results of studies conducted by NCI scientists and other researchers support a relationship between extended use of the pill (5 or more years) and a slightly increased risk of cervical cancer. However, the exact nature of the association between OC use and risk of cervical cancer remains unclear.

One reason that the association is unclear is that two of the major risk factors for cervical cancer (early age at first intercourse and a history of multiple sex partners) are related to sexual behavior. Because these risk factors may be different between women who use OCs and those who have never used them, it is difficult for researchers to determine the exact role that OCs may play in the development of cervical cancer.

Also, many studies on OCs and cervical cancer have not accounted for the influence of human papillomaviruses (HPVs) on cervical cancer risk. HPVs are a group of more than 70 types of viruses, some of which are known to increase the risk of cervical cancer. Compared to non-OC users, women who use OCs may be less likely to use barrier methods of contraception (such as condoms). Since condoms can prevent the transmission of HPVs, OC users who do not use them may be at increased risk of becoming infected with HPVs. Therefore, the increased risk of cervical cancer that some studies found to be caused by prolonged OC use may actually be the result of HPV infection.

There is evidence that pill users who never use a barrier method of contraception or who have a history of genital infections are at a higher risk for developing cervical cancer. This association supports the theory that OCs may act together with sexually transmitted agents (such as HPVs) in the development of cervical cancer. Researchers continue to investigate the exact nature of the relationship between OC use and cancer of the cervix.

OC product labels have been revised to inform women of the possible risk of cervical cancer. The product labels also warn that birth control pills do not protect against human immunodeficiency virus (HIV) and other sexually transmitted diseases such as HPV, chlamydia, and genital herpes.

Liver Tumors

There is some evidence that OCs may increase the risk of certain malignant (cancerous) liver tumors. However, the risk is difficult to evaluate because of different patterns of OC use and because these tumors are rare in American women (the incidence is approximately 2 cases per 100,000 women). A benign (noncancerous) tumor of the

137

liver called hepatic adenoma has also been found to occur, although rarely, among OC users. These tumors do not spread, but they may rupture and cause internal bleeding.

Reducing Risks

After many years on the U.S. market, the overall health effects of OCs are still mixed. The most serious side effect of the pill continues to be an increased risk of cardiovascular disease in certain groups, such as women who smoke; women over age 35; obese women; and those with a history of high blood pressure, diabetes, or elevated serum cholesterol levels. Information about the increased risk of cardiovascular disease is available from the National Heart, Lung, and Blood Institute (NHLBI). The NHLBI Information Center can be reached at:

NHLBI Information Center
Post Office Box 30105
Bethesda, MD 20824-0105
Telephone: 301-592-8573
Fax: 301-592-8563
E-mail: NHLBIinfo@rover.nhlbi.nih.gov
Internet Web site: http://www.nhlbi.nih.gov

The NCI (National Cancer Institute) recommends that women in their forties or older get screening mammograms on a regular basis, every 1 to 2 years. Women who are at increased risk for breast cancer should seek medical advice about when to begin having mammograms and how often to be screened. A high-quality mammogram, with a clinical breast exam (an exam done by a professional health care provider), is the most effective way to detect breast cancer early.

Women who are or have been sexually active or are in their late teens or older can reduce their risk for cervical cancer by having regular Pap tests. Research has shown that women who have never had a Pap test or who have not had one for several years have a higher-than-average risk of developing cervical cancer.

For More Information

Women who are concerned about their risk for cancer are encouraged to talk with their doctor. More information is also available from the Cancer Information Service.

Telephone: Cancer Information Service (CIS) provides accurate, up-to-date information on cancer to patients and their families, health professionals, and the general public. Information specialists translate the latest scientific information into understandable language and respond in English, Spanish, or on TTY equipment.
Telephone 1-800-4-CANCER (1-800-422-6237)
TTY: 1-800-332-8615 (for deaf and hard of hearing callers)

Internet: These web sites may be useful:

NCI's primary web site; contains information about the Institute and its programs. http://www.nci.nih.gov/

CancerNet; contains material for health professionals, patients, and the public, including information from PDQ about cancer treatment, screening, prevention, genetics, supportive care, and clinical trials, and CANCERLIT, a bibliographic database. http://cancernet.nci.nih.gov/

cancerTrials; NCI's comprehensive clinical trials information center for patients, health professionals, and the public. Includes information on understanding trials, deciding whether to participate in trials, finding specific trials, plus research news and other resources. http://cancertrials.nci.nih.gov/

E-mail: CancerMail includes NCI information about cancer treatment, screening, prevention, genetics, and supportive care. To obtain a contents list, send e-mail to cancermail@icicc.nci.nih.gov with the word "help" in the body of the message.

Fax: CancerFax includes NCI information about cancer treatment, screening, prevention, genetics, and supportive care. To obtain a contents list, dial 301-402-5874 or 1-800-624-2511 from a touch-tone telephone or fax machine hand set and follow the recorded instructions.

References

Breast Cancer

Brinton LA, Daling JR, Liff JM, et al. Oral contraceptives and breast cancer risk among younger women. *Journal of the National Cancer Institute* 1995; 87(13):827-835.

The Centers for Disease Control and the National Institute of Child Health and Human Development. Oral contraceptive use and the risk of breast cancer: The Centers for Disease Control and the National Institute of Child Health and Human Development Cancer and Steroid Hormone Study. *New England Journal of Medicine* 1986; 315:405-411.

Chilvers C, McPherson K, Pike MC, et al. Oral contraceptive use and breast cancer risk in young women. *Lancet* 1989; 1:973-982.

McPherson K, Vessey MP, Neil A, et al. Early oral contraceptive use and breast cancer: results of another case-control study. *British Journal of Cancer* 1987; 56:653-660.

Meirik O, Lund E, Adami HO, et al. Oral Contraceptive use and breast cancer in young women: a joint national study in Sweden and Norway. *Lancet* 1986; 2:650-654.

Miller DR, Rosenberg L, Kaufman DW, et al. Breast cancer before age 45 and oral contraceptive use: new findings. *American Journal of Epidemiology* 1989; 129:269-280.

Olsson H, Olsson ML, Moeller TR, et al. Oral contraceptive use and breast cancer in young women in Sweden. *Lancet* 1985; 1:748-749.

Paul C, Skegg DCG, Spears GFS. Oral contraceptives and risk of breast cancer. *International Journal of Cancer* 1990; 46:366-373.

Pike MC, Henderson BE, Krailo MD, et al. Breast cancer in young women and use of oral contraceptives: possible modifying effect of formulation and age at use. *Lancet* 1983; 2:926-930.

Romiu I, Berlin JA, Colditz G. Oral contraceptives and breast cancer: review and meta-analysis. *Cancer* 1990; 66:2253-2263.

Rookus MA, Van Leeuwen FE. Oral contraceptives and risk of breast cancer in women aged 25-54 years: The Netherlands Oral Contraceptives and Breast Cancer Study Group. *Lancet* 1994; 344:844-851.

Thomas DB. Oral contraceptives and breast cancer: review of the epidemiologic literature. *Contraception* 1991; 43(6):597-642.

White E, Malone KE, Weiss NS, et al. Breast cancer among young U.S. women in relation to oral contraceptive use. *Journal of the National Cancer Institute* 1994; 86: 505-514.

Wingo PA, Lee NC, Ory HW, et al. Age-specific differences in the relationship between oral contraceptive use and breast cancer. *Cancer Supplement* 1993; 71(4):1506-1517.

Ovarian and Endometrial Cancers

Brinton LA, Huggins GR, Lehman HF, et al. Long-term use of oral contraceptives and risk of invasive cervical cancer. *International Journal of Cancer* 1986; 38:339-344.

The Centers for Disease Control. Oral contraceptive use and the risk of ovarian cancer: The Centers for Disease Control Cancer and Steroid Hormone Study. *Journal of the American Medical Association* 1983; 249:1596-1599.

The Centers for Disease Control. Combination oral contraceptive use and the risk of endometrial cancer: The Cancer and Steroid Hormone Study of the Centers for Disease Control and the National Institute of Child Health and Human Development. *Journal of the American Medical Association* 1987; 257(6):796-800.

The Centers for Disease Control and the National Institute of Child Health and Human Development. The reduction in risk of ovarian cancer associated with oral contraceptive use: The Cancer and Steroid Hormone Study of the Centers for Disease Control and the National Institute of Child Health and Human Development. *New England Journal of Medicine* 1987; 316:650-655.

Stanford JL, Brinton LA, Berman ML, et al. Oral contraceptives and endometrial cancer: do other risk factors modify the association? *International Journal of Cancer* 1993; 54(2):243-248.

Cancer of the Cervix

Brinton LA. Epidemiology of cervical cancer—overview. *IARC Scientific Publications* 1992; 119:3-23.

Brinton LA. Oral contraceptives and cervical neoplasia. *Contraception* 1991; 43(6):581-595.

Brinton LA, Huggins GR, Lehman HF, et al. Long-term use of oral contraceptives and risk of invasive cervical cancer. *International Journal of Cancer* 1986; 38(3):399-444.

Daling JR, Madeleine MM, McKnight B, et al. The relationship of human papillomavirus-related cervical tumors to cigarette smoking, oral contraceptive use, and prior herpes simplex virus type 2 infection. *Cancer Epidemiology, Biomarkers, and Prevention* 1996; 5(7):541-548.

Gram IT, Macaluso M, Stalsberg H. Oral contraceptive use and the incidence of cervical intraepithelial neoplasia. *American Journal of Obstetrics and Gynecology* 1992; 167(1):40-44.

Munoz N, Bosch FX, de Sanjose S, et al. The causal link between human papillomavirus and invasive cervical cancer: a population-based case-control study in Colombia and Spain. *International Journal of Cancer* 1992; 52(5):743-749.

Liver Cancer

Rooks JB, Ory HW, Ishak KG, et al. Epidemiology of hepatocellular adenoma: the role of oral contraceptive use. *Journal of the American Medical Association* 1979; 242:644-648.

Tao, LC. Oral contraceptive-associated liver cell adenoma and hepatocellular carcinoma. *Cancer* 1991; 68:341-347.

Palmer J, Rosenberg L, Kaufman DW, et al. Oral contraceptive use and liver cancer. *American Journal of Epidemiology* 1989; 130:878-882.

Chapter 16

Phytoestrogens and the Risk of Breast Cancer

Many people want to know whether the estrogen-like compounds found in certain plant-based foods, particularly soy foods, may help reduce their risk of developing breast cancer. These compounds, called phytoestrogens, are also the focus of much research. Although there is still a lot of work to be done before we know whether phytoestrogen-rich foods reduce breast cancer risk, this chapter presents some of the most current information available and indicates where more research would help.

What are phytoestrogens?

Phytoestrogens are compounds found in plants that act like weaker versions of the hormone estrogen. Estrogen is necessary for childbearing and for bone and heart health in women. However, a woman's lifetime exposure to estrogen may influence her breast cancer risk. Isoflavonoids, coumestans, and lignans are all types of phytoestrogens that are currently being studied for their potential health benefits.

From "Phytoestrogens and the Risk of Breast Cancer," by Julie A. Napieralski, Ph.D. Research Associate, Dana Hibner, and Carol Devine, Ph.D., R.D. Division of Nutritional Sciences and Education Project Leader, Cornell University, Program on Breast Cancer and Environmental Risk Factors in New York State (BCERF), *FACT SHEET* #1, Institute for Comparative and Environmental Toxicology, Cornell Center for the Environment, Revised March 2000; reprinted with permission.

What foods contain phytoestrogens?

Whole grains, dried beans, peas and seeds, vegetables, fruits and soybeans and soy-foods, such as tofu, all contain phytoestrogens. Soybeans and foods made from soybeans are the most significant dietary source of some of the most active phytoestrogens, the isoflavonoids. Genistein and daidzein are two of the most well studied isoflavonoids. Information on the isoflavonoid content of specific foods can be found at the following United States Department of Agriculture website: http://www.nal.usda.gov/fnic/ foodcomp/Data/isoflav/isoflav.html

The phytoestrogen content of soy-food products varies with conditions such as the processing and preparation of the food; processing generally decreases the isoflavone content of soy products. When we eat soy-foods, the bacteria naturally present in our intestine changes the isoflavonoids in the soy into hormone-like compounds with estrogen activity.

Do phytoestrogens reduce breast cancer risk?

There is indirect evidence from both human and laboratory studies that phytoestrogens may help reduce a woman's risk of developing breast cancer. Women in Asian countries, such as Japan, who traditionally consume more soy products than most women in Western countries, such as the U.S., have a higher concentration of phytoestrogens in their blood and urine and a lower risk of breast cancer. In other studies, women who had soy products added to their diets, had lower levels of estrogen and other hormones in their bodies compared to women on regular diets. Since a lower level of estrogen has been associated with a lower risk of breast cancer, these results suggest that the consumption of soy products may help reduce a woman's risk of developing breast cancer.

There are few epidemiologic studies that have looked at whether the consumption of soy products is associated with a decrease in the risk of breast cancer. Studies that would provide direct evidence have mixed results. Four recent case-control studies were conducted in China, Japan and among Asian-American women living in California and Hawaii. One Chinese study reported that the intake of soy protein and soy products was associated with a significant decrease in the risk of breast cancer among premenopausal women, but not postmenopausal women. In contrast, the second Chinese study reported no association between the intake of soy and breast cancer risk in either premenopausal or postmenopausal women. In the Japanese study, there was no association between the consumption of soup made from miso (a fermented paste of ground soybeans, rice and barley) and the risk of breast cancer in either pre-or postmenopausal women. In the study of Asian-American women, consumption of tofu was associated with a significant decrease in the risk of breast cancer in premenopausal women and a slight decrease among postmenopausal women. One problem with the current studies is that they were not designed to specifically investigate the role of soy products in the development of breast cancer. Also, the intake of fruits and vegetables may be associated with the intake of soy and should be considered in all analyses. More studies that accurately measure a woman's consumption of phytoestrogens would help clarify whether or not they reduce breast cancer risk.

In two other studies, researchers reported that women with high levels of isoflavones in their urine had a significant reduction in their risk of breast cancer. These results suggest that women with a high intake of phytoestrogens, as measured by how much is excreted by the body, may have a reduced risk of breast cancer. However, since other researchers have reported that the metabolism and excretion of isoflavones varies considerably among women, excretion levels may not be an accurate measure of consumption.

Studies in animals and in isolated breast cells suggest that phytoestrogens may affect the growth of breast tumors. In the laboratory, isolated human breast cancer cells were exposed to different concentrations of genistein. The researchers found that a low concentration of genistein stimulated the growth of the cells, but that a high concentration inhibited growth. These results were dependent on whether or not the cells had estrogen receptors. The growth of cells with estrogen receptors depends on the concentration of genistein, while the growth of cells without estrogen receptors is always inhibited by genistein. These kinds of studies suggest that phytoestrogens have different effects on different types of cells and that they may be influencing growth in several different ways.

In addition, some studies in breast cells have reported that isoflavones such as genistein act as either estrogen receptor "agonists" or estrogen receptor "antagonists" depending on their concentration. However this has not been shown in animals or humans. An estrogen receptor agonist causes a cell to respond as it would respond to estrogen. An antagonist blocks the receptor and causes a response different from estrogen, or no response. Although the results from these studies cannot be directly transferred to humans because the form of the phytoestrogen and its metabolism may affect its role in the body, they do help researchers design studies in humans to answer these questions.

What amount of phytoestrogens would I have to eat to reduce my risk of breast cancer?

There is not enough information to make a recommendation on the amount or frequency of soy (isoflavone) intake necessary to protect against the development of breast cancer. Women in Asian countries such as China, where the incidence of breast cancer is low, consume about 25-100 mg per day of isoflavones. In Western countries such as the U.S., where the incidence of breast cancer is high, women consume less than 5 mg per day of isoflavones. It is important to remember that the isoflavone consumption in Asian women is based on soy-food consumption, not supplements. Also, the lifetime diets, physical activity and weight patterns of women in Asian countries differ in many ways from those of women in Western countries. Finally, the metabolism and excretion of isoflavones varies considerably among women. These differences in the way the body handles estrogen may need to be considered before any recommendations can be made on the amount of isoflavones required to prevent the development of breast cancer. Clinical studies are needed to obtain correct information on the consumption of soy-foods and the amount of isoflavones required to produce health benefits without causing harm to the body (see below).

Is there any harm in taking phytoestrogen supplements or eating more foods that contain phytoestrogens?

Since phytoestrogens act like weaker versions of the hormone estrogen, they may interact and affect the same parts of the body as estrogen. Studies in animals have shown that high concentrations of phytoestrogens can cause infertility and produce developmental changes. In addition, one study reported that women taking concentrated soy supplements had an increase in the rate of proliferation (cell division) of normal breast cells, and another reported breast cell hyperplasia (cells that grow too much) in premenopausal women taking concentrated soy supplements. Although not cancer, these changes also occur in early stages of cancer.

Although certain risks may be associated with the consumption of very high concentrations of phytoestrogens, it would be difficult for an adult to consume enough food containing phytoestrogens to achieve the levels that result in the toxicological responses seen in the laboratory. However, consuming very high doses from concentrated supplements may be more likely to cause these effects. Until more is known about the appropriate dose of phytoestrogens required for maximal health and low risk, it would be safer to add more soy-foods into the diets rather than relying on the use of supplements. Also, there is some evidence that other components of soybeans, not just the phytoestrogens, may have additional benefits. Some of the other components being studied include saponins and phytosterols.

Is there a certain age or time during a woman's life that is the best time to eat phytoestrogens?

No human studies that have been designed to assess when during a woman's life the consumption of phytoestrogens is most important to affect the risk of breast cancer. According to some animal studies, pre-adolescent exposure may be very important for full cancer-protection benefits. When given during the early prepubertal period of life (adolescence), phytoestrogens can enhance the differentiation of cells. These more mature cells are less susceptible to carcinogens. Other researchers have suggested that it may be lifetime exposure to phytoestrogens that is most important for decreasing the risk of developing breast cancer.

Should breast cancer survivors eat more phytoestrogens?

Currently, there are no human studies that have assessed the health effects of phytoestrogens among breast cancer patients. Also, there are no human studies that have studied the effects of combining tamoxifen (an anti-estrogenic drug prescribed for many breast cancer survivors and some women at high risk for breast cancer) and phytoestrogens on the outcomes of breast cancer. Until more is known, women taking tamoxifen are usually not included in studies where concentrated supplements of phytoestrogens are given.

Researchers have studied and compared the actions of tamoxifen and genistein in the laboratory using isolated breast cancer cells. These studies reported that tamoxifen and genistein have a similar attachment to the estrogen receptor. However, when isolated human breast cells are exposed to both genistein and tamoxifen at the same time, genistein can stimulate cell growth and override the growth inhibitory effect of tamoxifen. The results of these studies suggest that it is important for researchers to try to understand what happens when tamoxifen, genistein and naturally occurring estrogen are all together at the same time in the human body.

The only human studies available are correlation studies which report that Japanese breast cancer patients who typically consume more phytoestrogens than Western women with breast cancer, have a better prognosis. However, these studies did not ask about whether or not the women were also taking tamoxifen.

Should I eat more phytoestrogens if I am currently taking other hormones, such as hormone replacement therapy or birth control pills?

Since phytoestrogens act like weak versions of the hormone estrogen, they may interact with other types of estrogens, such as those in hormone replacement therapy or birth control pills. Currently there are no studies of the effects of combining phytoestrogens with other forms of estrogen.

Should infants and young children eat more phytoestrogens?

Soy infant formulas may contain about ten times the amount of phytoestrogens compared to human breast milk. However, there are no studies in humans on the consequences or benefits of high levels of soy consumption early in life. Long-term studies that look at the health benefits and risks of soy-based infant formulas are needed.

Should I eat more phytoestrogens if I am pregnant or breast-feeding?

There is no evidence that the children of women in China and Japan who regularly consume phytoestrogen containing foods during pregnancy and while breast-feeding have any adverse health affects. Also, several studies have reported that breast milk does not contain high levels of phytoestrogens. However, animal studies have reported that high levels of phytoestrogens consumed during pregnancy may affect the development of the fetus or possibly susceptibility to carcinogens in offspring. One study showed that physiological amounts (levels that could result from dietary intake) of genistein in the diet given to rats early in life may reduce, rather than enhance, the incidence of cancer in rats. The results of these studies may differ because of differences in study design, such as the method of administration and the size and timing of the phytoestrogen dose given to animals during development. Much more research is needed in this area.

How might phytoestrogens influence the risk of breast cancer?

There are several different ways that phytoestrogens may help reduce the risk of breast cancer. Phytoestrogens may:

- Suppress or inhibit normal estrogen production. Lower levels of estrogen have been associated with a decreased risk of breast cancer.
- Prevent the formation of new blood vessels by acting as anti-angiogenesis factors. This would prevent any tumor from obtaining a blood supply that is necessary for its continued growth.
- Act as antioxidants, like vitamin E. Antioxidants are compounds that absorb free radicals that may damage cells. Free radicals are produced by cells as natural by-products of normal cell activities, or in response to harmful contact with something in its environment.
- Prevent tumor cells from dividing and growing.
- Increase the excretion of estrogens into the urine and feces, leading to lower blood estrogen levels.

Are there more studies being done?

There are clinical trials underway to assess the protective effect of soy-foods. More research is needed to determine how much food containing phytoestrogens are needed to reduce breast cancer risk. Also, research is needed to determine how phytoestrogens may interact with other forms of estrogens used as drugs such as tamoxifen and those found in hormone replacement therapy and oral contraceptives.

Do phytoestrogens have other health benefits?

The consumption of foods containing phytoestrogens may also help reduce the risk of coronary heart disease and osteoporosis, and may help reduce the severity of menopausal symptoms.

What should women do now?

Women can help themselves stay healthy by eating plenty of fruits, vegetables and whole grains, and by getting plenty of exercise and maintaining a healthy weight.

Cornell University Program on Breast Cancer and Environmental Risk Factors in New York State

We hope you find this text informative. We welcome your comments. When reproducing this material, please credit the Program on Breast Cancer and Environmental Risk Factors in New York State.

An extensive bibliography on "Phytoestrogens and the Risk of Breast Cancer" is available on the BCERF web site: http://www.cfe.cornell.edu/bcerf/

Funding for this project was made possible by the US Department of Agriculture/Cooperative State Research, Education and Extension Service, the New York State Department of Health and Cornell University.

Cornell University
Program on Breast Cancer and Environmental
Risk Factors in New York State
112 Rice Hall
Ithaca, NY 14853-5601
Phone:(607) 254-2893
Fax:(607) 255-8207
email:breastcancer@cornell.edu
Internet: http://www.cfe.cornell.edu/bcerf/

—Prepared by: Julie A. Napieralski, Ph.D. Research Associate, BCERF; Dana Hibner, Cornell '99 and Carol M. Devine, Ph.D., R.D. Division of Nutritional Sciences and Education Project Leader, BCERF

Chapter 17

Dietary Fat and the Risk of Breast Cancer

Early studies suggested that high dietary fat intake was associated with a higher incidence of breast cancer. Other studies have failed to show a clear relationship between fat intake and breast cancer risk. These conflicting reports have left some women feeling frustrated. A closer look at the information available provides us with some idea of how fat in our diet might influence breast cancer risk and why the research results in this area are not in agreement. Also, some recommendations can be made for fat intake that would help promote general health. Although researchers may currently disagree on the role fat plays in the development of breast cancer, they do agree that the results of previous studies indicate that this relationship is worthy of further study.

Does the consumption of fat increase the risk of breast cancer?

The evidence on the relationship between the consumption of fat and the risk of breast cancer is mixed. According to international correlation studies, in countries with a high incidence of breast cancer such as the U.S., fat contributes about 34% of the total calories. In

From "Dietary Fat and the Risk of Breast Cancer," by Julie A. Napieralski, Ph.D. Research Associate, and Carol Devine, Ph.D., R.D. Division of Nutritional Sciences and Education Project Leader, Cornell University, Program on Breast Cancer and Environmental Risk Factors in New York State (BCERF), *FACT SHEET* #27, Institute for Comparative and Environmental Toxicology, Cornell Center for the Environment, May 1999; reprinted with permission.

countries with a low incidence of breast cancer such as China, fat contributes much less, about 15%-20% of the total calories. The limitation of this kind of study is that it can demonstrate only that dietary fat and breast cancer are related in the population, not that dietary fat causes breast cancer in particular women. These studies look at estimates of food intake for whole populations and do not provide information about the dietary habits of individual women. Also, they typically do not take into account the effects of other risk factors for breast cancer such as early age at menarche (a girl's first menstrual period) or family history in their analysis.

In numerous case-control studies, women with breast cancer and women without breast cancer were asked about their dietary habits during the previous year or two. Results from 25 studies that looked at the effect of total fat intake on breast cancer risk are inconsistent. Only two of those studies reported that a high fat diet was significantly associated with an increased risk of breast cancer. However, several of the studies reported a modest, but not significant increase in the incidence of breast cancer in women who had the highest levels of fat intake compared to women at the lowest levels of fat intake.

In cohort studies, a large group of women without breast cancer is asked about their usual dietary habits, including their consumption of foods containing fats and oils. These same women are contacted years later to see how many developed breast cancer. None of the available cohort studies reported a significant increase in the risk of breast cancer associated with a high fat intake. All of these studies were done in Western countries where the average total fat intake was usually well above 30% of total calories. Also, they include only current dietary habits and do not consider changes in the diet and/or diet during childhood.

In contrast, there are more than 95 studies, using four different animal models of breast cancer that reported that dietary fat increased the development of breast tumors in laboratory animals. This effect appears to be dependent on the type of fat in the diet, as discussed in more detail below.

Why are the results of studies of dietary fat and breast cancer contradictory?

The following is a list of some possible reasons why it has been so difficult to establish whether there is a link between dietary fat and breast cancer.

- It is difficult to study the relationship between specific nutrients and breast cancer. We consume foods, not individual nutrients. Therefore, the whole diet may be what is most important.

- There are differences among studies in design and in how dietary fat intake was measured.

- In many studies, the range of fat intake in the population studied is very narrow. For example, most of the women in the U.S. studies have a fat intake of about 30%-40% of total calories compared to 15%-35% in China. It may be that there are not enough women at the very low levels of fat intake in western countries like the U.S. to show a difference in breast cancer rates.

- Studies of diet and breast cancer risk usually include information about current dietary habits only. These studies are not able to determine if a high dietary fat intake during early childhood or adolescence influences breast cancer risk.

- Diet, exercise and obesity are all very closely related and may influence breast cancer risk independently or together.

- The effect of a high fat diet on the risk of breast cancer may not be as important as the effect of the different kinds of dietary fat, including saturated, monounsaturated and polyunsaturated fat.

How do dietary fats differ in ways that are important to breast cancer risk?

Many studies have also tried to determine if saturated, monounsaturated and polyunsaturated fats have different effects on the development of breast cancer. Both saturated fats and polyunsaturated fats, particularly those containing omega-6 fatty acids have been shown to increase the growth of breast tumors in laboratory animals. In human studies of saturated and polyunsaturated fats, the results are mixed and it is not possible to draw a conclusion.

The results of the human studies may differ because the different types of fatty acids mentioned above are present in many different kinds of foods and oils that may also have independent effects on breast cancer risk. Also, there may be differences in the structure of the saturated, monounsaturated and polyunsaturated fatty acids present in the different types of foods and oils. These structural differences include differences in the length of the fatty acid chain and the location of the saturation along that chain. Polyunsaturated fatty acids are called "omega-6" or "omega-3" to indicate the location of the saturation in the fatty acid chain. Omega-6 fatty acids are plentiful in vegetable oils and omega-3 fatty acids are plentiful in fish and fish oils. A measurement of polyunsaturated fatty acids may include both of these types of fatty acids without considering that they may have different effects on breast cancer risk.

Dietary fat contains different types of fatty acids. These fatty acids can be saturated, monounsaturated, or polyunsaturated. Saturated fatty acids are found in higher concentrations in foods of animal origin such as meats and dairy products in which the fat is solid at room temperature. Polyunsaturated fatty acids are found in higher concentrations in foods of plant origin such as vegetable oils and foods made from them in which the fat is liquid at room temperature. Sometimes when food is processed, vegetable oils are made more saturated as in the manufacture of margarine or food products such as cookies or snack foods. Monounsaturated fatty acids are intermediate between the other two types and are found in highest concentrations in foods such as olive oil and canola oil. These different types of fatty acids may have different effects on the development of breast cancer.

A complete analysis of dietary fat includes all food sources, condiments such as butter, and cooking practices such as frying.

Is there any evidence that some types of fats may help reduce the risk of breast cancer?

The results from some studies suggest that in addition to trying to limit our intake of fat for overall health, it might also be helpful to replace certain fats in our diet with others. While these studies do not show conclusively that specific types of fats can prevent breast cancer, they do offer promise for dietary steps that may reduce breast cancer risk.

Olive Oil: In three out of five studies, the consumption of olive oil was associated with a significant decrease in the risk of breast cancer. Of the two remaining studies, one reported that the consumption of olive oil was associated with a lower incidence of breast cancer and the other reported no association between olive oil consumption and breast cancer. These studies were done in Mediterranean countries such as Greece, Italy and Spain, where women may have a total fat intake of about 42% of total calories. This total fat intake is comparable to or even higher than that seen in the U.S. However, the incidence of breast cancer is lower in these countries compared to the U.S. Although the total fat intake of these Mediterranean women is similar to that of American women, an important difference may be that most of the fat in their diets comes from olive oil.

The possible relationship between the consumption of olive oil (which contains a lot of monounsaturated fat) and breast cancer risk has led to studies of monounsaturated fat. Meat and canola oil also contain a lot of monounsaturated fat. In studies of the relationship between monounsaturated fat and breast cancer risk, the results are mixed. Most of the studies report that there is no association between the consumption of monounsaturated fat and the risk of breast cancer. A few studies report that monounsaturated fat increases risk, and others report that it decreases the risk of breast cancer. One possible reason for the discrepancy in results may be that there is something about olive oil specifically, and not the monounsaturated fat, that is influencing breast cancer risk. Olive oil also contains vitamins, flavanoids, and phenolic compounds that may help slow the development of breast cancer. It is also possible that it is something else in the diet of the women who were studied that helps reduce their risk of breast cancer.

Fish Oil: There is very strong evidence from several animal studies that fish oils slow the development and decrease the growth of breast tumors. The evidence from human studies is not as conclusive, with about half of the studies reporting a decrease in the risk of breast cancer associated with a high intake of fish. Although international correlation studies have also reported that fish consumption is associated with a lower incidence of breast cancer, the limitations of these studies, as described earlier, need to be considered.

Ratio of fatty acids: According to several animal studies and the results of some human studies, the ratio of fatty acids in the diet may be as important as the type of fatty acids. This is the ratio of "omega-3" fatty acids (plentiful in fish and fish oil) to "omega-6" fatty acids (plentiful in vegetable oils). Women who eat a lot of fish usually have a high omega-3/omega-6 ratio. In animal studies, a high omega-3/omega-6 ratio decreased the incidence, size and growth of breast tumors.

Why do I need fat in my diet?

We need to obtain certain types of essential polyunsaturated fatty acids in our diets because our bodies cannot make them, and they are necessary to help our bodies maintain cellular activities and function properly. Fat in the diet functions as an energy source. Dietary fat carries flavor, tenderizes food, and is necessary for the absorption of fat-soluble vitamins A, D and E. Fat stored in the body insulates the body against temperature extremes and protects vital organs from trauma.

What are the current recommendations for the consumption of fat in a healthy diet?

The uncertainty of the specific nature of the relationship between dietary fat and breast cancer makes it difficult to set guidelines on fat consumption with respect to breast cancer. However, the national recommendation for general health according to *Healthy People 2000*, is for a diet that is less than 30% total calories from fat, less than 10% total calories from saturated fat, and 1-2% linoleic (one of the essential polyunsaturated fatty acids). For example, under these guidelines, in a diet of 2000 calories, fat would make up fewer than 600 calories, which is equivalent to 67 grams of fat. In addition to these specific guidelines on fat intake, women should eat a healthful diet consisting of plenty of fruits, vegetables, and whole grains, and remain physically active. It is important to note that eating reduced fat foods does not necessarily mean that the diet is balanced and healthy. For example it would be more beneficial for women to incorporate more fruits and vegetables and whole grains into their diets, rather than increasing their consumption of "low-fat" or "reduced-fat" snacks and prepared foods.

Are more studies being done?

Because of the important health implications regarding dietary fat and breast cancer risk and the current controversy over the influence of fat on breast cancer risk, this relationship is still the focus of much study. Clinical or intervention trials offer hope for an answer. Several clinical trials that are currently underway to study the relationship between dietary fat, other components of the diet, and the risk of breast cancer, other diseases, and mortality are, 1) The Women's Health Initiative (WHI), 2) The Women's Intervention Nutrition Study (WINS) and 3) The Women's Healthy Eating and Lifestyle Study (WHEL).

Should breast cancer survivors consume less fat?

There is evidence from some animal studies that a high fat diet increases the progression of breast cancer and decreases survival.

There are also differences between the mortality rates from breast cancer in countries with a low fat intake, such as Japan, compared to countries with a high fat intake, such as the U.S. Overall calorie intake, to which dietary fat is one contributor, may increase body weight. An increase in body weight may influence the recurrence of breast cancer and survival.

How might dietary fat influence the risk of breast cancer?

There are some biologically plausible mechanisms that continue to fuel the debate on the role of dietary fat in breast cancer. Some studies suggest that a high fat diet may raise the concentration of hormones such as estrogen. A diet that is high in fat may lead to increases in body weight, an established risk factor for postmenopausal breast cancer. Some researchers think that a high fat diet in childhood may lead to faster growth and an earlier menarche, an established risk factor for breast cancer. Others are studying the possibility that a high fat intake may alter the expression of genes involved in the growth of mammary tumors (breast cancer).

Some fats (olive oil and fish oil) may decrease the risk of breast cancer because they are less susceptible to free-radical peroxidation. This means that fewer cell-damaging free radicals are formed.

What Can Women Do Now?

- Get plenty of exercise and maintain a healthy weight.
- Eat more fruits, vegetables and grains.
- When sautéing fresh vegetables, or making salad dressing, try olive oil.

Cornell University Program on Breast Cancer and Environmental Risk Factors in New York State (BCERF)

We hope you find this chapter informative. We welcome your comments. When reproducing this material, credit the Program on Breast Cancer and Environmental Risk Factors in New York State.

An extensive bibliography on *Dietary Fat and the Risk of Breast Cancer* is available on the BCERF web site: http://www.cfe.cornell.edu/bcerf/

Funding for this fact sheet was made possible by Cornell University, the U.S. Department of Agriculture/Cooperative State Research,

Education and Extension Service and the New York State Department of Health.

Cornell University
Program on Breast Cancer and Environmental
Risk Factors in New York State
112 Rice Hall
Ithaca, NY 14853-5601
Phone: (607) 254-2893
Fax: (607) 255-8207
email: breastcancer@cornell.edu
Internet: http://www.cfe.cornell.edu/bcerf/

*—Julie A. Napieralski, Ph.D. Research Associate, BCERF
and Carol Devine, Ph.D., R.D. Division of Nutritional
Sciences and Education Project Leader, BCERF*

We would like to acknowledge the valuable contributions of Elaine Yee-Tak Cheng (Cornell 2000) and Dana Hibner (Cornell 1999) to this fact sheet.

Chapter 18

Consumer Concerns about Hormones in Food

This text addresses some of the consumer concerns that have been brought to BCERF regarding health effects of hormones used by the meat and dairy industries. Evidence available so far, though not conclusive, does not link hormone residues in meat or milk with any human health effect.

What are hormones?

Hormones are chemicals that are produced naturally in the bodies of all animals, including humans. They are chemical messages released into the blood by hormone-producing organs that travel to and affect different parts of the body. Hormones may be produced in small amounts, but they control important body functions such as growth, development and reproduction.

Hormones can have different chemistry. They can be steroids or proteins. Steroid hormones are active in the body when eaten. For example, birth control pills are steroid hormones and can be taken orally. In contrast, protein hormones are broken down in the stomach, and lose their ability to act in the body when eaten. Therefore, ordinarily, protein hormones need to be injected into the body to have

From "Consumer Concerns about Hormones in Food," by Renu Gandhi, Ph.D. Research Associate and Suzanne M. Snedeker, Ph.D. Research Project Leader, Cornell University, Program on Breast Cancer and Environmental Risk Factors in New York State (BCERF), *FACT SHEET* #37, Institute for Comparative and Environmental Toxicology, Cornell Center for the Environment, June 2000; reprinted with permission.

an effect. For example, insulin is a protein hormone. Diabetic patients need to be injected with insulin for treatment.

Why are hormones used in food production?

Certain hormones can make young animals gain weight faster. They help reduce the waiting time and the amount of feed eaten by an animal before slaughter in meat industries. In dairy cows, hormones can be used to increase milk production. Thus, hormones can increase the profitability of the meat and dairy industries.

Why are consumers concerned about hormones in foods?

While a variety of hormones are produced by our bodies and are essential for normal development of healthy tissues, synthetic steroid hormones used as pharmaceutical drugs, have been found to affect cancer risk. For example, diethylstilbestrol (DES), a synthetic estrogen drug used in the 1960s was withdrawn from use after it was found to increase the risk of vaginal cancer in daughters of treated women. Lifetime exposure to natural steroid hormone estrogen is also associated with an increased risk for breast cancer. Hence, consumers are concerned about whether they are being exposed to hormones used to treat animals, and whether these hormones affect human health. We try to address this complex issue based on scientific evidence that is currently available.

History of Hormone Use in Food Production

As early as the 1930s, it was realized that cows injected with material drawn from bovine (cow) pituitary glands (hormone secreting organ) produced more milk. Later, the bovine growth hormone (bGH) from the pituitary glands was found to be responsible for this effect. However, at that time, technology did not exist to harvest enough of this material for large-scale use in animals. In the 1980s, it became possible to produce large quantities of pure bGH by using recombinant DNA technology. In 1993, the Food and Drug Administration (FDA) approved the recombinant bovine growth hormone (rbGH), also known as bovine somatotropin (rbST) for use in dairy cattle. Recent estimates by the manufacturer of this hormone indicate that 30%of the cows in the United States (US) may be treated with rbGH.

The female sex hormone estrogen was also shown to affect growth rates in cattle and poultry in the 1930s. Once the chemistry of estrogen was understood, it became possible to make the hormone synthetically in large amounts. Synthetic estrogens started being used to increase the size of cattle and chickens in the early 1950s. DES was one of the first synthetic estrogens made and used commercially in the US to fatten chickens. DES was also used as a drug in human medicine. DES was found to cause cancer and its use in food production was phased out in the late 1970s.

What are the different hormones used now by the meat and dairy industries?

There are six different kinds of steroid hormones that are currently approved by FDA for use in food production in the US: estradiol, progesterone, testosterone, zeranol, trenbolone acetate, and melengestrol acetate. Estradiol and progesterone are natural female sex hormones; testosterone is the natural male sex hormone; zeranol, trenbolone acetate and melengesterol acetate are synthetic growth promoters (hormone-like chemicals that can make animals grow faster). Currently, federal regulations allow these hormones to be used on growing cattle and sheep, but not on poultry (chickens, turkeys, ducks) or hogs (pigs). The above hormones are not as useful in increasing weight gain of poultry or hogs.

As mentioned earlier, FDA allows the use of the protein hormone rbGH to increase milk production in dairy cattle. This protein hormone is not used on beef cattle.

How are the hormones introduced into the animals?

Steroid hormones are usually released into the animal from a pellet (ear implant) that is put under the skin of the ear. The ears of the animals are thrown away at slaughter. Improper use of pellet implants in other parts of the animal can result in higher levels of hormone residues to remain in the edible meat. Federal regulations prohibit their use in this manner. Melengestrol acetate is also available in a form that can be added to animal feed.

Dairy cattle may be injected under the skin with rbGH. This hormone is available in packages of single dose injections to reduce chances of accidental overdose.

Do federal agencies monitor for the presence of these hormones in food?

Estradiol, progesterone and testosterone are sex hormones that are made naturally by animals. No regulatory monitoring of these hormones is possible, since it is not possible to separate or tell the difference between the hormones used for treatment from those made by the animal's own body. However, it is possible to detect residues of zeranol and trembolone acetate in the animal's meat. FDA has set the tolerance levels for these hormones. A tolerance is the maximum amount of a particular residue that may be permitted in or on food. The Food Safety Inspection Service (FSIS) of the US Department of Agriculture (USDA) monitors meat from cattle for zeranol residues. FSIS also monitors meats for DES residues from any illegal use (DES use is no longer permitted). In response to concern about cases of early puberty in Puerto Rico described below, a large number of meat samples were tested for hormone residues in the mid-to late 1980s. No zeranol or DES residues were found in the meat samples in this survey.

Do hormones remain in the milk or meat of treated animals?

The levels of naturally produced hormones vary from animal to animal, and a range in these levels is known to be normal. Because it is not possible to differentiate between the hormones produced naturally by the animal and those used to treat the animal, it is difficult to determine exactly how much of the hormone used for treatment remains in the meat or the milk. Studies indicate that if correct treatment and slaughter procedures are followed, the levels of these hormones may be slightly higher in the treated animal's meat or milk, but are still within the normal range of natural variation known to occur in untreated animals. Scientists are currently trying to develop better methods to measure steroid hormone residues left in edible meat from a treated animal.

Can steroid hormones in meat affect the age of puberty for girls?

Early puberty in girls has been found to be associated with a higher risk for breast cancer. Height, weight, diet, exercise, and family history have all been found to influence age of puberty. Steroid hormones in food were suspected to cause early puberty in girls in some reports. However, exposure to higher than natural levels of steroid hormones through hormone-treated meat or poultry has never been documented. Large epidemiological studies have not been done to see whether or not early puberty in developing girls is associated with having eaten growth hormone-treated foods.

A concern about an increase in cases of girls reaching puberty or menarche early (at age eight or younger) in Puerto Rico, led to an

162

investigation in the early 1980s by the Centers for Disease Control (CDC). Samples of meat and chicken from Puerto Rico were tested for steroid hormone residues. One laboratory found a chicken sample from a local market to have higher than normal level of estrogen. Also, residues of zeranol were reported in the blood of some of the girls who had reached puberty early. However, these results could not be verified by other laboratories. Following CDC's investigation, USDA tested 150 to 200 beef, poultry and milk samples from Puerto Rico in 1985, and found no residues of DES, zeranol or estrogen in these samples.

In another study in Italy, steroid hormone residues in beef and poultry in school meals were suspected as the cause of breast enlargement in very young girls and boys. However, the suspect beef and poultry samples were not available to test for the presence of hormones. Without proof that exposure to higher levels of steroid hormones occurred through food, it is not possible to conclude whether or not eating hormone-treated meat or poultry caused the breast enlargement in these cases.

Can eating meat from hormone-treated animals affect breast cancer risk?

Evidence does not exist to answer this question. The amount of steroid hormone that is eaten through meat of a treated animal is negligible compared to what the human body produces each day. The breast cancer risk of women who eat meat from hormone-treated animals has not been compared with the risk of women who eat meat from untreated animals.

Can drinking milk, or eating dairy products from hormone-treated animals affect breast cancer risk?

Once again, evidence does not exist to answer this question. Use of rbGH for dairy cattle has been in practice in US for only six to seven years. Breast cancer can take many years to develop. It is too early to study the breast cancer risk of women who drink milk and eat milk products from hormone-treated animals.

Can hormones that remain in milk affect human health?

Scientists at FDA's Center for Veterinary Medicine have reviewed the studies submitted by the manufacturers of rbGH. FDA scientists have concluded that eating foods with slightly higher levels of rbGH would not affect human health. This is because the amount of rbGH that is in milk or milk products as a result of treatment of the animals is insignificant compared to the amount of growth hormone that is naturally produced by our bodies. Also, rbGH is a protein hormone and is digested into smaller fragments (peptides and amino acids) when eaten. The rbGH hormone used on dairy cattle is effective in promoting growth in cows, but does not work in humans. Scientists know that rbGH is not recognized as a hormone by human cells.

There are gaps in our knowledge about whether rbGH used to treat dairy cattle can cause indirect effects. These gaps lead to uncertainties and debates, some of which are addressed below.

What do we know about growth factors in milk of treated animals?

The wholesomeness of milk is not affected by rbGH treatment. However, some subtle changes do take place in the treated animal. The growth hormone typically acts by triggering the cells to make other chemicals, called growth factors. These growth factors actually cause the increase in growth rate and milk production. Milk from rbGH-treated cattle has been found to have slightly higher levels of the naturally produced protein called insulin-dependent growth factor-1 (IGF-1). IGF-1 is a protein, and is digested into smaller pieces in the stomach.

Scientists at FDA have considered the evidence from studies of cancer risk in people who have naturally high body levels of IGF-1. Higher levels of IGF-1 in blood have been found in women with breast cancer compared to women without breast cancer in the Harvard-based Nurses' Health Study. Scientists are investigating if IGF-1 is just present at higher levels in breast cancer patients or if it has a role in increasing the risk for the disease. In laboratory studies, breast cancer cells growing on a plastic dish, grow at a faster rate when bathed in a solution containing IGF-1. However, IGF-1 also plays an important role in helping normal cells grow. Hence, from these few studies, we cannot conclude whether or not IGF-1 increases breast cancer risk.

FDA scientists have concluded that IGF-1 in milk is unlikely to present any human food safety concern for the following reasons: 1) IGF-1 levels in cow's milk from untreated animals vary in nature, depending on the number of calves and the lactation stage; 2) IGF-1 is also present in human breast milk, at levels higher than in hormone-treated cow's milk; 3) IGF-1 in milk is not expected to act as a growth factor in people who drink it because it gets digested in the stomach; 4) IGF-1 needs to be injected into the blood to have a growth-promoting effect; and 5) increased IGF-1 levels in food are not expected to result in higher blood levels of IGF-1 in humans who eat the food.

Concern about Milk-related Allergies

A detailed discussion of this topic is beyond the scope of this chapter. A brief outline of the issue is presented here, along with references for more information.

Digested or broken down fragments of proteins absorbed through the stomach can cause the immune system to produce antibodies, which sometimes can lead to milk-related allergies. There have been studies done to investigate whether the immune system can react to fragments of rbGH and IGF-1 absorbed through the stomach. Reviewers of these studies at Health Canada (the Canadian counterpart to FDA) expressed a concern that in one study, some of the laboratory rats that were fed high levels of rbGH for 90 days developed antibodies against it (http://www.hc-sc.gc.ca/english/archives/rbst). Scientists at FDA evaluated these studies in rats and concluded that only animals that were fed a very large amount of rbGH in food produced antibodies against it. Such large amounts of rbGH are not expected to occur in the milk that humans drink ("Report on the Food and Drug Administration's Review of the Safety of Bovine Somatotropin" available at: http://www.fda.gov/cvm;a copy of this report can be requested by calling:310-574-1755).

Studies have also looked at whether IGF-1 fed to laboratory rats and digested in the stomach can affect the immune system. No immune effects were observed in these studies, but the animals were fed IGF-1 for only two weeks. No studies have been done on the effects of feeding rats or other experimental animals with IGF-1 over longer periods of time.

Are hormone-treated animals healthy?

There is a concern that because of increased milking, hormone-treated cows may become more prone to infection of the udders, called mastitis. This could lead to more antibiotics being used to treat the cows, in turn leading to more residues of antibiotics to remain in the milk. Frequent exposure to antibiotic residues through milk or dairy products is a health concern for people over the long term. In the normal body, there are bacteria that live in the gut and mouth and help in the digestion of food in the gut. These "friendly" bacteria do not normally cause disease since the immune system keeps them in check. However, if the immune system is weak, these "friendly" bacteria can invade tissues and cause infection. Bacteria in the normal body that come across small amounts of antibiotics frequently, can develop ways to survive the antibiotics and become "antibiotic resistant." In cases of infection and illness, it then becomes more difficult to control such resistant bacteria with the available antibiotics.

Some increase in incidence of antibiotic residues was observed in cow's milk following the use of rbGH. At the same time as rbGH started being used, some of the major dairy states in US switched over to a new and improved method to test for antibiotic residues. It is difficult to determine whether the increase in incidence of antibiotic residues in milk was due to increased use, or better testing methods. New York State (NYS) was one of the states that had not changed its method to test for antibiotic residues in milk at that time. The incidence of antibiotic residues in milk from NYS was not found to be higher after the approval of rbGH use. This suggests that the increased incidence of antibiotic residues observed in some states may have been due to better testing methods rather than an increase in use of antibiotics for treatment of mastitis. An Expert Committee at FDA's Center for Veterinary Medicine has concluded that while rbGH use may cause a slight increase in mastitis, dairy management practices that are currently in use should prevent any increase in antibiotic residues in milk.

Are growth hormones used elsewhere in the world?

The debate on whether growth hormones should or should not be used for food production has become a very political issue. In 1989, the European Community (now European Union) issued a ban on all meat from animals treated with steroid growth hormones, which is still in effect. The use of steroid hormones for beef cattle is permitted in Canada.

Countries within the European Union do not allow the use of the protein hormone rbGH, for dairy cattle. In 1999, the Canadian government refused approval for the sale of rbGH for dairy cattle, based on concerns about the health effects including mastitis in treated animals.

Conclusions

Studies done so far do not provide evidence to state that hormone residues in meat or dairy products cause any human health effects. However, a conclusion on lack of human health effect can only be made after large-scale studies compare the health of people who eat meat or dairy products from hormone-treated animals, to people who eat a similar diet, but from untreated animals.

Where is more research needed?

Some of the consumer concerns in this chapter cannot be answered conclusively without further studies:

- Exposure to hormones in meat was suspected as the cause for early puberty in girls in Puerto Rico and Italy, but was never verified. To conclusively answer the question, large-scale epidemiological studies would be needed to compare the age of puberty in girls who eat meat from hormone-treated animals to those who eat meat from untreated animals. Such studies would need to make sure that other known influences that affect the age of puberty in girls are not playing a role.

- Short-term studies in laboratory rats have not indicated a concern about milk-related allergies or immune effects from exposure to rbGH or IGF-1 in milk or dairy products. However, short-term studies cannot be used to rule out all possibilities of any immune, or unexpected health effects after long-term exposure. Studies in laboratory animals on effects of life-long exposure to milk from rbGH-treated cows may help answer this question.

Some healthy diet tips that also help reduce exposure to hormones used in food production

While currently available evidence does not indicate a link between eating meat, milk or dairy products from hormone-treated animals and any health effects, adopting some known healthy diet habits can help reduce exposure to hormones used in meat, poultry and dairy production.

- Eat a varied diet, rich in fruits, grains and vegetables.
- Eat meats in moderation, well cooked, but not charred.
- Eat more lean muscle meat, less liver and fat.

167

Cornell University Program on Breast Cancer and Environmental Risk Factors in New York State

We hope you find this text informative. We welcome your comments. When reproducing this material, credit the Program on Breast Cancer and Environmental Risk Factors in New York State.

An extensive bibliography on *Consumer Concerns About Hormones in Food* is available on the BCERF web site: http://www.cfe.cornell.edu/bcerf/

Funding for this fact sheet was made possible by the US Department of Agriculture/Cooperative State Research, Education and Extension Service and the New York State Department of Health.

Cornell University
Program on Breast Cancer and Environmental Risk Factors in New York State
112 Rice Hall
Ithaca, NY 14853-5601
Phone:(607) 254-2893
Fax:(607) 255-8207
email:breastcancer@cornell.edu
Internet: http://www.cfe.cornell.edu/bcerf/

— by Renu Gandhi, Ph.D. BCERF Research Associate and Suzanne M. Snedeker, Ph.D. BCERF Research Project Leader

Chapter 19

Childhood Life Events and the Risk of Breast Cancer

Researchers are asking whether women and young girls may be able to reduce breast cancer risk by early adoption of healthful behaviors, such as eating plenty of fruits, vegetables, whole grains and beans, and getting regular exercise. Also, minimizing young girls' exposure to cancer-causing agents may be important in reducing their risk of breast cancer.

Why are researchers investigating breast cancer risk factors during childhood and adolescence?

Breast cancer is a disease that may develop and progress over the course of a woman's entire life. During puberty, breast cells are rapidly dividing. Since cells undergoing rapid division are more likely to be damaged by cancer-causing agents, environmental exposures before or during puberty may be important in determining a woman's lifetime risk of developing breast cancer. Also, researchers are beginning to assess whether healthful diet and exercise habits in young girls may help to prevent the development of breast cancer later in life.

From "Childhood Life Events and the Risk of Breast Cancer," by Julie A. Napieralski, Ph.D. Research Associate, and Carol Devine, Ph.D., R.D. Division of Nutritional Sciences and Education Project Leader, Cornell University, Program on Breast Cancer and Environmental Risk Factors in New York State (BCERF), *FACT SHEET* #8, Institute for Comparative and Environmental Toxicology, Cornell Center for the Environment, March 1998; reprinted with permission.

Although it is possible that factors in early life affect the risk of breast cancer, we have very little information on what those factors are and how we should alter them. In the meantime, understanding influences on established risk factors for breast cancer, such as age at menarche (a girl's first menstrual period), may provide hints about early influences on breast cancer risk.

Why is age at menarche a risk factor for breast cancer?

Breast cancer is a disease that is thought to be related to high lifetime exposure to the hormone estrogen. Estrogen is needed for normal reproductive development and estrogen levels in the body rise at menarche. The earlier a girl starts menstruating, the more menstrual cycles she will have, and the greater will be her exposure to estrogen during her child-bearing years. Height, weight, diet, exercise, and family history have all been found to influence age at menarche.

How do height, weight and body fat distribution affect the age at menarche?

There is a trend towards an earlier age at menarche among girls living in industrialized countries. Taller, heavier girls generally start menstruating earlier than shorter, lighter girls. In addition, the distribution of fat on a girl's body is related to the levels of hormones circulating in her body and may affect her age at menarche. Girls with fat localized around their hips (pear shaped), may have an earlier menarche than girls with abdominal fat (apple shaped). However, girls with abdominal fat are more likely to be obese and have higher levels of another hormone called insulin. Increases in insulin and growth hormone influence the levels of insulin-like growth factor (IGF-1), which may promote cancer in breast tissue. Height, weight and the distribution of body fat are influenced by heredity. However, diet and exercise behaviors that help maintain healthy weight may prevent changes in hormone levels that could promote the development of breast cancer.

How might childhood diet influence breast cancer risk?

Diet may affect age at menarche. In some reports, girls who ate more fiber, vegetables, nuts and seeds had a later age at menarche. However, these findings did not take into account. weight and height, which could also have influenced age at menarche. In other studies, which did take weight and height into consideration, the results differed.

170

Three studies found no influence of diet on age at menarche while one reported that a high intake of fat was associated with an early age at menarche. There is no compelling evidence that any particular food group has a strong influence on a girl's age at menarche.

Other possible ways that childhood diet might influence breast cancer risk include: 1) protection or repair of developing breast cells by nutrients from foods such as vitamin E and beta-carotene, 2) enhanced effects of carcinogenic (cancer-causing) components in food during early breast development, 3) the influence of diet on hormone levels, particularly estrogen, and 4) maintenance of overall health and a strong immune system.

Very few studies have assessed the influence of diet during childhood on the risk of developing breast cancer as an adult. In these studies, women were asked to remember what they ate as children, a difficult task for anyone. Also, memories may differ in women who have been diagnosed with cancer compared to those who have not. Several different types of food have been studied.

Fat intake: There is conflicting evidence on whether fat intake during childhood and adolescence is a risk factor for the development of breast cancer. Two studies reported no association between fat consumption during childhood and the development of breast cancer. Two other studies reported an increased breast cancer risk associated with the consumption of the fat on meat or fried meat.

Diets lower in calories and animals products: One recent study reported a decrease in the incidence of breast cancer among Norwegian women who were adolescents during World War II. During the war they had a decrease in total food consumption and a diet which consisted of less meat and milk, and more fish, vegetables and potatoes than before or after the war.

Vegetable and fruit intake: A recent U.S. study reported a slight, but non-significant association between high fruit and vegetable intake in childhood and reduced breast cancer risk in adults.

Vegetarian diet: Two studies did not show any association between a vegetarian diet during adolescence and the risk of breast cancer in adults. Two others demonstrated that girls who ate a vegetarian diet or had high intakes of dietary fiber had lower levels of circulating estrogens. This suggests that a diet high in vegetables, fruits, and whole grains may contribute to a reduction in body estrogen levels.

171

Dairy products: In animal studies and in studies using human breast cells, a component of milk called conjugated linoleic acid was found to be an anticarcinogen (protects against the development of cancer). However, this finding has not been adequately confirmed in humans.

Currently, there is no strong evidence supporting a role for childhood nutrition in the development of breast cancer. Most studies did not take into account the effect of established risk factors for breast cancer, such as age at menarche or height and weight. Future studies need to more carefully account for other breast cancer risk factors. However, it is important to establish healthy eating habits early in life to promote long term health.

How might exercise during adolescence influence breast cancer risk?

Several studies have reported a decrease in breast cancer risk associated with regular exercise. Exercise may reduce a girl's risk of breast cancer by decreasing the level of estrogen in her body, decreasing her weight, decreasing her insulin resistance, strengthening her immune system, or increasing her age at menarche.

Generally, athletes have a later age at menarche compared to non-athletes. The influence of moderate exercise on age at menarche is less clear. Some researchers have reported that girls who are moderately active (non-athletes) have differences in hormone levels and a delay in the onset of menstruation compared to inactive girls. Others have reported no effect of moderate physical activity on the age at menarche. Differences in the way the researchers assessed physical activity or problems with recall of earlier exercise practices may account for the differences in results. Later age at menarche in athletes may also be due to heredity.

Does obesity during childhood and/or adolescence affect breast cancer risk?

There are no data to suggest that adolescent obesity is a risk factor for the development of breast cancer. In fact, a few studies have suggested that a heavier weight in adolescence may be protective. However, gaining weight and being obese as an adolescent may be important for other reasons. Overweight. adolescents are more likely to be overweight adults, and it is harder for people to lose weight as they get older. Gaining weight and being overweight as an adult are thought to be risk factors for postmenopausal breast cancer. Therefore, it is important to establish a healthy lifestyle and healthy weight during adolescence.

Are there risks to promoting healthy eating and exercise among young girls?

Although age at menarche is an established risk factor for breast cancer, attempts to delay a girl's menarche are not advisable. The normal establishment of regular menstrual cycles is critical for reproduction. Delaying a girl's menarche via dieting, extreme weight loss and/or vigorous and stressful exercise may affect her ability to have children later. Also, emphasis on dieting and weight may contribute to eating disorders such as anorexia and bulimia. Girls who have started to menstruate, and exercise and diet too vigorously can actually cause their periods to stop, and can experience severe bone loss. Therefore, an active lifestyle that allows normal development should be the goal during adolescence.

Adolescent life-style factors and the risk of breast cancer:

Smoking cigarettes: Few studies have examined smoking during adolescence as a risk factor for breast cancer. However, some researchers think that smoking at a young age may be important because the carcinogens in cigarette smoke may cause more damage during adolescence when the breast cells are rapidly dividing.

Alcohol consumption: Alcohol consumption has been identified as a likely risk factor for breast cancer, but the influence of alcohol consumption in adolescence is not clear. It is not yet clear whether drinking at an early age, lifetime alcohol consumption or the intensity of drinking is most important. Encouraging teenagers not to drink may lessen their lifetime consumption of alcohol.

Oral contraceptives: Studies of oral contraceptive use and breast cancer risk have focused on adult women who started taking birth control pills when they were in their 20's. Today, the pill is a much more popular form of birth control among teenagers. Since there are natural hormonal differences between adolescent girls and adult women, the use of the pill in teenagers deserves special consideration. Indeed, a couple of studies have reported that there might be a slight increase in risk associated with early use of oral contraceptives. However, more studies that take into account the lower dose of hormones present in today's birth control pills are needed.

Are there any other risk factors that girls and their mothers should be aware of when thinking about breast cancer?

Radiation: The first clue that exposure to radiation during adolescence may increase the risk of breast cancer came from studies of atomic bomb survivors, especially those who were less than 15 years old at the time of the bomb. Recent studies have demonstrated that children who received radiation treatment for a type of cancer called Hodgkin's disease or children who received x-ray treatment for scoliosis (abnormal curvature of the spine) showed an increased incidence of breast cancer. Today, doctors use a lower dose of radiation, take the x-rays of the spine from the back, and cover the breasts with a lead apron to decrease the risk of exposing the breasts to x-rays. Sometimes a girl needs to have an x-ray. However, parents should take an extra precaution by asking if the x-ray is necessary.

Pesticides: There are no studies that look at the influence of pesticide exposure in children on the development of breast cancer. However, some research has shown that children, because of their smaller size, take in more contaminants from air, water and food, than adults. In addition, they absorb and retain more of certain contaminants and are less efficient at detoxifying them or repairing the damage the contaminants may have caused.

Once studies currently underway regarding pesticide exposure in adults and the risk of breast cancer are complete, the issue of time of exposure can be addressed. Until then, in the absence of definite information regarding this potential risk, it would be a good idea to keep children away from pesticides and other chemicals.

What should I do now?

There are a lot of factors that may influence a person's risk of developing breast cancer. Some of these, like age at menarche and genetic factors, are beyond our control. However, others like diet, exercise, smoking and alcohol intake are under our control. By setting a good example and encouraging our daughters and other young girls to eat well, stay physically fit and avoid smoking and drinking,

174

we may give them a better chance of avoiding breast cancer later in life.

Cornell University Program on Breast Cancer and Environmental Risk Factors in New York State (BCERF)

BCERF would like to acknowledge the members of the Educational Advisory Board and the Technical Advisory Reviewers for their critical review of this fact sheet. An extensive bibliography on *"Childhood Influences on Breast Cancer Risk"* is available on the BCERF web site http://www.cfe.cornell.edu/bcerf/

This text is a publication of the Cornell University Program on Breast Cancer and Environmental Risk Factors in New York State (BCERF). The Program is housed within the university-wide Institute for Comparative and Environmental Toxicology (ICET) in the Cornell Center for the Environment. BCERF strives to better understand the relationship between breast cancer and other hormonally-related cancers to environmental risk factors and to make this information available on an on-going basis to the citizens of New York State. The program involves faculty and staff from the Cornell Ithaca campus (College of Agriculture and Life Sciences, College of Arts and Sciences, the College of Human Ecology, the College of Veterinary Medicine, the Division of Biological Sciences and the Division of Nutritional Sciences), Cornell Cooperative Extension, and the Cornell Medical College and Strang Cancer Prevention Center.

If you would like to be added to our mailing list to receive future copies of our newsletter, *THE RIBBON*, please contact the Administrative/Outreach Coordinator at the address below. Also included in the newsletter is a tear-off sheet listing other fact sheets.

We hope you find this text informative. We welcome your comments. When reproducing this material, credit the Program on Breast Cancer and Environmental Risk Factors in New York State.

Funding for this fact sheet was made possible by the New York State Department of Health.

Cornell University
Program on Breast Cancer and Environmental Risk
Factors in New York State
112 Rice Hall
Ithaca, NY 14853-5601
Phone: 607 254-2893
FAX: 607-255-8027 *(continued on next page)*

email: breastcancer@cornell.edu
Internet: http://www.cfe.cornell.edu/bcerf/

—Julie A. Napieralski, Ph.D. Research Associate, BCERF and Carol M. Devine, Ph.D., R.D. Education Project Leader BCERF

Chapter 20

Diagnostic X-Rays and Breast Cancer Mortality

Researchers have found that women with scoliosis, or abnormal curvature of the spine, who were exposed to multiple diagnostic X-rays during childhood and adolescence may be at increased risk of dying of breast cancer. The study appears in the Aug. 15, 2000, issue of the journal *Spine*. Authors included scientists from the National Cancer Institute (NCI) in Bethesda, Maryland; the Twin Cities Spine Center in Minneapolis, Minnesota; the University of Texas M.D. Anderson Cancer Center in Houston, Texas; Information Management Services in Silver Spring, Maryland; and the U.S. Scoliosis Cohort Study Collaborators, a group of physicians from 14 orthopedic medical centers across the country. The study is entitled "Breast Cancer Mortality After Diagnostic Radiography: Findings from the U.S. Scoliosis Cohort Study." The authors are Michele Morin Doody, John E. Lonstein, Marilyn Stovall, David G. Hacker, Nickolas Luckyanov, and Charles E. Land. *Spine*, Aug. 15, 2000, Vol. 25, No. 16.

The 5,466 women in the study, who received an average of 24.7 X-rays, were found to have a 70 percent higher risk of breast cancer than women in the general population. There were 77 breast cancer deaths among the patients, compared to 46 expected deaths based on U.S. mortality rates. Patients were younger than 20 years old when they were diagnosed with scoliosis between 1912 and 1965. The mean age

"Scientists Find Link between Pre 1970s Diagnostic X-rays for Scoliosis and Breast Cancer Mortality," National Institutes of Health, Office of Cancer Communications, Building 31, Room 10A24, Bethesda, MD 20892; Press Release dated August 15, 2000.

for scoliosis diagnosis in this study was 10.6 years, and the average length of follow-up was 40.1 years. Follow-up was complete for 89 percent of patients.

"These findings provide yet another indication that radiation exposure, especially in childhood, is associated with increased breast cancer risk later in life, and that the amount of risk is proportional to radiation dose," said Michele M. Doody, M.S., from NCI's Radiation Epidemiology Branch and the principal investigator of the study. Reported risks for exposures after age 40 are much lower.

Scoliosis occurs in approximately 2 percent of girls and 0.5 percent of boys. It is commonly diagnosed in early adolescence and may gradually progress as rapid growth occurs. Scoliosis patients typically undergo routine X-rays of the spine throughout their adolescent growth spurt to monitor curvature progression so that corrective action may be taken.

The researchers found that the risk of dying from breast cancer increased significantly with the number of X-rays. The vast majority (89 percent) of exams in this study involved definite or probable radiation exposure to the breast. Patients who had 50 or more exams had nearly four times the risk of dying from breast cancer as women in the general population. The number of exams per patient ranged from zero to 618. Six hundred forty-four patients had no recorded exams.

Similarly, the risk of dying of breast cancer increased with increasing estimated cumulative radiation dose to the breast. Patients who received doses of greater than 20 centigray (cGy) had more than three times the chance of dying from breast cancer than women in the general population. The estimated cumulative dose of radiation ranged from zero to 170 cGy; the average was 10.8 cGy.

The amount of radiation energy absorbed by irradiated tissue is measured in centigray (cGy). The estimated breast dose for a single full spine X-ray with the patient facing the X-ray machine (anteroposterior view) during the 1940s was about 0.6 cGy. For comparison, the estimated breast dose today for a single full spine anteroposterior exam is on the order of 0.1 to 0.2 cGy, whereas the dose for the same examination with the patient's back facing the machine (posteroanterior view) is 0.02 cGy.

This is by far the largest group of scoliosis patients followed to date. The number of X-rays that each patient received was tabulated through detailed review of the medical records and films, and the breast doses were estimated using actual machine parameters derived from one medical center (University Hospital Rehabilitation Center,

Hershey, Pa.). Information was available during most of the calendar time periods covered.

Part of the increased risk of dying from breast cancer may be due to other breast cancer risk factors, said Doody. Breast cancer risk in the general population tends to be higher for women who have not experienced a full-term pregnancy or whose first full-term pregnancy was at age 30 or older. Based on questionnaire responses by 3,100 women in the study who were alive at the end of the follow-up period, it appears that women with more severe scoliosis were less likely to have given birth than those with less severe disease. Since severity of scoliosis also correlates with number of X-rays and radiation dose to the breast, it is possible that some of the observed breast cancer excess could be related to reproductive history.

Almost all of the X-rays received in this study were taken before 1976, when the dose to patients was considerably higher than with current techniques. For example, the estimated breast dose from a full-spine anteroposterior view (facing the X-ray machine) in 1940 to 1959 was about six times higher than an anteroposterior view in 1976 to 1989 and 200 times higher than a posteroanterior (turned with back facing the X-ray machine) view in 1976 to 1989. Although radiation exposures to breast tissue are much lower today than during the time period covered by this study, they are not insignificant. The authors recommend that efforts to reduce exposures continue by having patients stand with their backs to the X-ray machine, carefully limiting the portion of the body exposed to the radiation beam, and shielding the breasts. Repeat exposures should also be minimized wherever possible.

Chapter 21

Abortion and Breast Cancer: Controversial Reports

The relationship between abortion and breast cancer has been the subject of extensive research. However, evidence of a direct relationship between breast cancer and either induced or spontaneous abortion is inconsistent. Some studies have indicated small elevations in risk, while others have not shown any risk associated with either induced or spontaneous abortions.

A large-scale epidemiologic study of this question, reported in *The New England Journal of Medicine* in 1997, determined that the risk of developing breast cancer for women with a history of induced abortion was not different from the risk for women without such a history. The authors, Melbye and others, used data from Danish health registries. Registry data on abortions was collected before the diagnosis of breast cancer was made. Using information on abortions that was collected before breast cancer developed avoids recall or reporting bias, which may occur in retrospective studies when information about abortions is collected after the diagnosis of breast cancer. The authors concluded that "induced abortions have no overall effect on the risk of breast cancer."

Earlier studies that attempted to evaluate the association between abortion and breast cancer were limited in many cases by small numbers of women in the studies, questions of comparability between the study groups, inability to separate induced from spontaneous abortions, and incomplete knowledge of other potentially pertinent lifestyle factors.

Cancer Facts, National Cancer Institute, June 1999.

Also, most early studies were retrospective; that is, they relied on women's reports of their reproductive history. A significant potential problem in the interpretation of retrospective studies is related to the possibility of recall bias (inaccurate reporting of abortions in retrospect by study participants). Women with breast cancer may be more likely to accurately report sensitive reproduction issues, such as having had an abortion, than women without breast cancer. This type of reporting bias could make abortion appear to be more common among women with breast cancer, possibly leading to the false conclusion that abortion increases the risk of breast cancer.

One earlier study, published in the *Journal of the National Cancer Institute* in 1996, found a 90 percent increase in risk for breast cancer after an induced abortion (the risk of breast cancer among women who reported having had an abortion was 1.9 times the risk among those who did not report a history of abortion). However, the authors, Rookus and van Leeuwen of The Netherlands Cancer Institute, suggested that this figure may have been influenced by inaccurate recall associated with the underreporting of abortion by healthy control subjects in the religiously conservative southeastern region of The Netherlands. In the more liberal western regions of the country, the association between abortion and breast cancer was statistically insignificant. Rookus and van Leeuwen concluded that their study "does not support an appreciably increased risk for breast cancer after an induced abortion."

Another article, published in the *Journal of the National Cancer Institute* in 1994, illustrates the difficulty of drawing conclusions. In this study, Daling and others evaluated the risk of breast cancer among young women with a history of abortion. The results, based on self-reports of abortions, indicated that induced abortion was associated with a 50 percent increase in the average risk of developing breast cancer (the women who reported abortions had 1.5 times the risk of those who did not). Risk did not vary consistently with number of abortions, the woman's age at abortion or length of pregnancy, nor did the study show an increase in risk associated with spontaneous abortions. An accompanying commentary by Rosenberg, in the same journal, concluded that "While the findings of Daling et al. add to the limited evidence that induced abortion increases the risk of breast cancer, neither a coherent body of knowledge nor a convincing biologic mechanism has been established." Because the evidence is weak and inconsistent, researchers cannot be sure that there is a direct or causal relationship between abortion and breast cancer. At the time of publication, the National Cancer Institute released a press statement, concluding that "Taken together, the inconsistencies and scarcity of existing research do not permit scientific conclusions."

The most common risk factor for breast cancer is increasing age: In this country, this disease affects 1 out of 2,525 women in their thirties and 1 out of 11 in their seventies. Other well-established risk factors include a family history of breast cancer, early age at menarche, late age at menopause, late age at the time of the first full-term birth of a child, and certain breast conditions. Obesity is a risk factor for breast cancer in postmenopausal women. The increased risk of developing breast cancer associated with each factor varies, from 1.5 to 4 times the average risk.

References

Brinton LA, Hoover R, Fraumeni JF. Reproductive factors in the aetiology of breast cancer. *Br J Cancer* 1983;47:757–762.

Daling JR, Malone KE, Voigt LF, et al. Risk of breast cancer among young women: Relationship to induced abortion. *J Natl Cancer Inst* 1994;86:1584–1592.

Gammon MD, Bertin JE, Terry MB. Abortion and the risk of breast cancer: Is there a believable association? *JAMA* 1996;4:275:321–322.

Kelsey JL, Gammon MD, John EM. Reproductive factors and breast cancer. *Epidemiol Rev* 1993;15:36–47.

Kelsey JL. Breast cancer epidemiology: Summary and future directions. *Epidemiol Rev* 1993;15:256–263.

Lindefors-Harris BM, Eklund G, Adami HO, et al. Response bias in a case-control study: Analysis utilizing comparative data concerning legal abortions from two independent Swedish studies. *Am J Epidemiol* 1991;134:1003–1008.

Melbye M, Wohlfahrt M, Olsen JH, et al. Induced abortion and the risk of breast cancer. *N Engl J of Med* 1997;336:81–85.

Parazzini F, La Vecchia C, Negri E. Spontaneous and induced abortions and risk of breast cancer. *Int J Cancer* 1991;48:816–820.

Remennick LI. Induced abortion as cancer risk factor: A review of the epidemiological evidence. *J Epidemiol Community Health* 1990;44:259–264.

Rookus, MA, van Leeuwen, FE. Induced abortion and risk for breast cancer: Reporting (recall) bias in a Dutch case-control study. *J Natl Cancer Inst* 1996;88:1759–64.

Rosenberg L, Palmer JR, Kaufman DW, et al. Breast cancer in relation to the occurrence and the time of the induced and spontaneous abortion. *Am J Epidemiol* 1988;127:981–989.

Rosenberg L. Induced abortion and breast cancer: More scientific data are needed. *J Natl Cancer Inst* 1994;86:1569–1570.

Tavani A, Vecchia C, Franceshi S, et al. Abortion and breast cancer risk. *Int J Cancer* 1996;65:401–405.

Chapter 22

Silicone Breast Implants and Breast Cancer: Study Finds No Link

In one of the largest studies on the long-term health effects of silicone breast implants, researchers from the National Cancer Institute (NCI) in Bethesda, Maryland, found no association between breast implants and the subsequent risk of breast cancer. The study is titled, "Breast Cancer Following Augmentation Mammoplasty (United States)." The authors are Louise A. Brinton, Jay H. Lubin, Mary Cay Burich, Theodore Colton, S. Lori Brown, and Robert N. Hoover. It is published in the November 2000 issue of *Cancer Causes and Control*, Vol.11(9):819-827.

Breast Implant Study

Breast implants first appeared on the market in 1962. Manufacturers initially assumed that the implants were biologically inactive and, therefore, would have no harmful effects. However, over the past two decades there have been a number of reports of connective tissue disorders and cancers among implant patients.

In 1992, because of the lack of sufficient evidence on the long-term safety of implants, the Food and Drug Administration (FDA) restricted the use of silicone breast implants to women seeking breast reconstruction in controlled clinical trials, and Congress directed the National Institutes of Health to undertake a large follow-up study to evaluate the long-term health effects of the implants.

"Silicone Breast Implants Are Not Linked to Breast Cancer Risk," National Institutes of Health, Office of Cancer Communications, Building 31, Room 10A19, Bethesda, MD 20892; Press Release dated October 2, 2000.

"This is the first part of our analysis of the health risks from the study," said Louise A. Brinton, Ph.D., principal investigator from NCI's Division of Cancer Epidemiology and Genetics (DCEG) in Bethesda, Maryland. "For women followed for more than 10 years, there was no change in breast cancer risk. Our results do not confirm the findings from several other studies that exposure to implants reduces a woman's risk for breast cancer. This may relate to the longer follow-up in this study as compared with most others."

The average length of follow-up was 12.9 years among the implant patients and 11.6 years among the comparison patients. In previous studies, women with implants were generally followed for less than 10 years.

The participants included 13,500 women who had implant surgery for cosmetic reasons in both breasts sometime between 1962 and 1989 and, for comparison, about 4,000 women similar in age who had some other type of plastic surgery, such as removal of fat from the stomach, or wrinkles from the face and neck. Both groups of women were selected from 18 plastic surgery practices in which the surgeons had performed large numbers of cosmetic breast implant surgeries prior to 1989 and were willing to give the investigators access to their records. The practices were located in six geographic areas: Atlanta, Georgia; Birmingham, Alabama; Charlotte, North Carolina; Miami and Orlando, Florida; and Washington, D.C.

In order to carry out the study, researchers reviewed the medical records from the plastic surgery practices and collected data about the surgical procedures, types of implants, and complications, if any, as well as factors affecting health status, such as weight and medical history. Patients who were located were asked to complete a mailed questionnaire in order to collect information about their health status, factors that might affect their health, and short- and long-term complications that might be associated with the implants. No clinical exams were done on the patients, but attempts were made to verify patient reports of cancer and connective tissue disease from the medical records of the physicians who diagnosed or treated the diseases. For patients who had died, death certificates were collected to verify the causes of death.

Study Groups

Besides the size of the study and the length of follow-up, another unique feature of the NCI study is that the researchers compared the breast implant patients to both the general population and to women who had received other types of plastic surgery. In previous reports, the general population was used as the control group. However, NCI investigators found in an earlier study that women with implants tend to share more breast cancer risk factors with women who had received other types of plastic surgery than with the general population. (The study is titled: "Characteristics of a Population of Women with Breast Implants Compared with Women Seeking Other Types of Plastic Surgery." The authors are Louise A. Brinton, S. Lori Brown, Theodore Colton, Mary Cay Burich, Jay H. Lubin. *Plastic and Reconstructive Surgery* 2000;105(3):919-27.) These risk factors include histories of previous gynecologic operations and operations for benign breast disease. Therefore, they believe that women who received other types of plastic surgery may be a more appropriate comparison group than the general population. However, when compared to either the general population or women with other types of plastic surgery, there was no evidence of a change in breast cancer risk in the implant group.

Typically, implants are soft silicone sacs, inflated with either saline solution (salt water) or a synthetic silicone gel. Both have been marketed since 1962. Before the 1992 FDA ban, 90 percent to 95 percent of the implants contained silicone gel because they had a more pleasing look and feel than the saline-filled implants. Since 1992, 90 percent to 95 percent of the implants have been saline-filled. It is not known how many women currently have silicone vs. saline implants.

Of the implant patients in the study, 49.7 percent received silicone gel implants, 34.1 percent double lumen implants, 12.2 percent saline-filled implants, 0.1 percent other types of implants, and 3.8 percent unspecified types of implants. (Double lumen implants have two shells; the inner sac is filled with silicone gel and the outer with saline.) The participants had cosmetic surgery during a time (between 1962 and 1988) when a great number of changes were taking place in the manufacturing of breast implants such as the shell thickness, the type of shell coating, and the gel composition. However, the researchers found there was no altered breast cancer risk associated with any of the types of implants.

Implants and Cancer Diagnosis

One of the controversial issues is whether women with breast implants have more advanced breast cancer at diagnosis than women without implants. In the current study, NCI researchers found a somewhat later stage at detection of breast cancer among the implant patients compared to the controls and a smaller percentage of *in situ* (early-stage) cancers among the implant patients. However, the differences were not statistically significant and there was no significant difference in breast cancer mortality between the implant and comparison group.

"This is an issue that needs further study," said Brinton. "This would include continuing to follow participants in this study to see if their breast cancer death rate changes with time."

About 80 percent of breast implants in the United States are for cosmetic reasons and 20 percent for breast reconstruction. This study does not include women undergoing breast reconstruction after breast cancer surgery, so it is not possible to predict whether similar results would be found for this population. The majority of the previous studies have also focused on women who received implants for cosmetic reasons.

It is estimated that between 1.5 million and 2 million U.S. women have had breast implants since they first appeared on the market in 1962.

Future analyses of the data will evaluate the risk of other cancers, connective tissue disorders, and causes of death.

Chapter 23

Antiperspirants and Deodorants Not Considered Cancer Risk

Recent articles in the press and on the Internet have warned that underarm antiperspirants or deodorants cause breast cancer. The original source of this misinformation is not clear.

Scientists at the National Cancer Institute are not aware of any research to support a link between the use of underarm antiperspirants or deodorants and the subsequent development of breast cancer. The U.S. Food and Drug Administration, which regulates food, cosmetics, medicines, and medical devices, also does not have any evidence or research data to support the theory that ingredients in underarm antiperspirants or deodorants cause cancer. Thus, there appears to be no basis for this concern.

People who are concerned about their cancer risk are encouraged to talk with their doctor. Also, U.S. residents may wish to contact the Cancer Information Service with any remaining questions or concerns about breast cancer.

National Cancer Institute Information Resources
Telephone 1-800-4-CANCER (1-800-422-6237)
TTY: 1-800-332-8615 (for deaf and hard of hearing callers)

Cancer Information Service (CIS) provides accurate, up-to-date information on cancer to patients and their families, health professionals, and the general public. Information specialists translate the latest scientific information into understandable language and respond in English, Spanish, or on TTY equipment.

Cancer Facts, National Cancer Institute, April 2000.

Inquirers who live outside the United States may wish to contact the International Union Against Cancer (UICC) for information about a resource in their country. The UICC Web site is located at http://www.uicc.org on the Internet. Also, some countries have organizations that offer services similar to those of the U.S. Cancer Information Service. A list of international cancer information services can be found at http://cis.nci.nih.gov/resources/intlist.htm on the Internet.

Part Four

Mammograms and Other Screening Tools

Chapter 24

Screening for Breast Cancer

What Is Screening?

Screening for cancer is examination (or testing) of people for early stages in the development of cancer even though they have no symptoms. Scientists have studied patterns of cancer in the population to learn which people are more likely to get certain types of cancer. They have also studied what things around us and what things we do in our lives may cause cancer. This information sometimes helps doctors recommend who should be screened for certain types of cancer, what types of screening tests people should have, and how often these tests should be done. Not all screening tests are helpful, and they often have risks. For this reason, scientists at the National Cancer Institute are studying many screening tests to find out how useful they are and to determine the relative benefits and harms.

If your doctor suggests certain cancer screening tests as part of your health care plan, this does not mean he or she thinks you have cancer. Screening tests are done when you have no symptoms. Since decisions about screening can be difficult, you may want to discuss them with your doctor and ask questions about the potential benefits and risks of screening tests and whether they have been proven to decrease the risk of dying from cancer.

If your doctor suspects that you may have cancer, he or she will order certain tests to see whether you do. These are called diagnostic

CancerNet, National Cancer Institute, November 2000.

tests. Some tests are used for diagnostic purposes, but are not suitable for screening people who have no symptoms.

Purposes of This Summary

The purposes of this summary on breast cancer screening are to:

- give information on breast cancer and what makes it more likely to occur (risk factors)
- describe breast cancer screening methods and what is known about their effectiveness

You can talk to your doctor or health care professional about cancer screening and whether it would be likely to help you.

Breast Cancer Screening

The breast consists of lobes, lobules, and bulbs that are connected by ducts. The breast also contains blood and lymph vessels. These lymph vessels lead to structures that are called lymph nodes. Clusters of lymph nodes are found under the arm, above the collarbone, in the chest, and in other parts of the body. Together, the lymph vessels and lymph nodes make up the lymphatic system, which circulates a fluid called lymph throughout the body. Lymph contains cells that help fight infection and disease.

When breast cancer spreads outside the breast, cancer cells are most often found under the arm in the lymph nodes. In many cases, if the cancer has reached the lymph nodes, cancer cells may have also spread to other parts of the body via the lymphatic system or through the bloodstream.

Risk of Breast Cancer

More women in the United States get breast cancer than any other type of cancer (except for skin cancer). The number of cases per 1,000 women has increased slightly every year over the last 50 years. It is the second leading cause of death from cancer in women (lung cancer causes the most deaths from cancer in women). Breast cancer occurs in men also, but the number of new cases is small.

Anything that increases a person's chance of developing a disease is called a risk factor. Some of these risk factors for breast cancer are as follows:

Age—Breast cancer is more likely to develop as you grow older. Beginning menstruation at an early age and late age at first birth may also increase the risk of development of breast cancer.

History of Breast Cancer—If you have already had breast cancer, you are more likely to develop breast cancer again.

Family History—If your mother or sister had breast cancer, you are more likely to develop breast cancer, especially if they had it at an early age.

Radiation Therapy—Radiation therapy to the chest that was given more than 10 years ago, especially in women younger than 30 years old, may increase a woman's risk of developing breast cancer.

Other Breast Diseases—If you have had a breast biopsy specimen that showed certain types of benign breast conditions, you may be more likely to develop breast cancer. For most women, however, the ordinary "lumpiness" they feel in their breasts does not increase their risk of breast cancer.

Studies have found that race, social status, income, education, and access to screening and treatment services may affect a woman's risk of developing breast cancer.

Screening Tests for Breast Cancer

Breast Self-Examination—When you examine your own breasts it is called breast self-examination (BSE). Studies so far have not shown that BSE alone reduces the number of deaths from breast cancer. Therefore, it should not be used in place of clinical breast examination and mammography.

Clinical Breast Examination—During your routine physical examination, your doctor or health care professional may do a clinical breast examination (CBE). During a CBE, your doctor will carefully feel your breasts and under your arms to check for lumps or other unusual changes.

Mammogram—A mammogram is a special x-ray of the breast that can often find tumors that are too small for you or your doctor to feel.

Your doctor may suggest that you have a mammogram, especially if you have any of the risk factors listed above.

The ability of mammography to detect cancer depends on such factors as the size of the tumor, the age of the woman, breast density, and the skill of the radiologist. Studies have found that screening mammography is beneficial in women aged 50 to 69. Screening in women younger than 50 years or older than 69 years may or may not be helpful.

Ultrasonography—During ultrasonography, sound waves (called ultrasound) are bounced off tissues and the echoes are converted into a picture (sonogram). Ultrasound is used to evaluate lumps that have been identified by BSE, CBE, or mammography. Studies have not shown that ultrasonography is of any proven benefit in detecting breast cancer.

Magnetic Resonance Imaging (MRI)—A procedure in which a magnet linked to a computer is used to create detailed pictures of areas inside the body. MRIs are used to evaluate breast masses that have been found by BSE or CBE and to recognize the difference between cancer and scar tissue. The role of MRI in breast cancer screening has not yet been established.

Other screening methods are being studied. Your doctor can talk to you about what screening tests would be best for you.

To Learn More

For more information, call the National Cancer Institute's Cancer Information Service at 1-800-4-CANCER (1-800-422-6237); TTY at 1-800-332-8615. The call is free and a trained information specialist is available to answer your questions.

Chapter 25

Screening Mammograms

What is a screening mammogram?

A screening mammogram is an x-ray of the breast used to detect breast changes in women who have no signs of breast cancer. It usually involves two x-rays of each breast. Using a mammogram, it is possible to detect a tumor that cannot be felt.

What is a diagnostic mammogram?

A diagnostic mammogram is an x-ray of the breast used to diagnose unusual breast changes, such as a lump, pain, nipple thickening or discharge, or a change in breast size or shape. A diagnostic mammogram is also used to evaluate abnormalities detected on a screening mammogram. It is a basic medical tool and is appropriate in the workup of breast changes, regardless of a woman's age.

What is the position of the National Cancer Institute (NCI) on screening mammograms?

The National Cancer Institute recommends that women in their forties or older get screening mammograms on a regular basis, every 1 to 2 years.

Women who are at increased risk for breast cancer should seek medical advice about when to begin having mammograms and how often to be screened. (For example, a doctor may recommend that a

Cancer Facts, National Cancer Institute, September 1999.

woman at increased risk begin screening before age 40 or change her screening intervals to every year.)

What are the factors that place a woman at increased risk for breast cancer?

Every woman has some risk for developing breast cancer during her lifetime, and that risk increases as she ages. However, the risk of developing breast cancer is not the same for all women. These are the factors known to increase a woman's chance of developing this disease:

- Personal History: Women who have had breast cancer are more likely to develop a second breast cancer.

- Family History: The risk of getting breast cancer increases for a woman whose mother, sister, or daughter has had the disease; or who has two or more close relatives, such as cousins or aunts, with a history of breast cancer (especially if diagnosed before age 40). About 5 percent of women with breast cancer have a hereditary form of this disease.

- Genetic Alterations: Specific alterations in certain genes, such as those in the breast cancer genes BRCA1 or BRCA2, make women more susceptible to breast cancer.

- Abnormal Biopsy: Women with certain abnormal breast conditions, such as atypical hyperplasia or LCIS (lobular carcinoma *in situ*), are at increased risk.

- Other conditions associated with an increased risk of breast cancer: Women age 45 or older who have at least 75 percent dense tissue on a mammogram are at elevated risk. (This is not only because tumors in dense breasts are more difficult to "see," but because, in older women, dense breast tissue itself is related to an increased chance of developing breast cancer.)

  Women who received chest irradiation for conditions such as Hodgkin's disease at age 30 or younger are at higher risk for breast cancer throughout their lives and require regular monitoring for breast cancer.

  A woman who has her first child at age 30 or older has an increased risk of breast cancer.

  Recent evidence suggests that menopausal women who have long-term exposure (greater than 10 years) to hormone replacement therapy (HRT) may have a slightly increased risk of breast cancer.

What are the chances that a woman in the United States might get breast cancer?

Age is the most important factor in the risk for breast cancer. The older a woman is, the greater her chance of getting breast cancer. No woman should consider herself too old to need regular screening mammograms. A woman's chance. . .

by age 30	1 out of 2,212
by age 40	1 out of 235
by age 50	1 out of 54
by age 60	1 out of 23
by age 70	1 out of 14
by age 80	1 out of 10

(Source: NCI's Surveillance, Epidemiology, and End Results Program & American Cancer Society, 1994–1996)

About 80 percent of breast cancers occur in women over the age of 50; the number of cases is especially high for women over age 60. Breast cancer is uncommon in women under age 40.

What is the best method of detecting breast cancer as early as possible?

A high-quality mammogram, with a clinical breast exam (an exam done by a professional health care provider), is the most effective way to detect breast cancer early. Using a mammogram, it is possible to detect breast cancer that cannot be felt. However, like any test, mammograms have both benefits and limitations.

When a woman examines her own breasts, it is called breast self-exam (BSE). Studies so far have not shown that BSE alone reduces the numbers of deaths from breast cancer. Therefore, it should not be used in place of clinical breast exam and mammography.

What are the benefits of screening mammograms?

Several studies have shown that regular screening mammograms can help to decrease the chance of dying from breast cancer. The benefits of regular screening are greater for women over age 50. For women in their forties, there is recent evidence that having mammograms on a regular basis may reduce their chances of dying from breast cancer by about 17 percent. For women between the ages of 50 and 69, there is strong evidence that screening with mammography on a regular basis reduces breast cancer deaths by about 30 percent.

Estimates show that if 10,000 women age 40 were screened every year for 10 years, about four lives would be saved. In comparison, regular screening of 10,000 women age 50 would save about 37 lives.

What are some of the limitations of screening mammograms?

- Detection does not always mean saving lives: Even though mammography can detect most tumors that are 5 millimeters in size (5 millimeters is about 1/4 inch), finding a small tumor does not always mean that a woman's life will be saved. Mammography may not help a woman with a fast-growing or aggressive cancer that has already spread to other parts of her body before being detected.

- False Negatives: False negatives occur when mammograms appear normal even though breast cancer is actually present. False negatives are more common in younger women than in older women. The dense breasts of younger women contain many glands and ligaments, which make breast cancers more difficult to spot in mammograms. As women age, breast tissues become more fatty and breast cancers are more easily "seen" by screening mammograms.

  Screening mammograms miss up to 25 percent of breast cancers in women in their forties compared with about 10 percent of cancers for older women.

- False Positives: False positives occur when mammograms are read as abnormal, but no cancer is actually present. For women at all ages, between 5 percent and 10 percent of mammograms are abnormal and are followed up with additional testing (a diagnostic mammogram, fine needle aspirate, ultrasound, or biopsy). Most abnormalities will turn out not to be cancer. Over a 10-year period, the chance that a woman will have a false positive mammogram is about 50 percent.

  False positives are more common in younger women than older women. About 97 percent of women ages 40 to 49 who have abnormal mammograms turn out not to have cancer, as compared with about 86 percent for women age 50 and older. But all women have to undergo followup procedures when they have an abnormal mammogram. Some will require breast biopsies.

What happens if mammography detects DCIS?

Over the past 30 years, improvements in mammography have resulted in an ability to detect a higher number of small tissue abnormalities called ductal carcinomas *in situ* (DCIS), abnormal cells confined to the milk ducts of the breast. Some of these can eventually go on to become actual cancers, but many do not.

It is not possible to predict which cases of DCIS will progress to invasive cancer. These tissue abnormalities are commonly removed surgically; some are treated with mastectomy, some with breast-sparing surgery and radiation therapy. Often, DCIS is also treated with tamoxifen.

Younger women have a higher proportion of DCIS than older women. Approximately 45 percent of breast cancers detected by screening mammograms in women ages 40 to 49 are DCIS compared with about 20 to 30 percent of those detected in women age 50 and older.

How much does a mammogram cost?

Most screening mammograms cost between $50 and $150. Most states now have laws requiring health insurance companies to reimburse all or part of the cost of screening mammograms. Details can be provided by insurance companies and health care providers.

Medicare pays 80 percent of the cost of a screening mammogram each year for beneficiaries ages 40 or older. There is no deductible requirement for this benefit, but Medicare beneficiaries are responsible for a 20 percent copayment of the Medicare-approved amount. Information on coverage is available through the Medicare Hotline at 1–800–MEDICARE.

Some state and local health programs and employers provide mammograms free or at low cost. Information on low-cost or free mammography screening programs is available through the NCI's Cancer Information Service at 1–800–4–CANCER.

Where can a woman get a high-quality mammogram?

Women can get high-quality mammograms in breast clinics, radiology departments o f hospitals, mobile vans, private radiology offices, and doctors' offices.

Through the Mammography Quality Standards Act, all mammography facilities are required to display certification by the Food and Drug Administration (FDA). To be certified, facilities must meet standards for the equipment they use, the people who work there, and the records they keep. Women should go to an FDA-certified facility and look for the certificate and expiration date. Women can ask their doctors or staff at the mammography facility about FDA-certification before making an appointment. Information about local FDA-certified mammography facilities is available through NCI's Cancer Information Service at 1–800–4–CANCER.

What technologies are under development for breast cancer screening?

The NCI is supporting the development of several new technologies to detect breast tumors. This research ranges from technologies under development in research labs to those that have reached the stage of testing in humans, known as clinical trials.

Efforts to improve conventional mammography include digital mammography, where computers assist in the interpretation of the x-rays. Other studies are aimed at developing teleradiology, sending x-rays electronically, for long-distance clinical consultations. Magnetic resonance imaging (MRI), which does not use x-rays, is another imaging technology under development.

In addition to imaging technologies, NCI-supported scientists are exploring methods to detect markers of breast cancer in blood, urine, or nipple aspirates that may serve as early warning signals for breast cancer.

What studies is NCI supporting to find better ways to prevent and treat breast cancer?

NCI is supporting many studies that are looking for improved prevention and treatment for breast cancer.

- Basic Research: Many studies are taking place to identify the causes of breast cancer, including an analysis of the role that alterations in the BRCA1 and BRCA2 genes play in the development of cancer. Scientists also are looking at how these genes interact with other genes and with hormonal, dietary, and environmental factors to determine what influences the development of breast cancer.

- Prevention: Researchers are looking for ways to prevent breast cancer in women who are at increased risk. In addition, studies currently under way involving diet, nutrition, and environmental factors could also lead to new prevention strategies.

- Treatment: Several studies are aimed at finding treatments for breast cancer that are more effective and less toxic than current methods.

Women who would like more information on cancer prevention, treatment, or screening studies can call NCI's Cancer Information Service at 1–800–4–CANCER.

Chapter 26

Mammography Statistics

Breast Cancer and Mammography Facts

Breast Cancer Incidence and Mortality

Incidence: The number of newly diagnosed cancers per 100,000 population during a specific period of time (usually one year).

Mortality: The number of deaths due to a cancer per 100,000 population during a specific period of time (usually one year).

Table 26.1. Breast Cancer Incidence Rates, 1988–1992

Korean	29	Alaska Natives	79
American Indians	32	Japanese	82
Vietnamese	38	African American	95
Chinese	55	Hawaiian	106
Hispanic	70	White Non-Hispanic	116
Filipino	73		

Rates are average annual per 100,000 and age-adjusted to 1970 U.S. standard population.

Data Source: Racial/Ethnic Patterns of Cancer in the United States 1988–1992, National Cancer Institute.

Cancer Facts, National Cancer Institute, January 1998.

- White Non-Hispanic women have the highest incidence rate for breast cancer among the U.S. racial/ethnic groups shown in the Table 26.1; Korean women have the lowest.

- African American women have the highest mortality rate for breast cancer among these groups; Chinese women have the lowest.

Table 26.2. What are the Chances of a Woman Getting Breast Cancer as She Ages?

by age 30	1 out of 2,525
by age 40	1 out of 217
by age 50	1 out of 50
by age 60	1 out of 24
by age 70	1 out of 14
by age 80	1 out of 10

Source: NCI Surveillance, Epidemiology, and End Results (SEER) Program & American Cancer Society, 1993.

Table 26.3. Breast Cancer Mortality Rates, 1988–1992

Chinese	11
Filipino	12
Japanese	13
Hispanic	15
Hawaiian	25
White Non Hispanic	28
African American	31

Rates are average annual per 100,000 and age-adjusted to 1970 U.S. standard population.

Data Source: Racial/Ethnic Patterns of Cancer in the United States 1988–1992, National Cancer Institute.

Note: Rates for Alaska Natives, American Indians (New Mexico), Koreans, and Vietnamese not available.

Mammography Rates: Percentages were computed using SUDAAN, a statistical program for survey data analysis that incorporates the NHIS sample weights and complex survey design into its population estimates.

- Among African American, White Non-Hispanic, and Hispanic women ages 40 and older, the screening rates in 1992 are higher than in 1987.

- In every ethnic group, mammography rates for women age 65 and older are lower than for women who are under age 65.

Table 26.4. Mammography Rates Among African American Non-Hispanic, White Non-Hispanic, and Hispanic Women Ages 40 and Older, Who Ever Had a Mammogram, 1987 & 1992

	1987	1992
African American Non-Hispanic	31%	64%
White Non-Hispanic	40%	69%
Hispanic	28%	70%

Data Source: *MMWR* 1995; 45(3):57–61.

Table 26.5. Mammography Rates Among African American Non-Hispanic, White Non-Hispanic, and Hispanic Women Ages 40 and Older, Who Had a Mammogram Within the Year, 1987 & 1992

	1987	1992
African American Non-Hispanic	14%	32%
White Non-Hispanic	18%	36%
Hispanic	13%	38%

Data Source: *MMWR* 1995; 45(3):57–61.

Table 26.6. Mammography Rates Among African American Non-Hispanic, White Non-Hispanic, and Hispanic Women, Who Ever Had a Mammogram, 1992

	Ages 40-49	Ages 50-64	Ages 65+
African American Non-Hispanic	67%	75%	59%
White Non-Hispanic	72%	76%	65%
Hispanic	78%	73%	65%

Data Source: National Health Interview Survey, 1992.

Table 26.7. Mammography Rates Among African American Non-Hispanic, White Non-Hispanic, and Hispanic Women, Who Had a Mammogram Within the Year, 1992

	Ages 40-49	Ages 50-64	Ages 65+
African American Non-Hispanic	34%	43%	32%
White Non-Hispanic	39%	47%	36%
Hispanic	48%	42%	33%

Data Source: National Health Interview Survey, 1992.

Barriers to Getting Mammograms

- Lack of physician recommendation
- Misconception that, without symptoms, there is no need to get screened
- Lack of awareness about mammography
- Cost and/or lack of health insurance
- Lack of access to mammography facilities
- Fear of cancer detection
- Language
- Cultural beliefs and values that are not consistent with preventive medical care

Recommendations for Education and Outreach Programs

- Encourage routine mammography screening for women in their forties and older.

- Emphasize the importance of *routine* screening for the early detection of breast cancer—once is not enough.

- Highlight that early detection of breast cancer can increase women's options for treatment and increase survival rates. (See the following for information on specific audiences.)

- Develop breast cancer/mammography outreach and education efforts for minority and underserved audiences that address barriers to getting mammograms.

- Provide access to the latest information on risks for breast cancer, screening, diagnosis, treatment, and follow-up care. Resources include the National Cancer Institute's Cancer Information Service (CIS) at 1-800-4-CANCER and the Food and Drug Administration's mammography facility locator service available through the CIS.

- Provide underserved women information about low-cost and/or free mammography screening programs sponsored by the Centers for Disease Control and Prevention's Breast and Cervical Cancer Early Detection Program. Information on the program is available through the CIS.

- Provide women ages 65 or older information on Medicare's coverage of mammograms. Information is available through the Medicare Hotline at 1-800-638-6833.

- Early detection messages may be particularly important for:
  - African American women because they have the highest mortality and lowest survival rates for breast cancer.
  - Hispanic women because breast cancer incidence rates are increasing faster among Hispanics than other women.
  - American Indian or Alaska Native women because they have higher breast cancer incidence rates and lower survival rates than some other groups of women.
  - Asian or Pacific Islander women because some studies suggest that their cancer rates increase as they become acculturated.
  - Older women because as women age, their chances of getting breast cancer increase.

Chapter 27

Detection Rates by Race and Ethnicity Show Importance of Screening

Commemorating Breast Cancer Awareness Month, HHS Secretary Donna E. Shalala announced today the first race- and ethnic-specific rates of breast cancer detection. She also released public service announcements (PSAs) featuring Surgeon General David A. Satcher, M.D. that underscore the importance of early detection in the fight against breast and cervical cancer through health programs such as the Centers for Disease Control and Prevention's (CDC) National Breast and Cervical Cancer Early Detection Program.

"This year marks the 10th anniversary of the CDC's breast and cervical cancer program which has saved women's lives through early detection," said Secretary Shalala. "This milestone is the result of much effort and commitment from public health professionals in state and local governments throughout the country. I feel certain that the second decade will bring women even greater access to screening and follow-up services."

According to CDC data published in the October 2000 issue of *Cancer Causes and Control*, among women receiving their first National Breast and Cervical Cancer Early Detection Program (NBCCEDP)-funded mammogram, 7.7 cancers were detected per 1,000 white women; 6.4 cancers per 1,000 African-American women; 6.2 per 1,000 Asian/Pacific Islander women; 4.9 per 1,000 American Indian/Alaska Native women; and 4.9 per 1,000 Hispanic women.

"Breast Cancer Detection Rates by Race and Ethnicity Show Importance of Screening for All Age Groups," *HHS News*, U.S. Department of Health and Human Services, Press Release dated October 12, 2000.

Women who reported no mammography before their first NBC-CEDP mammogram were more likely to have abnormal results and cancers than women who reported previous mammography. Approximately three-fourths of white and African-American women had at least one mammogram before entering the NBCCEDP; the percentage was much lower for Asian/Pacific Islander, American Indian/Alaska Native and Hispanic women.

"These data remind us that women of every race and ethnic group need access to the potentially life-saving benefits of regular mammography screening," said CDC Director Jeffrey Koplan, M.D., M.P.H. "Although many thousands of women have received free mammograms through the NBCCEDP, there is an enormous need for additional resources to reach those who are still not able to afford routine breast cancer screening. We must continue to work to provide affordable breast cancer screening and follow-up services to all women."

Established in 1990, the screening and early detection program has grown from eight states in 1991 to 50 states, six U.S. territories, the District of Columbia, and 12 American Indian/Alaska Native organizations in 2000. During its first decade, the program has provided more than 2.5 million screening tests, nearly 1.2 million mammograms and more than 1.3 million Pap tests, and diagnosed nearly 8,000 breast and cervical cancers. The program also provides educational information to women and health care providers about the need for these life-saving screening tests.

"Even if you don't have health insurance or Medicare, you can still get free screening exams for breast and cervical cancer through this vital program," said Dr. Satcher about the main focus of the CDC program.

Breast cancer is the most common cancer, except for skin cancer, and is second only to lung cancer as a cause of cancer-related deaths among American women. Cervical cancer is one of the most preventable cancers that affect women, but women are still dying unnecessarily because the cancer is often caught too late. This year, 40,800 women will die from breast cancer and 4,600 women from cervical cancer.

Recognizing the value of screening and early detection in preventing unnecessary deaths, Congress passed the Breast and Cervical Cancer Mortality Prevention Act of 1990. The Act authorized CDC to provide breast and cervical cancer screening services to older women, women with low incomes, and underserved women of racial and ethnic minority groups.

To request copies of the Surgeon General's PSA or for more information about the study on race- and ethnic-specific rates of breast cancer detection, call 770-488-4751. To learn more about the National Breast and Cervical Cancer Early Detection Program, visit http://www.cdc.gov/cancer/NBCCEDP or call toll-free 1-888-842-6355.

Note: Audio of Surgeon General David Satcher reminding women that they can get free screening exams for breast and cervical cancer even if they do not have health insurance is available on the Internet at: http://www.hhs.gov/news/broadcast/20001012.wav.

Chapter 28

Mammography Guidelines, Limitations, and Standards

Breast Cancer and Mammography

Overview

The Department of Health and Human Services supports a wide variety of programs in research, treatment and screening for breast cancer. Total HHS spending on breast cancer in FY 1997 is $513 million for public health programs, in addition to an estimated $280 million for mammography services paid for by Medicare and Medicaid.

Early detection of breast cancer is crucial for successful treatment, and HHS programs promote mammography and clinical breast exams. This is especially true for older women: about 80 percent of breast cancers occur in women age 50 or older, yet 40 percent of women age 50 and older have reported not having a mammogram in the past two years. HHS agencies support a number of efforts to inform women about mammography, assure high quality service, and help provide access:

- The National Cancer Institute, and other NIH institutes, provide information outreach and support broad research on breast cancer and on new breast imaging technologies.

HHS Backgrounder, U.S. Department of Health and Human Services, March 27, 1997.

- The Food and Drug Administration establishes quality standards for mammography facilities and certifies facilities.

- The Agency for Health Care Policy and Research has issued guidelines on the quality and delivery of mammography, and does research on mammography services.

- The Centers for Disease Control and Prevention supports an early detection program providing access to mammography for uninsured and low-income women.

- Medicare and Medicaid cover treatment for breast cancer and for screening services. President Clinton has proposed improvements in Medicare and Medicaid coverage for mammography.

The National Cancer Institute provides science-based guidance on the use of mammography. NCI now recommends that women age 40 and over be screened with mammography every one to two years. In addition, the institute recommends that women at higher risk of breast cancer get expert medical advice even before they are 40 about when to begin screening and about the frequency of their screening.

Breast Cancer

Breast cancer is the most frequently diagnosed non-skin cancer in women in the United States. It is second only to lung cancer in cancer-related deaths. Approximately 180,000 new cases of breast cancer will be diagnosed in 1997, and about 44,000 women are expected to die from the disease.

Between 1982 and 1987, breast cancer incidence (rate of new cases) for women increased about 4 percent per year, but recently has leveled off. The death rate for women with breast cancer declined 6.3 percent between 1991 and 1995. The greatest reductions in death rates were among younger women (9.3 percent) and white women (6.6 percent), with more modest reductions among African Americans (1.6 percent) and women age 65 and older (2.8 percent).

There are a variety of effective treatments for breast cancer, including surgery, radiotherapy, hormonal therapy, and chemotherapy.

Risk Factors

Elevated risk of breast cancer is associated with the following conditions:

- Having had a previous breast cancer.

- Laboratory evidence that the woman is carrying a specific genetic mutation or change that increases susceptibility to breast cancer.

- Having a mother, sister, or daughter with a history of breast cancer or having two or more close relatives, such as cousins, with a history of breast cancer.

- Having had a diagnosis of other types of breast disease (not cancer but a condition that may predispose to cancer) or having had two or more breast biopsies for benign disease, even if no atypical cells were found.

- Having so much dense breast tissue on a previous mammographic examination that clear reading was difficult.

- Having a first birth at age 30 or older.

Breast cancer is more prevalent in older age groups. The risk of breast cancer increases with age. About 80 percent of breast cancers occur in women age 50 or older. The risk is especially high in women over age 60. Breast cancer is uncommon under age 35. Present rates project that each year, out of 100,000 women:

- in their 30s, 43 women will be diagnosed with breast cancer and 8 will die of the disease;

- in their 40s, 163 women will be diagnosed with breast cancer and 29 will die of the disease;

- in their 50s, 263 women will be diagnosed with breast cancer and 59 will die of the disease;

- in their 60s, 374 women will be diagnosed with breast cancer and 91 will die of it.

Early Detection

Screening is a means to detect breast cancer before the onset of symptoms. High-quality mammography, with or without clinical breast exams, is the most effective technology presently available to detect breast tumors.

Several studies have shown that regular mammography screening can decrease the chance of dying from breast cancer. In addition, early detection may prevent the necessity of removing lymph nodes and in some cases may prevent the need for removing the entire breast or for undergoing chemotherapy.

Current NCI Guidance on Mammography

On February 25, the National Cancer Advisory Board (NCAB), a presidentially appointed committee that advises, assists, and consults with the NCI Director with respect to NCI activities and policies, began a discussion of the findings from the NIH Consensus Development Conference. NCAB members recognized the importance and complexity of the topic and decided to form a Working Group to develop clear recommendations to NCI. In late March, members of the full Board concurred with the Working Group's recommendations. These recommendations were also accepted by the National Cancer Institute.

The National Cancer Institute, following the advice of the NCAB, recommends:

- Women in their 40s who are at average risk of breast cancer should be screened every one to two years with mammography.

- Women aged 50 and older should be screened every one to two years.

- Women who are at higher risk of breast cancer should seek expert medical advice about whether they should begin screening before age 40 and the frequency of screening.

Along with mammograms, a clinical breast examination by a health care provider should be included as part of regular, routine health care.

Limitations of Mammography

While mammography is the best screening tool available now, early detection does not necessarily mean lives will be saved. Mammography may not help a woman with a small but fast growing tumor that has already spread at the time of detection. And about 50 percent of women whose breast cancer is detected by mammography would not have died from the cancer even if they had waited until a lump could be felt because the tumors are slow-growing and easy to treat.

Breasts of younger women contain many glands and ligaments that appear dense on a mammogram, so it is sometimes difficult to spot tumors in their breasts. About 25 percent of breast tumors are missed in women in their 40s compared to 10 percent for women in their 50s.

Also, between 5 percent and 10 percent of mammograms are abnormal. Of those in younger women that are followed up with additional tests (another mammogram, fine needle aspiration, ultrasound, or biopsy) most will not be cancer. Over the past 30 years, mammography has been able to detect a higher proportion of small tissue abnormalities called ductal carcinoma *in situ* (DCIS), abnormal cells confined to the milk ducts of the breast. Some believe these tumors are not life threatening, while others think they are. Because there is so little data to support either view, the abnormalities are commonly removed surgically.

HHS Programs Supporting Mammography

Mammography Quality Standards

Under the Mammography Quality Standards Act, the FDA sets high standards for mammography facilities and certifies those which meet the standards. The roughly 10,000 mammography facilities nationwide certified by the FDA must meet quality standards for both equipment and personnel, and are inspected annually. MQSA regulations require facilities to hire capable technicians, use quality equipment that produces clear images, and employ skilled radiologists to interpret the results. The rules also require that doctors and patients be fully and quickly informed of results so that any follow-up testing or treatment can begin immediately. Resources devoted to the Mammography Quality Standards Act is $26.4 million for FY 1997.

The names and locations of FDA certified mammography facilities are available by calling the Cancer Information Service at 1-800-4-CANCER. In addition, the FDA has included a list of all FDA certified mammography facilities in the United States on its internet home page. The address is http://www.fda.gov/cdrh/faclist.html.

Research to Develop Better Screening

New imaging technologies under development for breast cancer screening include magnetic resonance imaging, breast ultrasound, and breast-specific positron emission tomography. In addition to imaging technologies, NCI-supported scientists are exploring methods to detect breast cancer using simple tests of the blood, urine, or nipple aspirates, and to detect genetic alterations that place women at increased risk for breast cancer.

In addition, HHS is working with the Department of Defense, the CIA, NASA, and other public and private entities to explore ways in which imaging technologies from other fields may be applied to the early detection of breast cancer. In particular, the computer technologies that have been used to improve spy satellites may help improve breast cancer detection as well. In October, 1996, HHS awarded $1.98 million to the University of Pennsylvania to conduct a multi-site clinical trial of imaging technology from the intelligence community—originally used for missile guidance and target recognition—to improve the early detection of breast cancer.

Mammography Clinical Practice Guidelines

Recognizing the importance of the quality of screening mammograms in the early detection of breast cancer, HHS' Agency for Health Care Policy and Research developed a *Clinical Practice Guideline: Quality Determinants of Mammography* with separate versions for mammography providers, health care professionals, and consumers. The guideline provides information on the roles and responsibilities of each health care professional involved in mammography services, as well as information and recommendations for women.

Medicare and Medicaid Coverage of Mammography

Since 1991, Medicare has covered mammography screening for the early detection of breast cancer. For women age 40-49, Medicare currently covers one screening mammogram every two years, except for women with a high risk (for example, a woman with a mother, sister or daughter who has had breast cancer), in which case annual mammograms are covered. For women age 50-64, annual screening mammograms are covered; and for women 65 and older, Medicare covers one screening mammogram every two years.

President Clinton is proposing to expand Medicare coverage to include annual mammograms for all Medicare beneficiaries age 40 and over, with no copayment or deductible requirement.

Under Medicaid, diagnostic mammograms are a mandated service and states must cover them. Screening mammograms, however, are provided by states as an optional service, with most states covering screening mammograms in fee-for-service Medicaid. In addition, virtually all Medicaid managed care plans offer preventive services, including mammography, to their enrollees.

The Health Care Financing Administration has urged states to provide annual mammography screening to Medicaid beneficiaries at age 40; HCFA will continue to provide federal matching payments for annual mammography screening services.

National Breast and Cervical Cancer Early Detection Program

The CDC's National Breast and Cervical Cancer Early Detection Program offers free or low-cost mammography screening to uninsured, low-income, elderly, minority, and Native American women nationwide. The resources devoted to breast cancer screening services have increased from $42 million in FY 1993, to $81 million in FY 1997. The program, which has been operating in an increasing number of states over the past six years, has provided screening tests to almost one million medically underserved women. In October, 1996, the program went nationwide, with funding for all 50 states.

Chapter 29

Higher Standards for Mammography

Janie Pfefferkorn knows all too well the value of having a mammogram. She believes the procedure saved her life.

"I owe a great deal to the American Cancer Society for educating me and other women about the importance of having regular mammograms and doing self-examinations," says the 47-year-old Sikeston, Missouri, resident.

Following a routine mammogram in June 1996, Pfefferkorn received a call from her physician saying there was an area of concern in one of her breasts. A follow-up visit and second mammogram the next day both identified an abnormal area. A biopsy taken shortly after revealed that Pfefferkorn was in the early stages of breast cancer.

The Key to Early Detection

Mammography is the best method for detecting breast cancer in its earliest stages, when the disease is most successfully treated and there are more treatment options. Mammograms can find 85 to 90 percent of breast cancers in women over 50, and can discover a tumor up to two years before a lump can be felt. In some cases, finding a breast tumor early may mean a woman can choose breast-saving surgery, and she may not need chemotherapy.

"FDA Sets Higher Standards for Mammography," by Carol Lewis, *FDA Consumer*, (January-February 1999).

Although Pfefferkorn wasn't so fortunate—she was hospitalized for two days in 1996 for a mastectomy and underwent chemotherapy over the next five months—the mother of four daughters feels lucky to be alive.

"Early detection saved my life," she insists. "My girls have the mind-set now to take care of themselves after what we've been through."

The Mammography Quality Standards Act

As important as mammograms are, they are only worthwhile if the equipment is properly maintained and the personnel properly trained. The primary objective of the Mammography Quality Standards Act (MQSA) of 1992 is to ensure that mammography is safe and reliable and that breast cancer is detected in its most treatable stages. The Food and Drug Administration has the responsibility for implementing and enforcing MQSA, which requires that all mammography facilities in the United States meet certain stringent quality standards, be accredited by an FDA-approved accreditation body, and be inspected annually.

The final regulations for MQSA, which went into effect April 28, 1999, toughen the 1994 interim standards for personnel, equipment, quality assurance and quality control, and requirements for accreditation bodies. For example, physicians who interpret mammograms must now be board certified or have three months of training in mammography, technologists must keep their skills current by doing an average of 200 mammograms every two years, and medical physicists, who survey mammography equipment and facilities, must meet initial and continuing education and experience requirements.

Of significant importance to women is the MQSA regulation that requires mammography facilities to give patients an easy-to-read report on the results of their mammogram. Prior to MQSA, mammography facilities were not required to communicate results directly to patients and, instead, sent results only to the referring physician. Referring physicians will continue to receive the results. Self-referred patients with no designated health-care provider will receive both the simplified report and the one doctors normally receive.

MQSA also clarifies a facility's responsibility to retain and transfer mammograms to a patient's physician or to the patient directly, regardless of whether the transfer is permanent or temporary. This is important because it aids diagnosis by allowing doctors to compare old mammograms with new ones.

In addition, the final regulations:

- better define equipment capabilities needed for high-quality mammography
- require more quality control of mobile mammography units
- set standards for imaging breast tissue in women who have implants
- provide for additional clinical review and patient notification when a facility's images are determined to be substandard and a risk to health
- balance cost with need for mammography to be accessible
- require each facility to have a way for consumers to file complaints or voice concerns about the facility.

To be MQSA-certified, a mammography facility must be accredited by a federally approved private, nonprofit or state accreditation body. FDA has approved the American College of Radiology (ACR) and the states of Arkansas, California and Iowa as accreditation bodies. The agency will announce additional states that become approved.

To be accredited, the facility must apply to an FDA-approved accreditation body, undergo periodic review of its clinical images, have an annual survey by a medical physicist, and meet federally developed quality standards for personnel qualifications, equipment quality assurance programs, and record keeping and reporting. The facility must also undergo an annual inspection conducted by federally trained and certified federal or state personnel. A certificate is required to be displayed at the facility. FDA encourages women getting mammograms to look for this certificate.

What Is a Mammogram?

A mammogram is an x-ray picture of the breast. It uses a dedicated x-ray machine specifically designed for that purpose, as opposed to machines that take x-rays of the bones or other body parts.

Mammograms that look for breast changes in women who have no signs of breast cancer are called "screening" mammograms. The standard screening mammogram includes two views of each breast, one from above and one angled from the side. A trained technologist places the breast on a plastic plate. A second piece of plastic is placed on top and for a few seconds, some pressure is applied to flatten the breast and get a picture. This may be temporarily uncomfortable, but it is necessary to flatten the breast as much as possible because spreading

225

out the tissue makes it easier to spot any abnormal details. The doses of radiation used for mammography are very low and considered safe. The entire mammography procedure lasts about 15 minutes, and the average cost is between $100 and $150. After the procedure, a radiologist reads and interprets the x-ray image of the breast tissue that the mammogram produces.

The M1000 ImageChecker, a computerized device that analyzes the content of mammograms and highlights suspicious areas on the images after the radiologist has done the initial evaluation, is the latest FDA-approved mechanism for improving cancer detection. The device, made by R2 Technology, Inc., Los Altos, California., and approved in June 1998, scans the image with a laser beam, then converts it into a digital signal that a computer can process. After the computer marks suspicious areas on a video display of the image, the radiologist can compare the image to the original mammogram to see if any of these areas escaped notice and require further evaluation. The device has been shown to improve radiologists' detection rate from approximately 80 out of 100 cancers to almost 88 out of 100.

If problems are noted, a second "diagnostic" mammogram may be needed. Diagnostic mammograms are also used to assess specific symptoms or unusual breast changes such as a lump, pain, nipple thickening or discharge, or changes in breast size or shape.

Ensuring High-Quality Mammography

FDA first turned its focus on mammography following a 1974 Pennsylvania report. A state inspector had found that some mammography techniques used in different facilities had resulted in a few extremely high doses of radiation.

"That was the first time there had ever been any real attention paid to mammography—how it was being conducted and what was happening," says Richard Gross, recently retired from FDA's Center for Devices and Radiological Health.

In an effort to reduce the exposures, two voluntary programs were developed between 1975 and 1985 that involved industry working to improve the equipment. Mammography techniques began to change and radiation doses began to decrease.

"But we were concerned that much of the pressure to reduce the dose might have the effect of compromising image quality," Gross says. One program conducted, for example, showed that some images were found to be so bad that it would have been very difficult to detect anything. And these were issues over which FDA, at the time, had no regulatory authority and which had to be corrected within the facility. The American College of Radiology agreed to try to help correct the problem and in 1987 established its voluntary mammography accrediting program. FDA regulated the equipment, and ACR policed the facilities.

Limitations of Mammography

Despite its usefulness, mammography is not foolproof. The National Cancer Institute (NCI) says that some breast changes, including lumps that can be felt, do not always show up on a mammogram. Meg Long's tumor was one of them.

When the 56-year-old Norman, Oklahoma, resident found a lump in one of her breasts in the middle of the night in 1988, a mammogram only hours later failed to detect any signs of the mass. NCI says if a woman's tumor at the particular time she has a mammogram is the same density as the surrounding breast tissue, it may not show up on the x-ray. Fortunately for Long, the tumor appeared on an ultrasound taken immediately following the mammogram.

In short, occasionally mammograms may miss cancer that is present or may indicate something that can turn out not to be cancerous. Because the procedure is not as sensitive for the denser breast tissue in younger women, these false readings, according to NCI, occur more often in women under age 50.

Breast implants can also impede accurate mammogram readings because silicone implants are not transparent on x-rays and can block a clear view of the tissues behind them, especially if the implant has been placed in front of, rather than beneath, the chest muscles. But NCI says that experienced technologists and radiologists know how to carefully compress the breasts to improve the view without rupturing the implant. When making an appointment for a mammogram, women with implants should ask if the facility uses special techniques designed to accommodate them. And before the mammogram is taken, they should make sure the technologist is experienced in x-raying patients with breast implants.

When Should a Woman Get a Mammogram?

Breast cancer strikes about 180,000 American women yearly and kills about 44,000, according to both the American Cancer Society (ACS) and NCI. Next to skin cancer, breast cancer is the most frequently diagnosed cancer in women in the United States. It is second only to lung cancer in cancer-related deaths. Although the risk of developing the disease increases as a woman gets older, it can occur in young women and even in a small number of men.

While there has never been a disagreement on the health benefits of annual screening mammograms for women age 50 to 69 according to ACS, there has been a split among health-care organizations about when and how often women in other age groups should get a mammogram. Current guidelines from ACS recommend women age 40 to 49 have a routine screening mammogram every one to two years, with the first one beginning at age 40.

NCI agrees that women in their 40s who are at average risk for breast cancer should have a screening mammogram every one to two years. In addition, the institute says women who are at increased risk due to a genetic history of breast cancer, or who have had breast cancer, may need to get mammograms at an earlier age and more frequently.

For example, women who carry either of two genetic mutations called BRCA1 and BRCA2 were advised in 1997 guidelines by the National Genome Research Institute to begin getting annual mammograms between the ages of 25 and 35. These women, ACS advises, should seek medical advice about when to begin having mammograms and how often to be screened.

According to NCI, many women claim they have—or don't have—mammograms based on whether or not their doctors routinely recommend them. NCI advises that if your doctor fails to remind you about routine mammograms, it is important for you to take charge of your own health care and remember to raise the issue.

"Cutting life short because I did not take charge of my health would have been such a waste," says Pfefferkorn. "The advances in treatment and early detection are there until we find a cure."

Preparing for a Mammogram

Before you schedule a mammogram, the American Cancer Society recommends that you discuss any new findings or problems in your breasts with your doctor. In addition, inform your doctor of any pertinent history, including prior surgeries, hormone use, or family or personal history of breast cancer.

When you're ready to set up your appointment, don't schedule your mammogram for the week before your period if your breasts are usually tender during this time. In that case, the best time is one week following your period.

ACS also has these recommendations:

- Do not wear deodorant, talcum powder, or lotion under your arms on the day of the exam. This can interfere with the mammogram by appearing on the x-ray film as calcium spots.

- Describe any breast symptoms or problems to the technologist performing the exam.

- If possible, obtain prior mammograms and make them available to the radiologist at the time of the current exam.

- Ask when your results will be available.

How to Find a Certified Mammography Facility

Food and Drug Administration: A list of certified facilities is available on FDA's website at www.fda.gov/cdrh/faclist.html. The listing, which can be accessed by state and zip code, is updated periodically based on information received from the four FDA-approved accreditation bodies. While FDA has certified the facilities listed, providing this information does not mean the agency or any other organization recommends one facility over another. FDA recommends you check the facility's current status and look for the FDA certificate.

The National Cancer Institute: The Mammography Information Service line at 1-800-422-6237 (TTY: 1-800-332-8615) will provide a list of the certified mammography facilities in your geographic area. An NCI Information Specialist is available to answer cancer-related questions and to make referrals for free or low-cost mammography exams. You may also visit NCI's main website at www.nci.nih.gov.

American Cancer Society: You can obtain information from local ACS chapters by calling 1-800-227-2345.

Veterans Administration: While not certified under MQSA, VA facilities operate under a similar program. For information about VA facilities, call their Mammography Help Line at 1-888-492-7844.

—by Carol Lewis

Carol Lewis is a staff writer for FDA Consumer. Judith Willis, a member of FDA's public affairs staff, contributed to this article.

Chapter 30

False Positives on Mammograms

The Story

About 1 time in 10, the dread statement "Your mammogram looks suspicious" turns out to be a false alarm. For a woman who has routine mammograms, there's a pretty good chance she'll eventually get a result that looks like cancer but actually isn't. These so-called false positives create unfounded anxiety and often require more tests.

A study in the April 16, 1998 *New England Journal of Medicine* looked at the records of 2,400 women between the ages of 40 and 69. Over a 10 year period, the women had, on average, four mammograms and five clinical breast exams.

Close to one third of the women had abnormal results that prompted further evaluation, even though they did not have breast cancer. False positive tests were mammograms or clinical breast exams that were difficult to interpret, aroused a suspicion of cancer, or led to recommendations for additional testing in women who subsequently were not found to have breast cancer within a year of the initial test.

According to the researchers' estimates, nearly half of all women will have a false positive over the course of 10 mammograms. Fewer than a quarter will have a false positive among 10 clinical breast exams.

Most of the additional testing the women underwent was fairly simple. For instance, they had a repeat mammogram or a second opinion review of the screening film. Only a small number—188 women—ended up having surgical biopsies. But that still means that, over the course of 10 mammograms, about 19 percent of women without breast cancer will end up having a biopsy, the study authors say.

—The Editors, HealthNews

The Physician's Perspective

The results of this study do not surprise me, nor should they undermine women's confidence in the test. Although mammography is the best way to diagnose early breast cancer, we've long known it's not foolproof.

In fact, millions of women have already lived through a mammogram scare, only to find out after a closer look that everything was just fine.

Realize that no screening test is absolutely perfect. One of the most important attributes of a test is how accurately it picks up disease in people who have it; these are called "true positives." This new study looked at the flip side of the coin: It evaluated the number of times mammography suggests that a woman has breast cancer when, in fact, she does not—a false positive. One way of lowering the number of false positives of any test is to raise the threshold for calling the results abnormal. But this means missing more cancers. It's a trade-off. In the U.S. we accept higher rates of false positive tests to make sure we're not missing cases of disease.

False positives are troubling for two reasons. First, they can provoke considerable anxiety. One study suggests that nearly half of women who have a false positive mammogram still have substantial anxiety three months later. Secondly, false positives also lead to unnecessary testing—further mammography, ultrasound scans, and biopsies—at considerable expense.

These issues are particularly pertinent to women in their 40s. Because fewer cancers are found in this group, the drawbacks of mammography weigh more heavily than they do in the over-50 crowd. How a woman in her 40s feels about the "cost" of living with false positive exams versus potentially finding cancer early should help her determine, in conversation with her physician, exactly how often she should be screened.

In one sense, these study results are reassuring. If women better understand that mammography is just the first step—and not a perfect one—in diagnosis, then perhaps fewer will be anxiety stricken when they first hear of a questionable finding. But doctors can take action too. Physicians need to better explain the risk of false positive tests when discussing the pros and cons of mammograms. And testing facilities should reduce the time it takes for women to get results. I'm appalled when I hear that some women wait for days; at the clinic I attend, a radiologist reads the films before the woman leaves.

A final note: This study was conducted between 1983 and 1995. Technology has improved, so these figures probably aren't entirely accurate for testing today. The false positive rate may be lower, and it promises to drop further with the introduction of new diagnostic technologies. But in the meantime, don't let the chance of a false positive test keep you from getting a mammogram. It's still the best test we have.

—Holly Atkinson, MD, Editor, HealthNews

Chapter 31

Mammograms vs. Physical Examination

Long-term results from a major mammography screening trial were released this week, contributing more data on what continues to be a major research question at NCI and elsewhere: What is the best way to screen for breast cancer?

The Canadian National Breast Screening Study-2 found that annual mammograms combined with physical breast examination did not reduce breast cancer deaths compared with physical examination alone. The results, reflecting a median 13 years of follow-up in nearly 40,000 women age 50-59, appear in the Sept. 20, 2000 issue of the *Journal of the National Cancer Institute (JNCI)*.

Previous large trials have shown that mammograms reduce breast cancer mortality compared to no screening in women age 50 and over. The new findings "do not negate" those earlier, positive results said the Canadian investigators, who were led by Anthony Miller, M.D., from the University of Toronto.

However, their trial is the first to compare mammography to physical examination. The exam to which mammography was compared was an extremely thorough, 10-minute-long clinical breast examination by specially trained staff. Women randomized to receive this exam plus mammography had more small, node negative tumors discovered than those in the physical-exam-only group. Nevertheless, mortality rates in the two groups were not significantly different.

"Latest Study: Mammograns vs. Physical Examination: Survival Same," Cancer Trials, National Cancer Institute, September 19, 2000.

Like earlier trials, this one does not represent the end of the research process. Studies continue to explore both new screening technologies and new ways to assess and interpret conventional mammograms.

For example, the National Cancer Institute (NCI) is sponsoring a large trial to assess the use of magnetic resonance imaging for screening of high-risk women. Another NCI-sponsored trial, due to open early next year, will compare digital mammography to conventional film-screen mammography. NCI also funds individual investigators who are developing a variety of potential new screening devices, such as the use of laser light (optical techniques), microwaves, or electrical impedance, as well as measurement of the heat or electrical fields generated by breast tissues and breast cancer.

Chapter 32

Improving Imaging Methods for Breast Cancer Detection and Diagnosis

For breast cancer screening, high-quality mammography, an X-ray technique to visualize the internal structure of the breast, is the most effective technology presently available.

Efforts to improve conventional mammography center on refinements of the technology and quality assurance in the administration and interpretation of the X-ray films. To advance breast imaging, the National Cancer Institute (NCI) is funding research to reduce the already low radiation dosage; enhance image quality; and develop and evaluate digital mammography as an improvement over the conventional, film-based technique; develop statistical techniques for computer-assisted interpretation of digitized images; and enable long-distance image transmission technology, or teleradiology, for clinical consultations. NCI also funds research on non-X-ray based technologies such as magnetic resonance imaging (MRI), and breast-specific positron emission tomography (PET) to detect the disease.

This chapter includes excerpts from "Improving Imaging Methods for Breast Cancer Detection and Diagnosis," CancerNet, National Cancer Institute (NCI), March 1997; "FDA Approves New Breast Imaging Device," FDA Talk Paper, U.S. Food and Drug Administration, April 19, 1999; and "FDA Approves First Digital Mammography System," FDA Talk Paper, U.S. Food and Drug Administration, January 31, 2000.

Research and Imaging Technology

Digital Mammography

Digital mammography, a computerized technique that displays images using an infinite scale of gray tones, is of keen research interest. Mammography X-ray films can contain subtle information not easily discernible to the radiologist. Digital images potentially could enhance the quality of the image and even magnify the view of specific areas of the breast. This technology is expected to improve the sensitivity of mammography, especially in radiographically "dense" breast tissue which renders visualization of cancer problematic, and to decrease the radiation dose per mammogram. Digital mammography also will allow computer-aided diagnosis and teleradiology.

Novel Non-Ionizing Radiation (Non-X Ray) Imaging

Scientists are exploring novel non-ionizing imaging technologies including magnetic resonance imaging (MRI), ultrasound, optical imaging, and other technologies. The NCI-funded studies encompass basic technology and instrumentation development through pre-clinical and clinical testing. They aim to define the precise role of the technologies in detecting and characterizing breast tumors.

MRI and Ultrasound

Of novel non-ionizing technologies, MRI and ultrasound have been the most studied as ways to improve the sensitivity of breast cancer detection and staging. Both have shown potential for improving differentiation between benign, and malignant lesions and in detecting tumors in dense breast tissue. Furthermore, MRI appears unique in its ability to define local anatomic tumor extent, or staging, critical for treatment planning.

MRI and ultrasound have their limitations, too. MRI cannot detect microcalcifications, minute calcium deposits that may indicate a small cancer. About half of cancers detected by mammography appear as a cluster of microcalcifications. Ultrasound does not consistently detect microcalcifications, nor can it detect very small tumors.

Breast Biopsies

Imaging is also being tested as an aid in performing biopsies. The majority of women in the United States (80 percent) who undergo surgical breast biopsies do not have cancer. As an alternative to surgical tissue removal, image-guided, needle breast biopsy is being studied for women with non-palpable lesions. (Women who have large, palpable lesions usually undergo needle aspirations to determine if their lesions are fluid-filled benign cysts). Image-guided needle biopsy offers the potential advantages of minimized tissue damage, reduced waiting time until diagnosis, and cost savings. A multi-institutional research program is now testing the efficacy and cost-effectiveness of the large-core and fine-needle biopsies compared with more extensive surgical biopsies.

Other Areas of Study

In addition to research on imaging technologies, other research is developing methods to detect products of breast cancer (antigens) in blood, urine, or nipple aspirates, and to detect genetic alterations in women who are at increased risk for breast cancer. Once cancer is diagnosed, studies of these types contribute to characterization of breast tumors and can be useful in treatment planning. Still other NCI-funded projects seek to increase the utilization of mammography among women in age groups for which mammography has proven benefit. An emphasis is increasing utilization among minority and medically underserved women.

Breast Imaging Device Gains Approval

The Food and Drug Administration (FDA) has approved a new imaging device that will help radiologists determine whether a woman should be evaluated further when the results of her mammograms are ambiguous. It is not intended for use in patients with clear mammographic or non-mammographic indications for biopsy.

The device has the potential to reduce the number of negative biopsies, thus saving women worry about breast lesions that turn out to be non-cancerous. It also has the potential to increase the identification of women who should be referred for early biopsy.

The T-Scan 2000, manufactured by TransScan Medical, Inc., of Ramsey, N.J., is intended for use as a follow-up step to mammography for patients whose mammograms are ambiguous.

It does not replace conventional methods of detecting or diagnosing breast cancer, such as mammography, clinical breast examination, ultrasound, or biopsy evaluation, but is intended to be used along with conventional methods.

The T-Scan uses a hand-held scan probe placed on the breast to evaluate certain suspicious areas detected on the mammogram. The probe is connected to a computer, which displays an image of the involved areas of the breast.

The T-Scan images are based on differences in the electrical impedance between malignant tumor tissue and surrounding normal tissue. Impedance is a measure of how any material affects the flow of electricity.

The device measures impedance by passing a small electrical signal through the body and displaying on a computer the result from sensors in the probe contacting the breast. The computer image contains bright spots where the impedance values are consistent with a possible malignancy.

Approval of the device was based on the results of three clinical studies of safety and effectiveness performed by TransScan Medical and on the recommendation of an advisory panel of outside experts.

In the first study, the radiologists evaluated the screening mammograms and T-Scan images of the entire breast from each of 504 women without knowing which patient's images they were reviewing or whether the women were suspected of having cancer. The results showed that in women with ambiguous mammograms, the additional use of T-Scan images improved diagnostic accuracy, that is, detection of potentially cancerous lesions and discrimination from non-cancer.

A second study of 657 patients, under conditions more closely resembling actual use, showed that targeting the T-Scan examination to suspicious areas of the breast can improve diagnostic accuracy to a greater degree than imaging the entire breast.

In a third study, of 36 women with mammograms with ambiguous results, the T-Scan was targeted at the equivocal mammographic lesion and reviewed simultaneously with the mammogram. This third study, which reflects the approved intended use for the T-Scan, showed even greater improvement in diagnostic accuracy.

Together the three studies showed that, when used along with screening mammography, T-Scan gives doctors a useful tool to enhance care of women whose mammogram results are ambiguous.

As a condition of approval, TransScan Medical is being required to conduct a post-market study on the effects of hormonal changes during the menstrual cycle on the device's ability to detect and distinguish among breast abnormalities.

FDA Approves First Digital Mammography System

FDA has approved the Senographe 2000D, the first mammography system that produces digital images on a solid state receptor instead of analog images on a radiographic film. Film/screen (analog) mammography along with physical examination and breast self-examination is the standard method for breast cancer screening in women.

The Senographe 2000D, made by General Electric Medical Systems, was approved on the basis of clinical data showing its safety and effectiveness and on the recommendation of FDA's Radiological Devices Panel. The study compared digital mammography films with analog mammography films of 625 women, 44 of whom had breast cancer. The digital and film/screen images were analyzed and evaluated by five qualified radiologists specializing in mammography and found to have comparable clinical performance in screening and diagnosis of breast cancer.

From the patient's point of view, mammography with a digital system is essentially the same as with the film/screen system. The radiologist will look at analog and digital films in the same way under this approval.

The evidence presented so far does not show that the digital images are more helpful in finding cancer than the analog/film images. The digital technology, however, offers several potential advantages over the standard use of radiographic film. Unlike images on radiographic film, digital images:

- can be stored and transferred electronically, which facilitates their quick and easy retrieval as well as remove evaluation by distant specialists;

- can be manipulated to correct for under- or over-exposure without the necessity of taking another mammogram;

- have a large dynamic range that allows examination of all areas of the breast, despite their varying density. The limited dynamic range of the film/screen systems sometimes requires additional exposures at different settings to reveal very high or very low density areas of the breast.

For the immediate future, digital mammography may only be used in facilities certified to practice film/screen mammography.

Chapter 33

Ductal Lavage: A New Evaluation Procedure for High-Risk Women

Over 95% of all breast cancers begin in the cells lining the milk ducts. By the time these cells grow into a tumor large enough to see on a mammogram or feel in a physical exam, eight to 10 years have passed, on average.

Knowing that breast cancer develops over time has raised an important question: Why not look for pre-cancerous and cancerous breast cells before they become visible on a mammogram or are able to be felt on physical exam? Ductal lavage allows physicians to conduct this very search.

Ductal lavage is a minimally invasive method of collecting samples of cells from the milk ducts. These cells are analyzed under a microscope and determined to be normal, pre-cancerous or cancerous. As noted breast cancer authority, company co-founder, and author Dr. Susan Love has said, "With ductal lavage, we can find cells that are just thinking about becoming cancer."

Who Is High Risk?

Research shows that the two most significant risk factors for developing breast cancer are being female and getting older. A woman

"The Fight Against Breast Cancer—Past, Present, and Future." © 2000 Susan G. Komen Breast Cancer Foundation; reprinted with permission. Preliminary data was presented at the American Society of Clinical Oncology Annual Meeting, May 2000, and at the Second Annual Lynn Sage Breast Cancer Symposium, September 2000.

may be at an even higher risk if she has experienced any of the following:

- A personal history of breast or ovarian cancer
- A close relative who has had breast cancer before menopause or in both breasts
- Menstruation starting at an early age (before 12)
- Late menopause (after 55)
- The birth of a first child after the age of 30 or not having children at all
- A previous breast biopsy showing abnormal cells, such as lobular carcinoma *in situ* (LCIS) or atypical hyperplasia

Procedure Overview

Ductal lavage is well-tolerated. The majority of the high-risk women enrolled in the Pro-Duct Health clinical trial reported no significant discomfort during or after ductal lavage. Ductal lavage involves three steps and can be performed either in a physician's office or an outpatient clinic.

Step 1: An anesthetic cream is applied first to the nipple area. Gentle suction is used to help draw tiny amounts of fluid from the milk ducts up to the nipple surface. The fluid droplets that appear help locate the milk ducts' natural openings on the surface of the nipple.

Step 2: A hair-thin catheter is inserted into a milk duct opening on the nipple. A small amount of anesthetic is infused into the duct. Saline then is slowly introduced through the catheter to gently "rinse" the duct and collect cells. The ductal cell fluid is withdrawn through the catheter and deposited into a collection vial.

Step 3: The sample is sent to a cytology laboratory for analysis to detect normal, pre-cancerous and cancerous cells.

Clinical Trial Information

In a recent clinical study, ductal lavage was performed on over 500 high-risk women at 19 prestigious breast cancer centers. All of the women had normal mammograms and physical exams within 12 months prior to study enrollment. In this group of women, ductal lavage detected:

- Abnormal/pre-cancerous cells in 15% of the breasts studied

- Suspected/known cancerous cells in 5% of the breasts studied

If abnormal/pre-cancerous cells are detected through ductal lavage, it does not necessarily mean that breast cancer will follow. In fact, it is believed that, in most cases, these cells don't progress to cancer. However, a number of clinical studies have shown that finding abnormal/pre-cancerous cells predicts which women are more likely to develop breast cancer.

What Ductal Lavage Offers High-Risk Women

Ductal lavage must be used with standard breast cancer detection methods such as mammography, clinical breast exam and monthly breast self-exam. For high-risk women, it can offer:

- Power of information. Ductal lavage provides unique, early information at the cellular level.

- Repeatable testing. Specific ducts can be regularly re-tested to check the status of cells.

- Informed prevention decisions. Many high-risk women face difficult choices about whether or when to pursue particular breast cancer prevention options. Ductal lavage offers additional information that can be used in the decision-making process.

- An opportunity for earlier intervention. There are a number of strategies high-risk women can discuss with their physicians. Ductal lavage information may help them in considering whether to pursue closer monitoring, drug prevention (i.e. tamoxifen), or other options.

Part Five

Treatment Options

Chapter 34

Better Treatments Save More Lives

Two different women. The same deadly disease. One thought she couldn't get it. The other was told she didn't have it. Both opinions were wrong.

In 1994, one week before turning 35, Cathy Young received the devastating news. "I thought people had to be in their 50s to get cancer," the Oak Grove, Mo., resident says. "And then it happened to me."

Linda Hunter, 42, recalls that in January 1995, her mammogram results came back normal. But skin changes on one of her breasts compelled her to seek a second, third and fourth opinion—all of which supported the initial mammogram findings. Her tenacity finally paid off when a fifth doctor she visited detected a rare form of the disease.

Every three minutes a woman in the United States learns she has breast cancer. It is the most common cancer among women, next to skin cancers, and is second only to lung cancer in cancer deaths in women. Only 5 to 10 percent of breast cancers occur in women with a clearly defined genetic predisposition for the disease. The overall risk for developing breast cancer increases as a woman gets older.

Although treatment is initially successful for many women, the American Cancer Society (ACS) says that breast cancer will return in about 50 percent of these cases.

"Breast Cancer: Better Treatments Save More Lives," by Carol Lewis, *FDA Consumer*, July-August 1999; this version is from Publication No. (FDA) 00-1306 and contains revisions made in October 1999 and June 2000.

"It's hard to say that things are back to normal when one survives breast cancer," says Young, "because a survivor always has a fear that one day the cancer may return."

New drugs, new treatment regimens, and better diagnostic techniques have improved the outlook for many, and are responsible, according to ACS, for breast cancer death rates going down.

"Women have greater options in breast cancer treatment compared to a decade ago," says Harman Eyre, M.D., chief medical officer for ACS. "New drugs and procedures open up a whole new era of effective treatment."

Breast Cancer Treatments

Breast cancer can be treated with surgery, radiation and drugs (chemotherapy and hormonal therapy). Doctors may use one of these or a combination, depending on factors such as the type and location of the cancer, whether the disease has spread, and the patient's overall health.

Most women with breast cancer will have some type of surgery, depending on the stage of the breast cancer. (See "Stages of Breast Cancer.") The least invasive, lumpectomy (breast-conserving surgery), removes only the cancerous tissue and a surrounding margin of normal tissue. Removal of the entire breast is a mastectomy. A modified radical mastectomy includes the entire breast and some of the underarm lymph nodes. The very disfiguring radical mastectomy, in which the breast, lymph nodes, and chest wall muscles under the breast are removed, is rarely performed today because doctors believe that a modified radical mastectomy is just as effective.

While removing underarm lymph nodes after surgery is important in order to determine if the cancer has spread, this procedure may add chronic arm swelling and restricted shoulder motion to the discomforts of the overall treatment. But a new method, sentinel node biopsy, still under investigation, allows physicians to pinpoint the first lymph node into which a tumor drains (the sentinel node), and remove only the nodes most likely to contain cancer cells.

To locate the sentinel node, the physician injects a radioactive tracer in the area around the tumor before the mastectomy. The tracer travels the same path to the lymph nodes that cancer cells would take, making it possible for the surgeon to determine the one or two nodes most likely to test positive. The surgeon will then remove the nodes most likely to be cancerous.

Radiation therapy is treatment with high-energy rays or particles given to destroy cancer. In almost all cases, lumpectomy is followed by six to seven weeks of radiation, an integral part of breast-conserving treatment. Although radiation therapy damages both normal cells and cancerous cells, most of the normal cells are able to repair themselves and function properly.

Radiation therapy can cause side effects such as swelling and heaviness in the breast, sunburn-like skin changes in the treated area, and lymphedema (swelling of the arm due to fluid buildup) if the underarm lymph nodes were treated after a node dissection.

Drug Options Expand

Drugs are used to reach cancer cells that may have spread beyond the breast—in many cases even if no cancer is detected in the lymph nodes after surgery.

While doctors once believed that the spread of breast cancer could be controlled with extensive surgery, they now believe that cancer cells may break away from the primary tumor and spread through the bloodstream, even in the earliest stages of the disease. These cells cannot be felt by examination or seen on x-rays or other imaging methods, and they cause no symptoms. But they can establish new tumors in other organs or the bones. The goal of drug treatment, even if there's no detectable cancer after surgery, is to kill these hidden cells. This treatment, known as adjuvant therapy, is not needed by every patient. Doctors will make recommendations regarding specific types of therapy based on the stage of the breast cancer.

FDA has approved several new drugs and new uses for older drugs in recent years that improve the chances of successfully treating breast cancer. These drugs include:

Herceptin: About 30 percent of women with breast cancer have an excess of a protein called HER2, which makes tumors grow quickly. A genetically engineered drug, Herceptin (trastuzumab), binds to HER2 and kills the excess cancer cells, theoretically leaving healthy cells alone.

Herceptin, made by Genentech Inc., San Francisco, California., and approved by FDA in September 1998, is an intravenous treatment that is used alone in patients who have had little success with other drugs, or as a first-line treatment in combination with the drug Taxol (paclitaxel).

Recent follow-up research shows that Herceptin, in combination with chemotherapy, also may modestly extend the lives of terminal breast cancer patients. Updated survival figures reported from a two-year study by one of the drug's key developers from the University of California at Los Angeles showed an improvement in survival (about 4 months on average) in those getting Herceptin. Scientists say that while the improvement is small—about four months on average—it is especially noteworthy in a disease that until now has eluded many efforts to slow its progression to death.

Selection of patients who are most likely to benefit from Herceptin is important because of the possible serious risks from the drug, including weakening of the heart muscle that can lead to congestive heart failure. It is not known whether Herceptin has beneficial effects in women with normal levels of the HER2 protein.

FDA also approved in September 1998 a test called DAKO Hercep-Test to measure HER2 protein in tumors.

Nolvadex: A drug that has been used as a breast cancer treatment for more than 20 years, Nolvadex (tamoxifen citrate) was approved by FDA in October 1998 for breast cancer risk reduction in high-risk women.

Doctors know that estrogen promotes the growth of breast cancer cells. Tamoxifen interferes with the activity of estrogen by slowing or stopping the growth of cancer cells already present in the body. As adjuvant therapy, tamoxifen has been shown to help prevent both the original breast cancer from returning, and also the development of new cancers in the other breast.

A National Cancer Institute study showed that the drug reduced the short-term chance of getting breast cancer by 44 percent in women who were judged to be at increased risk for the disease. FDA emphasizes, however, that tamoxifen, manufactured by AstraZeneca Pharmaceuticals, Wilmington, Del., will not eliminate breast cancer risk completely, and should be used only following a medical evaluation of individual risk factors.

Due to potentially serious side effects, including endometrial (lining of the uterus) cancer and blood clots in major veins and the lungs, the American Society of Clinical Oncology recommends that patients talk with their regular health-care providers to determine whether individual medical circumstances and histories are appropriate for considering use of tamoxifen.

Xeloda: Xeloda (capecitabine), made by Hoffmann-La Roche, Nutley, New Jersey., was approved by FDA in April 1998 for the treatment of breast cancer that has spread to other parts of the body (metastasized) and is resistant to both paclitaxel and an anthracycline-containing regimen. Xeloda does not kill the cancer cells directly. Instead, once the drug enters the cancer cells, it is metabolized to 5-fluorouracil (5-FU), a drug routinely used for breast cancer. The advantage of Xeloda, in addition to the convenience of its pill form, is that cancer cells actively convert it to 5-FU, but normal cells convert very little to 5-FU.

Taxotere: In May 1996, FDA gave accelerated approval to Taxotere (docetaxel) to treat patients whose locally advanced or metastasized breast cancer has progressed despite treatment with other drugs. The approval was conditional on the manufacturer, Rhone-Poulenc Rorer Pharmaceuticals, Inc., Collegeville, Pa., conducting additional studies. In June 1998, after additional studies confirmed its safety and effectiveness, the drug was granted full FDA approval.

In addition to these newer drugs, combinations of the anticancer drugs Cytoxan (cyclophosphamide) and Adriamycin (doxorubicin), with or without Adrucil (fluorouracil), may be used to treat breast cancer.

Chemotherapy (drug treatment) is given in cycles, with each period of treatment followed by a recovery period. The total course of chemotherapy can last three to six months, depending on the drugs and how far the cancer has spread.

Kelly Munsell of Tucson, Arizona., took the combination Adriamycin and Cytoxan in six cycles, spaced three weeks apart, after doctors diagnosed her breast cancer in 1996 at age 27.

"Chemo for me was torture," Munsell recalls, describing profuse vomiting and severe weight gain as two of the serious side effects. But despite the discomfort, Munsell, whose mother and grandmother both died of breast cancer, is glad she underwent the grueling treatment two years ago. "My recent battery of tests came back negative for cancer," she says.

In addition to the drugs actually battling the disease, there also is help for patients in severe pain from cancer. FDA approved Actiq (oral transmucosal fentanyl citrate) in November 1998 as a treatment specifically for cancer patients with severe pain that breaks through their regular narcotic therapy. A narcotic more potent than morphine, Actiq is in the form of a flavored sugar lozenge that dissolves slowly in the mouth. Actiq is approved for patients already taking at least 60 milligrams of morphine per day for their underlying persistent cancer pain.

Looking Ahead

It is important for every woman to consider herself at risk for breast cancer, ACS says, simply because she's female. At the same time, however, studies continue to uncover lifestyle factors and habits that can alter that risk, and many new chemotherapy drugs and drug combinations continue to be developed and tested in clinical trials. Drugs and procedures currently under investigation include bisphosphonates (a group of drugs routinely used to treat osteoporosis), monoclonal antibodies (similar to Herceptin), and angiogenesis inhibitors (drugs that block the development of blood vessels that nourish cancer cells).

"While death rates from breast cancer are falling, and while there are a number of exciting new strategies being developed," says Michael A. Friedman, M.D., former FDA deputy commissioner and cancer research specialist, "we recognize that a great deal more needs to be done."

Mammography: A Lifesaving Step

The American Cancer Society says that the best strategy for successfully beating breast cancer is to follow guidelines for early detection. Currently, the most effective technique for early detection is screening mammography, an x-ray procedure that can detect small tumors and breast abnormalities up to two years before they can be felt and when they are most treatable.

Studies show that regular screening mammograms can help decrease the chance of dying from breast cancer. Finding a breast tumor early may mean that a woman can choose breast-saving surgery. Furthermore, she may not have to undergo chemotherapy.

To find a certified mammography facility near you, go to www.fda.gov/cdrh/mammography/certified.html on FDA's Website, or call the National Cancer Institute at 1-800-4-CANCER (1-800-422-6237).

Cancer Liaison Program

FDA's Cancer Liaison Program answers questions from patients, their friends and family members, and patient advocates about therapies for life-threatening diseases. The staff works closely with cancer patients, other federal agencies (including the National Cancer Institute), and cancer patient advocacy programs, listening to their concerns and educating them about the FDA drug approval process, cancer clinical trials, and access to investigational therapies.

For more information on the Cancer Liaison Program, call 301-827-4460 or visit www.fda.gov/oashi/cancer/cancer.html on FDA's Website.

Stages of Breast Cancer

Stages of breast cancer, according to the American Cancer Society, indicate the size of a tumor and how far the cancer has spread within the breast, to nearby tissues, and to other organs. Specific treatment is most often determined by the following stages of the disease:

Carcinoma *in situ*: Cancer is confined to the lobules (milk-producing glands) or ducts (passages connecting milk-producing glands to the nipple) and has not invaded nearby breast tissue.

Stage I: Tumor is smaller than or equal to 2 centimeters in diameter and underarm (axillary) lymph nodes test negative for cancer.

Stage II: Tumor is between 2 and 5 centimeters in diameter with or without positive lymph nodes, or tumor is greater than 5 centimeters without positive lymph nodes.

Stage III: This stage is divided into substages known as IIIA and IIIB:

- **IIIA:** Tumor is larger than 5 centimeters with positive movable lymph nodes, or tumor is any size with lymph nodes that adhere to one another or surrounding tissue.
- **IIIB:** Tumor of any size has spread to the skin, chest wall, or internal mammary lymph nodes (located beneath the breast and inside the chest).

Stage IV: Tumor, regardless of size, has metastasized (spread) to distant sites such as bones, lungs, or lymph nodes not near the breast.

Recurrent breast cancer: The disease has returned in spite of initial treatment.

— *by Carol Lewis*

Carol Lewis is a staff writer for FDA Consumer.

For More Information

Contact any of these organizations for more on breast cancer and support groups.

National Cancer Institute
31 Center Drive, MSC 2580
Bethesda, MD 20892-2580
1-800-4-CANCER (1-800-422-6237)
www.nci.nih.gov
cancertrials.nci.nih.gov

American Cancer Society
1599 Clifton Road, N.E.
Atlanta, GA 30329-4251
1-800-ACS-2345 (1-800-227-2345)
www.cancer.org

National Alliance of Breast Cancer Organizations (NABCO)
9 E. 37th St., 10th Floor
New York, NY 10016
1-888-806-2226
www.nabco.org

Y-ME National Breast Cancer Hotline
212 West Van Buren, 5th Floor
Chicago, IL 60607-3907
1-800-221-2141
www.y-me.org

Susan G. Komen Breast Cancer Foundation
5005 LBJ Freeway
Suite 370
Dallas, TX 75244
1-800-IM-AWARE or 1-800-462-9273
www.komen.org

Chapter 35

Understanding Breast Cancer Treatment

Each year in the United States, almost 180,000 women are told they have breast cancer.

Upon hearing this unexpected and overwhelming news, a woman is faced with having to make treatment choices within a short period of time.

This chapter can help her and her family understand what the diagnosis means and why treatment is necessary. It suggests questions to ask the doctor and identifies other resources for more information.

With this knowledge, a newly diagnosed breast cancer patient can more confidently participate with her doctor in planning the best possible treatment.

Introduction

This chapter is written especially for you if you have been diagnosed with breast cancer. You probably have many questions and concerns. You may be feeling confused, worried, or anxious. It may be hard for you to concentrate or make decisions. These reactions are normal.

The information in this chapter should help you understand your diagnosis and the treatments that are available. It is very important that you become a partner with your doctor in deciding what treatment is best for you. The following tips may make it easier for you to use this chapter:

Understanding Breast Cancer Treatment: A Guide for Patients, National Cancer Institute, NIH Pub. No. 98-4251, April 1998.

257

- Read the material as you need it. You may want to ask a family member or close friend, or someone on your health care team, to read this text along with you. Or ask them to read it, and talk about it with you when you are ready.

- Understanding the meaning of the words that you are hearing will help you understand what is happening and will help you make informed choices. The medical words that you hear as you go through treatment are explained throughout this chapter.

- Remember, there is no single treatment that is "right" for all women. New treatments are available today that were not even imagined a few years ago. Medical researchers continue to find better ways to treat breast cancer.

- You can always ask more than one doctor about your diagnosis and treatment plan. Your doctor can help you arrange an appointment with another specialist. Many health insurance companies pay for other opinions.

- As you go through treatment, you may find it helpful to write out questions before you meet with your doctors. Some questions are suggested in this chapter. You may want to make an audiotape recording of your discussions with your doctors. Consider asking a family member or close friend to go to your appointments with you and to take notes for you.

- Most important, you should never be afraid to ask people to repeat information or instructions, or to ask questions. There are no "dumb" questions when you are faced with cancer. When you know what to expect, you will feel more in control of your life.

- The choice about how much information you seek is yours. If you would like to know more about any of the topics in this chapter, call the National Cancer Institute's (NCI) Cancer Information Service (CIS) toll-free at 1-800-4-CANCER (1-800-422-6237). A cancer information specialist can answer your questions, send you more information, or help you find a breast cancer support group in your community.

About Breast Cancer

What Is Cancer?

Cancer is a group of more than 100 different diseases. Cancer occurs when, for unknown reasons, cells become abnormal and divide without control or order. All parts of the body are made up of cells that normally divide to produce more cells only when the body needs them. When cancer occurs, cells keep dividing even when new cells are not needed.

The change from normal to cancerous cells requires several separate, different gene alterations. Eventually, altered genes and uncontrolled growth may produce a tumor that can be benign (not cancer) or malignant (cancer). Malignant tumors can invade, damage, and destroy nearby tissues and spread to other parts of the body. A benign tumor won't spread to other parts of the body, but local tissue may be damaged and the growth may need to be removed.

Types of Breast Cancer

There are several types of breast cancer. The most common is ductal carcinoma, which begins in the lining of the milk ducts of the breast. Another type, lobular carcinoma, begins in the lobules where breast milk is produced. If a malignant tumor invades nearby tissue, it is known as infiltrating or invasive cancer.

How Cancer Spreads

A malignant tumor can invade surrounding tissue and destroy it. Cancer cells can also break away from a malignant tumor and enter the bloodstream or the lymphatic system. This is how cancer spreads within the body. When breast cancer spreads outside the breast, cancer cells often are found in the lymph nodes under the arm. Cancer cells may spread beyond the breast such as to other lymph nodes, the bones, liver, or lungs. (Although it is not common, some patients whose underarm lymph nodes are clear of breast cancer may still have cancer cells which have spread to other parts of the body.)

Cancer that spreads to other parts of the body is the same disease and has the same name as the original cancer. When breast cancer spreads, it is called metastatic breast cancer even though it is found in another part of the body. For example, breast cancer that has spread to the bones is called metastatic breast cancer, not bone cancer.

What Causes Breast Cancer?

Medical researchers are learning about what happens inside cells that may cause cancer. They have identified changes in certain genes within breast cells that can be linked to a higher risk for breast cancer. Breast cells contain a variety of genes that normally work cooperatively with a woman's natural hormones, diet, and environment to keep her breasts healthy. Certain genes routinely keep breast cells from dividing and growing out of control and forming tumors. When these genes become altered, changes occur and a cell no longer can grow correctly.

Genetic changes may be inherited from a parent or may accumulate throughout a person's lifetime. Breast cancer usually begins in a single cell that changes from normal to malignant over a period of time. Presently, no one can predict exactly when cancer will occur or how it will progress. When breast cancer is diagnosed—even if detected at the earliest stage—it is not yet possible to predict which cancer cells will be treated successfully and which will continue to grow and spread quickly to other parts of the body.

What is known:

- You should not feel guilty. You haven't done anything wrong in your life that caused breast cancer.

- You cannot "catch" breast cancer from other women who have the disease. It is not contagious.

- Breast cancer is not caused by stress or by an injury to the breast.

- Most women who develop breast cancer do not have any known risk factors or a history of the disease in their families.

Who Gets Breast Cancer?

Every woman has some chance of developing breast cancer during her lifetime. As women get older, their chances increase. Breast cancer is the most frequently diagnosed cancer in women in the United States today, other than skin cancer. Even though breast cancer is more common in older women, it also occurs in younger women and even in a small number of men.

Gene Testing

Medical researchers are now able to look within cells, and are making new discoveries that explain how genes are related to cancer and other diseases. They have identified specific genes linked to breast cancer and other cancers that run in families. Tests are becoming available for women and family members who choose to find out if they have inherited the genetic changes that increase their risk for cancer. There is still much uncertainty involved with gene testing. If you or your family members are considering testing, your doctor or a genetics counselor can give you guidance and help you make an informed decision. It's important to consider carefully the benefits, risks, limitations, and the far-reaching consequences of gene testing.

Making a Decision about Treatment

The only way to find out for sure if a breast lump or abnormal tissue is cancer is by having a biopsy. The suspicious tissue that is removed by a surgeon or radiologist during a biopsy is examined under a microscope by a pathologist who makes the diagnosis. If your biopsy result is positive, it means that the tumor or tissue from the suspicious area contains cancer and you will need treatment. Information on the following pages can help you understand the various treatments that are available and decide what is best for you. It is safe to begin treatment up to several weeks after diagnosis. This gives you time to:

- Have a complete study of your breast tissue and tests of other parts of your body.

- Get other opinions about your diagnosis and the suggested treatment plan.

- Talk with each of the specialists who will be on your treatment team.

- Call your health insurance plan before treatment begins.

- Call NCI's Cancer Information Service at 1-800-4-CANCER for the most up-to-date, accurate breast cancer treatment information.

- Contact breast cancer organizations to find support groups near you.

- Talk with other women who have had breast cancer and have gone through treatment.

- Prepare yourself and loved ones for your treatment.

Remember, you don't have to face breast cancer alone—there are knowledgeable and caring people who can help you.

Are All Breast Cancers Alike?

Breast cancer is a complex disease. All cases are not the same. Once breast cancer has been found, more tests will be done to find out the specific pattern (description) of your disease. This important step is called staging. Knowing the exact stage of your disease will help your doctor plan your treatment. Your doctor will want to know:

- The size of the tumor and exactly where it is in your breast.
- If the cancer has spread within your breast.
- If cancer is present in the lymph nodes under your arm.
- If cancer is present in other parts of your body.

Staging—Specific Patterns of Breast Cancer

Stage 0: Very early breast cancer. This type of cancer has not spread within or outside the breast. It is sometimes called DCIS, LCIS, or breast cancer *in situ* or noninvasive cancer.

Stage I: The cancer is no larger than about 1 inch in size and has not spread outside the breast. (Also described as early breast cancer.)

Stage II: The doctor may find any of the following:

- The cancer is no larger than 1 inch, but has spread to the lymph nodes under the arm.
- The cancer is between 1 and 2 inches. It may or may not have spread to the lymph nodes under the arm.
- The cancer is larger than 2 inches, but has not spread to the lymph nodes under the arm.

Stage III: Stage III is divided into stages IIIA and IIIB:

Stage IIIA: The doctor may find either of the following:

- The cancer is smaller than 2 inches and has spread to the lymph nodes under the arm. The cancer also is spreading further to other lymph nodes.
- The cancer is larger than 2 inches and has spread to the lymph nodes under the arm.

Stage IIIB: The doctor may find either of the following:

- The cancer has spread to tissues near the breast (skin, chest wall, including the ribs and the muscles in the chest).

262

- The cancer has spread to lymph nodes inside the chest wall along the breast bone.

Stage IV: The cancer has spread to other parts of the body, most often the bones, lungs, liver, or brain. Or, the tumor has spread locally to the skin and lymph nodes inside the neck, near the collarbone.

Inflammatory Breast Cancer: Inflammatory breast cancer is a rare, but very serious, aggressive type of breast cancer. The breast may look red and feel warm. You may see ridges, welts, or hives on your breast; or the skin may look wrinkled. It is sometimes misdiagnosed as a simple infection.

Recurrent Breast Cancer: Recurrent disease means that the cancer has come back (recurred) after it has been treated. It may come back in the breast, in the soft tissues of the chest (the chest wall), or in another part of the body.

Tumor size is usually reported in metric measurement: 1 centimeter = approximately ½ inch.

Breast Cancer in situ—*DCIS and LCIS*

Many breast cancers being found are very early cancers known as breast cancer *in situ* or noninvasive cancer. Most of these cancers are found by mammography. These very early cell changes may become invasive breast cancer. Two types of breast cancer *in situ* are:

1. DCIS (ductal carcinoma *in situ*), which means that abnormal cells are found only in the lining of a milk duct of the breast. These abnormal cells have not spread outside the duct. They have not spread within the breast, beyond the breast, to the lymph nodes under the arm, or to other parts of the body. There are several types of DCIS. If not removed, some types may change over time and become invasive cancers. Some may never become invasive cancers. (DCIS is sometimes called intraductal carcinoma.)

2. LCIS (lobular carcinoma *in situ*), which means that abnormal cells are found in the lining of a milk lobule. Although LCIS is not considered to be actual breast cancer at this noninvasive stage, it is a warning sign of increased risk of developing invasive cancer. LCIS is sometimes found when a biopsy is done

for another lump or unusual change that is found on a mammogram. Patients with LCIS have a 25 percent chance of developing breast cancer in either breast during the next 25 years.

Microcalcifications are very small specks of calcium that can't be felt, but can be seen on a mammogram. They are formed by rapidly dividing cells. When they are clustered in one area of the breast, this could be an early sign of breast cancer *in situ*. About half of the breast cancers found by mammography appear as clusters of microcalcifications. The other half appear as lumps.

To be sure that you have a correct diagnosis if breast cancer *in situ* is detected, an experienced pathologist should examine your biopsy slides. You may want to have your slides examined also by a second pathologist at a university hospital, cancer center, or breast clinic. This is important because it is sometimes difficult to make an accurate diagnosis. The pathologist needs to determine the types of cells that are present in the tissue sample, how fast the cells are changing, and whether it is likely to become invasive cancer. The diagnosis will help your doctor decide on the appropriate treatment from a wide range of choices. The decision could be to have frequent followup exams to watch the suspicious area, or surgery to remove only the affected tissue, or surgery to remove one or both breasts. Surgery removing only the affected area is sometimes followed by radiation therapy to the breast.

For more information about breast cancer *in situ*:

- Talk with your doctor.

- Get as many expert opinions as you need to feel confident in the accuracy of your diagnosis.

- Call the NCI's Cancer Information Service at 1-800-4-CANCER.

Prognosis (Chance of Recovery)

Most women who are treated for early breast cancer go on to live healthy, active lives. You may have more choices of treatment if your breast cancer is found early.

Treatments have changed over time. Today, many women who are diagnosed with breast cancer do not have to lose a breast. Because there are improved ways to treat breast cancer, it is more important than ever for you to learn all you can. Working with your team of medical specialists, you can play a key role in choosing the treatment that is best for you.

Once your doctor has determined your specific type and stage of breast cancer, you can begin to plan for your treatment and recovery. Your chance of recovery will depend on many factors, including:

- The type and stage of your cancer (what kind of cancer; the size of the tumor; and whether it is only in your breast, or has spread to any lymph nodes or to other parts of your body).

- How fast the cancer is growing. Special lab tests on the tissue can measure how fast the cancer cells are dividing and how different they are compared to normal breast cells.

- How much the breast cancer cells depend on female hormones (estrogen and progesterone) for growth which can be measured by hormone receptor tests. Patients whose tumors are found to be dependent on hormones (described as estrogen-positive or progesterone-positive) can be treated by hormonal therapy to prevent further growth or recurrence of breast cancer. (See section on hormonal therapy.)

- Your age and menopausal status (whether or not you still have monthly menstrual periods).

- Your general state of health.

Risk Factors for Recurrence

Your chance of surviving breast cancer will also depend upon your risk for return of cancer after treatment is completed. Some women are at higher risk for the spread or return of breast cancer. In many cases, doctors can't explain why one patient stays well and another does not. Remember, the risk factors for recurrence are complex. They are not absolute predictions of your future health. Some factors that affect the spread or the recurrence of breast cancer are:

Tumor size: The smaller your tumor, the lower the risk.

Lymph nodes: The fewer underarm lymph nodes that have cancer, the lower your risk.

Cell growth: Cancer cells that grow slowly are linked to a lower risk.

Hormones: If a tumor depends on hormones for growth, hormonal therapy can lower the risk of cancer spread or recurrence.

Questions to Ask Your Doctor After a Biopsy

- Please explain what is on the pathology report.

- What type of breast cancer do I have? What stage of breast cancer do I have?

- Did a pathologist who is experienced in diagnosing breast cancer examine my biopsy slides?

- Should my biopsy slides be examined again? Why or why not?

- What are the chances that the cancer has spread within or outside my breast?

- Were lab tests done on the tumor tissue? What do the results mean for me?

- Were estrogen and progesterone receptor tests done? What do the results mean for me? (See section on hormonal therapy.)

- What other tests do I need? (Chest x-ray, bone scan, etc.)

- What are my treatment choices? How can I get more information about them?

- What benefit can I expect from each kind of treatment?

- What are the risks and possible side effects of each treatment? Short-term? Long-term?

- What are the risks if I don't get treatment?

- What are my chances for recurrence?

- How can I get another opinion?

- Did you check NCI's PDQ® database for physicians to get the latest information about my type and stage of breast cancer?

- Is there any research being done on my kind of cancer? Did you check NCI's Web site for clinical trials on the Internet at http://cancertrials.nci.nih.gov?

Your Treatment Team

Once your doctor has all the specific information about your breast cancer, you will talk about all the treatments considered appropriate for your case. No one doctor is able to provide all the care and services you may need, and you will quickly learn about new people who will be on your treatment team. Some of the medical experts who may be part of your treatment team are:

Anesthesiologist: a doctor who gives drugs or gases that keep you comfortable during surgery.

Gynecologist: A doctor who specializes in the care and treatment of women's reproductive systems. This doctor or your primary care doctor can serve as the manager and main source of information among your treatment team members and you.

Nutritionist or dietitian: a health professional with specialized training in nutrition who can offer help and choices about the foods you eat.

Oncologist, medical oncologist, or cancer specialist: a doctor who uses chemotherapy or hormonal therapy to treat cancer. This specialist can put together all the information about your case and can discuss your treatment choices with you.

Oncology nurse: a nurse with special training in caring for cancer patients. You may also receive care from a clinical nurse specialist or nurse practitioner.

Oncology pharmacy specialist: a person who prepares anticancer drugs in consultation with the oncologist and can answer your questions about chemotherapy.

Pathologist: a doctor who examines tissues and cells under a microscope to determine if they are normal or abnormal.

Physical therapist: a health professional who teaches exercises that help restore arm and shoulder movement and build back strength after breast cancer surgery.

Plastic surgeon or reconstructive surgeon: a doctor who can surgically rebuild (reconstruct) your breast.

Primary care doctor: the doctor who usually manages your health care and can discuss cancer treatment choices with you.

Psychologist: a specialist who can talk with you and your family about emotional and personal matters, and can help you make decisions.

Radiation oncologist: a doctor who uses radiation therapy to treat cancer.

Radiation therapist: a health professional who gives radiation treatments.

Radiologist: a doctor with special training in reading x-rays and performing specialized x-ray procedures.

Social worker: a professional who can talk with you and your family about your emotional or physical needs and can help you find support services. An oncology social worker has specific training in working with cancer patients.

Surgeon or surgical oncologist: a doctor who performs biopsies and other surgical procedures such as removing a lump (lumpectomy) or a breast (mastectomy).

A Second Opinion

Once you receive your doctor's opinion about what treatments you need, you have the right to get more advice before you make up your mind. Other doctors' opinions can help you make one of the most important decisions of your life. Getting another doctor's advice is normal medical practice, and your doctor can help you with this effort. Many health insurance companies require and will pay for other opinions. Another opinion can help you:

- Confirm or adjust your treatment plan based on the diagnosis and stage of the disease.

- Get answers to your questions and concerns and help you become comfortable with your decisions.

- Decide about taking part in a research study of new breast cancer treatment methods. (See Clinical Trials)

To get a second opinion:

- Ask your doctor to refer you to another breast cancer specialist who is not already on your treatment team. Take along your mammogram films, biopsy slides, pathology report, and proposed treatment plan when you see this doctor.

- Call the NCI's Cancer Information Service (1-800-4-CANCER) for help in locating cancer centers that may be in your area.

- Talk with women in breast cancer organizations, cancer survivor groups, or other women who have been through breast cancer treatment. Keep in mind, however, that all breast cancer cases are not the same. Individual experiences and treatments may be different.

Treatment Options

Today, most women with breast cancer are diagnosed at an early stage and they benefit from newer, more effective treatments. There are treatments available for patients at all stages of breast cancer. Often, more than one type of treatment is needed. The treatments used today are listed below and described in detail later in this section.

Clinical Trials: where patients help scientists find new, improved treatments for cancer.

Surgery: taking out the cancer in an operation.

Radiation therapy: using high-dose x-rays to kill cancer cells or keep them from dividing and growing.

Chemotherapy: using anticancer drugs to kill or stop the growth of cancer cells.

High-dose chemotherapy: using high doses of anticancer drugs to kill cancer cells. High-dose drug treatments with peripheral stem cell transplantation and bone marrow transplantation are being tested in clinical trials.

Hormonal therapy: using hormones to stop cancer cells from growing.

Biological therapy (immunotherapy): using the immune system to fight cancer or to lessen the side effects that may be caused by some cancer treatments. Many biological therapies are being tested in clinical trials.

Breast reconstruction: surgery to rebuild a breast's shape.

Complementary therapies: you should discuss their possible value and side effects with your medical doctors.

Clinical Trials

Your doctor may suggest that you consider taking part in a breast cancer treatment clinical trial, where patients help scientists find new, improved treatments for cancer. You may want to ask your doctor if you should consider joining such a research study. It's important to make this decision before you start treatment because you may not be eligible if you have had certain treatments already. Every successful treatment used today started as a clinical trial, and the patients who participated were the first to benefit from improved therapy.

Research studies for breast cancer treatments take place in many hospitals and cancer centers across the country. In these clinical trials, doctors use the newest treatments to care for cancer patients. Each carefully planned study is designed to answer certain questions and to find out specific information about how well a new drug or treatment method works. All new treatments must go through three steps or "phases" of clinical trials:

Phase 1: Tests the best way to give a new treatment and how much can be given safely.

Phase 2: Finds out how well a treatment destroys cancer cells.

Phase 3: Compares two or more different treatments.

Each phase depends and builds on information from earlier phases. As time goes on, new and better ways to help cancer patients are being developed. It takes time, often several years, for clinical trials to prove the true value and effectiveness of a new treatment. All clinical-study patients receive the best care possible, and their reactions to the treatment are watched very closely. If the treatment doesn't seem to be helping, a doctor can take a patient out of a study. Also, a patient may choose to leave at any time. If a patient leaves a research study for any reason, standard care and treatment are still available.

If you are thinking about joining a breast cancer treatment clinical trial, your doctor can give you information that will help you decide if the choice is right for you. You should consider carefully what is involved and all possible benefits and risks of the treatment that is being offered.

Surgery

Surgery has an important role in the treatment of patients with breast cancer. Most women can choose between breast-conserving surgery (lumpectomy with radiation therapy) or removal of the breast (mastectomy). Clinical trials have proven that both options provide the same long-term survival rates for most types of early breast cancer. However, neither option guarantees that cancer will not recur. Whichever choice you make, you will need close medical followup for the rest of your life.

Breast Conserving Surgery

Figure 35.1. Lumpectomy: *The surgeon removes the breast cancer and some normal tissue around it (in order to get clear margins). This procedure usually results in removing all the cancer, while leaving you with a breast that looks much the same as it did before surgery. Usually, the surgeon also takes out some of the lymph nodes under the arm to find out if the cancer has spread. Women who have lumpectomies almost always have radiation therapy as well. Radiation therapy is used to destroy any cancer cells that may not have been removed by surgery.*

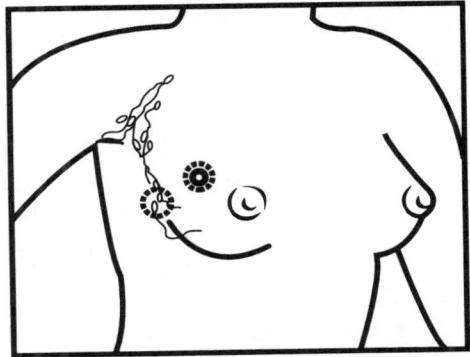

Figure 35.2. Partial or Segmental Mastectomy: *Depending on the size and location of the cancer, this surgery can conserve much of the breast. The surgeon removes the cancer, some of the breast tissue, the lining over the chest muscles below the tumor, and usually some of the lymph nodes under the arm. In most cases, radiation therapy follows.*

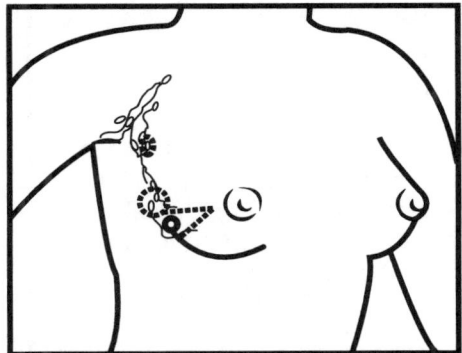

Mastectomy

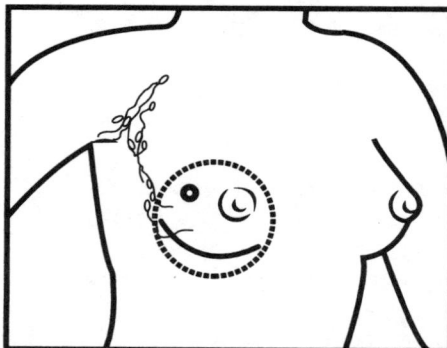

Figure 35.3. Total (or Simple) Mastectomy: *The surgeon removes the entire breast. Some lymph nodes under the arm may be removed, also.*

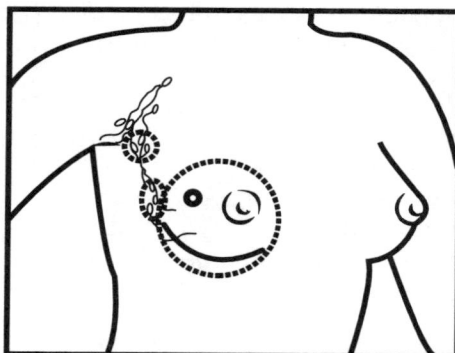

Figure 35.4. Modified Radical Mastectomy: *The surgeon removes the breast, some of the lymph nodes under the arm, and the lining over the chest muscles, and sometimes part of the chest wall muscles.*

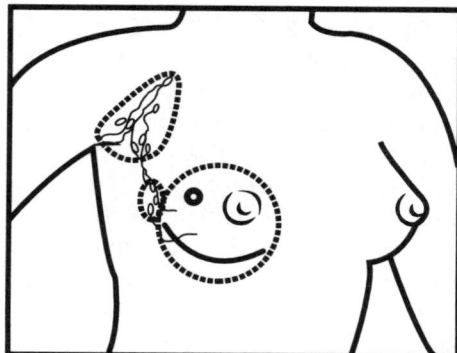

Figure 35.5. Radical Mastectomy: *The surgeon removes the breast, chest muscles, and all the lymph nodes under the arm. This was the standard operation for many years, but it is used now only when a tumor has spread to the chest muscles.*

A mastectomy may be recommended when:

- Cancer is found in more than one part of the breast.
- The breast is small or shaped so that a lumpectomy would leave little breast tissue or a very deformed breast.
- A woman chooses not to have radiation therapy.
- A woman prefers a mastectomy.

Possible Problems: As in any kind of surgery, there is a risk of infection, poor wound healing, bleeding, or a reaction to the anesthesia used in surgery. There may be a collection of fluid under the skin; or tingling, numbness, stiffness, weakness, or swelling of the arm. (See lymphedema.) Physical therapy and exercise can help to restore arm movement and strength.

After a mastectomy, a woman may choose to:

- Wear a breast form, called a prosthesis, that fits in her bra. To find stores that have breast forms and fitters, talk with your doctor, nurse, or a volunteer from the American Cancer Society Reach for Recovery program or other breast cancer organization, or other women who have had breast cancer.
- Have her breast reconstructed by a plastic surgeon.
- Do neither.

Some health insurance plans pay for all or part of the costs of a prosthesis or for breast reconstruction. However, there may be health insurance rules about where a woman can have breast reconstruction surgery or where to buy a prosthesis. For details about your health plan coverage, contact your insurance company.

Questions to Ask Your Surgeon Before Surgery

- What kind of surgery do you recommend for me?
- How much of my breast will be removed?
- If I have a mastectomy, will I be able to have breast reconstruction?
- Do you recommend it at the time of surgery or later?
- Will I meet with the plastic surgeon before surgery?

273

- Will you remove any of my lymph nodes?

- Where will the operation be done? Will I have local or general anesthesia?

- How should I feel after the operation? If I have pain, how can I get relief?

- What side effects should I report to you?

- Where will the scars be? What will they look like?

- Will a nurse or physical therapist teach me how to exercise and care for my arm?

- How long will I stay in the hospital? Will I need followup care?

- When can I get back to my normal activities? What activities should I avoid?

- What do I need to do to prepare for surgery?

Removal of Lymph Nodes

Whether you have a lumpectomy or mastectomy, your surgeon will probably remove some of the lymph nodes under your arm. This procedure is usually done at the same time as the breast surgery to check if the cancer has spread outside the breast. Clear lymph nodes are reported as negative nodes. If cancer is found, you have positive nodes. Your doctor will talk with you about any additional treatments needed to destroy and control cancer cells.

Lymphedema

The lymph nodes under your arm drain lymph fluid from your chest and arm. Both surgery and radiation therapy can change the normal drainage pattern. This can result in a swelling of the arm called lymphedema. The problem can develop right after surgery or months to years later.

Treatment of lymphedema depends on how serious the problem becomes. Options include an elastic sleeve, an arm pump, arm massage, and bandaging the arm. Exercise and diet also are important. If you have this problem, talk with your doctor and see a physical therapist as soon as possible. Many hospitals and breast clinics offer help with lymphedema. There is no cure for this condition, so you should do what you can to prevent it.

Sentinel Lymph Node Biopsy

Surgeons are investigating a new procedure in cancer patients used to detect lymph node involvement. In this procedure, either a blue dye or a small amount of radioactive material is injected around the tumor site. The surgeon performs a small incision in the axillary underarm area looking for a lymph node containing the blue dye or uses a scanner to locate the radioactive material. The lymph node(s) where the dye first accumulates after leaving the tumor region is called the "sentinel node(s)." This node(s) is then surgically removed and examined by a pathologist. If it is positive for cancer cells, then the rest of the nodes are usually removed; if it is negative, the remaining lymph nodes may not have to be removed.

After underarm lymph nodes are removed, your arm will have to be protected for the rest of your life.

To help prevent or control lymphedema and to protect your arm after treatment:

- Carry packages or handbags on the other arm or shoulder.
- Avoid sunburns and burns to your affected arm and hand.
- Have shots (including chemotherapy), blood draws, and blood pressure tests done on the other arm.
- Avoid cuts when shaving underarms; use an electric shaver.
- Wash cuts promptly, apply antibacterial medication, and cover with a bandage. Call your doctor if you think that you have an infection.
- Wear gloves to protect your hands when gardening and when using strong detergents.
- Avoid wearing tight jewelry on your affected arm; avoid elastic cuffs on blouses and nightgowns.
- Have careful manicures; avoid cutting your cuticles.

Questions to Ask Your Surgeon After Surgery

- What did you learn from the pathology report?
- Please explain what is in the pathology report.

- How many lymph nodes were removed? Were they free of cancer? If not, how many showed signs of cancer?

- Did the tumor have clear margins (normal tissue around the tumor)?

- Were hormone receptor tests done? What are the results?

- What other tests will be done on the tissue? When will I know the results?

- Do I need further treatment?

- Should I consider joining a clinical trial?

Radiation Therapy

A lumpectomy usually is followed by radiation therapy. During radiation therapy, high-energy x-rays are used to destroy cancer cells that still may be present in the affected breast or in nearby lymph nodes. Radiation therapy is sometimes used to shrink tumors before surgery. Doctors sometimes use radiation therapy along with chemotherapy, before or instead of surgery, to destroy cancer cells and shrink tumors.

Radiation Therapy After Lumpectomy

In radiation therapy after a lumpectomy, a machine delivers radiation to the affected breast and, in some cases, to the lymph nodes under the arm or at the collarbone (clavicle). The usual schedule for radiation therapy is 5 days a week for 5 to 6 weeks. The actual treatment, given by a radiation therapist, takes only a few minutes each day. Sometimes an additional "boost" or higher dose of radiation is given to the area where the cancer was found.

During your first visit for radiation treatment planning, your chest area will be marked with ink or with a few long-lasting tattoos. These marks must stay on your skin during the entire treatment period because they show exactly where the radiation will be given. Your radiation oncologist will plan your specific treatment based on a physical exam, mammograms, pathology and lab reports, and your medical history. Doctors carefully limit both the intensity of each treatment and the area being treated so that the least amount of normal tissue will be affected. Throughout your therapy, your radiation oncologist will check on the effects of your treatment, and you will have regular physical exams and blood tests to check your general health. To get the full benefit from radiation therapy, you need to complete all your treatments as scheduled.

Possible Problems: Feeling more tired than usual; skin problems such as itchiness, redness, soreness, peeling, darkening, or shininess of the skin; or decreased sensation in the breast. Radiation to the breast does not cause hair loss, vomiting, or diarrhea.

Long-term changes may include changes in the shape and color of the treated breast or a feeling of heaviness in the breast. Once a breast has been irradiated, it cannot be irradiated again. Any local recurrence or new tumor would have to be treated by mastectomy.

Radiation Therapy After Mastectomy

There are times when radiation therapy is used after a mastectomy. It may be used if:

- The tumor is larger than 2 inches.

- Cancer is found in many lymph nodes under the arm.

- The tumor is close to the rib cage or chest wall muscles.

Questions to Ask Your Radiation Oncologist

You will have time during your radiation treatment planning session and the daily treatments to ask questions and talk about your concerns. You may want to ask:

- What benefit will I get from radiation therapy? What are the side effects? What are the risks?

- When will my treatment begin? What is the schedule? When will treatment end?

- What should I do to prepare for each treatment? Who will give the actual radiation treatment? How long will each session take?

- What will happen during each treatment? Will I feel anything?

- How do I care for myself during the weeks of therapy? What side effects should I report to you?

- How will we know the treatment is working successfully?

- How will my breast look and feel when radiation therapy is completed?

- Will I be able to drive to and from the radiation center alone? Are there any restrictions to my normal activities?

- How long will I have to protect the irradiated skin from the sun?

- Will I need followup care?

- What if I don't have radiation therapy?

Chemotherapy

Research suggests that, even if a lump is small, cancer cells may have spread outside the breast. Doctors can use chemotherapy drugs to destroy cancer cells. Some chemotherapy drugs work better when combined with other chemotherapy drugs than when used alone.

The oncologist will recommend a treatment plan according to your individual case. The treatment will depend on your age, whether or not you still are having periods, the risk for spread or recurrence, and your general health. The drugs you take will depend on the type and stage of cancer, where it is located, how much or how fast it has grown, and how it is affecting you. Chemotherapy is used to:

- Decrease the chances that cancer will come back after breast cancer surgery.

- Shrink breast cancer before surgery, when the tumor is large or it is inflammatory cancer.

- Control the disease when breast cancer is found in the lungs, bones, liver, brain, or other parts of the body.

Chemotherapy drugs travel throughout the body to slow the growth of cancer cells or kill them. Often, the drugs are injected into the bloodstream through an intravenous (IV) needle that is inserted into a vein. Some drugs are given as pills. Treatment can be as short as a few months or as long as 2 years.

Chemotherapy is usually given in cycles during which you have treatment for a period of time, and then you have a few weeks to recover before your next treatment. Depending on the drugs you take, you may have your chemotherapy at home, in your doctor's office, in a clinic, in a hospital's outpatient department, or in a hospital. How often and how long you have chemotherapy will depend on the type and stage of breast cancer, the drugs that are used and how your body responds to them, and the goals of the treatment. You should follow the schedule prescribed by your doctor.

Throughout chemotherapy, your oncologist and nurse will watch how you respond to the therapy. You will have frequent physical exams and blood tests. You should check with your doctor before taking any other medications during your treatment.

Chemotherapy affects all fast-growing cells throughout the body. Therefore, in addition to killing cancer cells, it also kills fast-growing normal cells. This is what may cause side effects such as hair loss, mouth sores, and fatigue. Today, because of what has been learned in research studies, doctors are able to control, lessen, or avoid many side effects of chemotherapy.

Possible Problems: Chemotherapy can cause short-term and long-term side effects that are different for each patient, depending on the drugs used.

The most common short-term side effects that may appear during chemotherapy include: loss of appetite, nausea, vomiting, diarrhea, constipation, fatigue, infections, bleeding, weight change, mouth sores, and throat soreness. Some of these problems may continue for some time after chemotherapy ends.

Some drugs cause short-term hair loss. Hair will grow back either during treatment or after treatment is completed. Before you start chemotherapy, you may want to have your hair cut short, or buy a wig, hat, or scarves that you can wear while you are going through treatment.

Serious long-term side effects may include weakening of your heart, damage to your ovaries, infertility, early menopause, or second cancers such as leukemia (cancer of the blood). These side effects may not appear until later, some time after chemotherapy is completed.

Fighting Infections

You are more likely to get infections during chemotherapy, and your body is less able to fight infections during this time. You can help yourself stay healthy by following these steps:

- Finish dental work before starting chemotherapy. You cannot have dental work during chemotherapy.

- Eat a healthy diet and get plenty of rest.

- Stay away from large crowds and from anyone with a cold, infection, or contagious disease.

- Bathe daily, wash your hands often, and follow good mouth care.

- Wear work gloves to protect your hands against cuts and burns.

- If you cut yourself, keep the wound clean and covered. Talk with your doctor or nurse about applying antibiotics or medications.

Pregnancy

During chemotherapy, you may stop having monthly menstrual periods. You still can get pregnant, however, so talk with your doctor about birth control. The effect of chemotherapy on an unborn baby is unknown. After your treatment is over, your ability to get pregnant will depend on your age and the types of drugs you received. If you hope to become pregnant after treatment, talk with your doctor before starting chemotherapy.

Managing Nausea

Feeling nauseous, or as if you have to vomit, is a common side effect of chemotherapy. Your doctor can prescribe medication to help with this problem. Good nutrition is especially important during cancer treatment. The following suggestions may help:

- Eat small meals often; do not eat 3 to 4 hours before your treatment.

- Eat whatever you can tolerate; for example, popsicles, gelatin desserts, cream of wheat, oatmeal, baked potatoes, and fruit juices mixed with water.

- Chew your food thoroughly and try to relax during meals.

- Learn stress reduction exercises such as relaxation, meditation, and deep breathing.

Questions to Ask Your Medical Oncologist about Chemotherapy

- Why do I need chemotherapy?

- What drugs do you recommend? How successful is this treatment for my type and stage of breast cancer?

- What are the benefits and risks of taking these drugs?

- Are there any research studies that I should consider?

- How will you and I be sure that the drugs are working?

- Where and how will I receive these drugs? Will someone stay with me during treatments?

- How many treatments will I need, and how long will I be on chemotherapy?

- What are the common side effects of these drugs and how can I manage them?

- What side effects should I report to you?

- Are there any restrictions? Will I be able to maintain my normal activities?

- How should I prepare for the treatment?

- Will I be able to drive home alone afterwards?

- Will there be long-term side effects? Will I need followup care?

- What if I choose not to have chemotherapy?

High-Dose Chemotherapy

In breast cancer treatment clinical trials, researchers at NCI and other health institutions are testing high-dose chemotherapy to find out if it is better than standard chemotherapy. They are trying to learn if higher doses of drugs can prevent or delay the spread or return of breast cancer better than standard doses of drugs, and which type of treatment helps patients live longer.

Patients who receive high-dose chemotherapy are at great risk of suffering life-threatening side effects because the treatment damages their bone marrow and they no longer are able to produce needed blood cells. To help repair the damage done by high doses of drugs, the treatment includes peripheral blood stem cell transplantation and/or bone marrow transplantation.

Peripheral Blood Stem Cell Transplantation

Peripheral blood stem cell transplantation involves the removal of a certain type of blood cell (stem cell) from a patient's blood. Stem cells are immature cells from which all blood cells develop as they are needed. Stem cells are able to divide and form more stem cells (copies of themselves) or they can become fully mature red blood cells (erythrocytes), platelets, and white blood cells (leukocytes).

The removed stem cells are frozen and stored while the patient is treated with high-dose chemotherapy. After chemotherapy ends and the drugs are gone from the body, the stem cells are returned to the patient through a vein. The healthy stem cells can then begin to grow and produce all types of blood cells the patient needs to survive.

Bone Marrow Transplantation

Bone marrow is the sponge-like material found inside bones that produces blood cells. Autologous bone marrow transplantation is used in breast cancer treatment. In this procedure, some of a patient's own healthy bone marrow is removed with a needle before treatment begins. The bone marrow is then frozen and stored while the patient is treated with high-dose chemotherapy. Several days after the treatment ends and the drugs are gone from the body, the healthy bone marrow is given back to the patient through a vein. The healthy bone marrow can then begin to produce blood cells that the patient needs to survive. Peripheral blood stem cells and bone marrow transplantation may be used together as part of high-dose chemotherapy.

It hasn't been proven yet whether high-dose chemotherapy is better than standard chemotherapy, or which breast cancer patients need this treatment. It is best to have high-dose chemotherapy at an established transplant center or medical institution conducting a clinical trial. Some health insurance plans pay for some of the costs of peripheral blood stem cell or bone marrow transplantation.

Possible Problems: There are major risks involved with high-dose chemotherapy. Talk with your doctor about possible complications and severe side effects, and whether this would be an appropriate treatment for your type and stage of breast cancer.

Hormonal Therapy

Hormonal therapy is used to prevent the growth, spread, or recurrence of breast cancer. If lab tests show that your tumor depended on your natural hormones to grow, it will be described as estrogen-positive or progesterone-positive in the lab report. This means that any remaining cancer cells may continue to grow when these hormones are present in your body. Hormonal therapy can block your body's natural hormones from reaching any remaining cancer cells.

- You may be given a hormone drug. One of the most common drugs used for hormonal therapy for breast cancer is tamoxifen.

- You may have surgery to remove both ovaries that produce natural hormones.

Research has proven that hormonal therapy can extend the lifespan of a breast cancer patient who has cancer cells that depend on hormones to grow. Tamoxifen has been used for nearly 20 years to treat patients with advanced stage breast cancer. Now it is being used also as additional treatment for early stage disease after breast cancer is removed by surgery. Clinical trials show that taking tamoxifen as part of the treatment for breast cancer helps to reduce the chances of recurrence in the treated breast and of new cancer developing in the other breast.

Tamoxifen is taken daily by mouth as a pill. Your oncologist will decide on the dose and length of treatment according to current research findings. Like chemotherapy, hormonal therapy affects cells throughout your body. Studies have shown that there is some increased risk for cancer of the uterus. Blood clots have been reported in the veins of a small percentage of patients who take tamoxifen along with chemotherapy. These risks, however, are much lower than the benefits received from tamoxifen.

Of course, you will have frequent blood tests and physical exams while you are on hormonal therapy. Be sure your gynecologist and primary care doctor know you are taking this drug. You should have yearly pelvic exams while taking tamoxifen, and you should notify your doctor about any unusual bleeding or pain.

Possible Problems: Side effects could include hot flashes, nausea, vaginal spotting (small amounts of blood), or increased fertility in younger women. Less common side effects include depression; vaginal itching, bleeding, or discharge; loss of appetite; eye problems; headache; and weight gain.

Questions to Ask Your Medical Oncologist about Hormonal Therapy

- What benefit might I get from hormonal therapy?
- Which would be better for me, hormone medication or surgery to remove my ovaries? Why?
- What drug will I be taking? How will I know it is working?
- What are the side effects and how can I manage them?
- What side effects should I report to you?
- How long will I be on hormonal therapy?
- Will I need followup care?
- What if I don't have hormonal therapy?

Biological Therapy (Immunotherapy)

Your own immune system is your body's natural defense against diseases, including cancer. Your immune system also defends your body against infections and other side effects of cancer treatment. A strong immune system detects the difference between healthy cells and cancer cells, and it can get rid of those that become cancer. The immune system can be strengthened and improved by new biological therapies. These treatments are designed to repair, stimulate, or increase your body's natural ability to fight infections and cancer.

Medical researchers are looking at many types of biological therapies that use and boost the substances produced naturally by the body's own cells. They are also creating new substances that can imitate or help the body's natural immune system to work against infection and disease. These are being used in clinical trials with chemotherapy and radiation therapy.

Possible Problems: Biological therapies may produce side effects such as rashes or swellings at the site where shots are given; flu-like symptoms, including fever, chills and fatigue; digestive tract problems; or allergic reactions.

Breast Reconstruction

Breast reconstruction (surgery to rebuild a breast's shape) is often an option after mastectomy. Some health insurance plans pay for all or part of the cost of breast reconstruction and, also, for surgery to the other breast so that both breasts are about the same shape and size.

Reconstruction will not give you back your breast. Although the reconstructed breast will not have natural sensation, the surgery can give you a result that looks like a breast. If you are thinking about reconstruction, you should talk with a plastic surgeon before your mastectomy. Ask your surgeon for a referral to an experienced plastic surgeon. Some women begin reconstruction at the same time as the mastectomy is done; others wait several months or even years.

Breast Implants

A plastic surgeon is able to form a breast mound by using an implant or by using tissues from another part of your body. Breast implants are silicone sacs filled with saline (salt water) or silicone gel. The sacs are placed under your skin behind your chest muscle. Your body type, age, and cancer treatment will determine which type of reconstruction will give you the best result.

Saline and Silicone Implants

Saline-filled breast implants are available for anyone who wants them.

Some scientists are concerned about possible short-term and long-term health problems associated with silicone gel-filled breast implants. The Food and Drug Administration (FDA) has decided that breast implants filled with silicone gel may be used only in an FDA-approved clinical trial. Your surgeon can determine if you are eligible and can make arrangements for you to join the study.

Possible Problems: As with any surgery, you may have some pain, swelling, bruising, and tenderness. These problems should disappear as you recover. Scars will fade over time. You should let your doctor know immediately about any fever, infection, or bleeding.

Side effects that could appear later include rupture, leakage, deflation or shifting of the implant, or interference with mammography readings. Breast implants age over time and may need to be replaced.

For More Information about Breast Implants

- Contact plastic surgeons and other medical experts.
- Call NCI's Cancer Information Service (CIS), 1-800-4-CANCER.
- Call the Food and Drug Administration (FDA), 1-800-532-4440.
- Call the American Cancer Society (ACS), 1-800-ACS-2345.
- Talk to breast cancer survivors who have had reconstruction.
- Contact your health insurance company.

Reconstruction with Tissue Flaps

A flap (section) of skin, muscle, and fat can be moved from another part of the body to the chest area where it is formed to create a breast shape. This tissue can be taken from the lower abdomen, back, or buttocks.

Choose a plastic surgeon who has been trained in this procedure and has performed it successfully on many women. Of course, you will need to have regularly scheduled followup care and mammograms.

Possible Problems: Tissue flap reconstruction is a major operation, resulting in large surgical wounds. If there is a poor blood supply to the flap tissue, part or all of the tissue in the breast area may not survive the transplant. Infection and poor wound healing are possible problems.

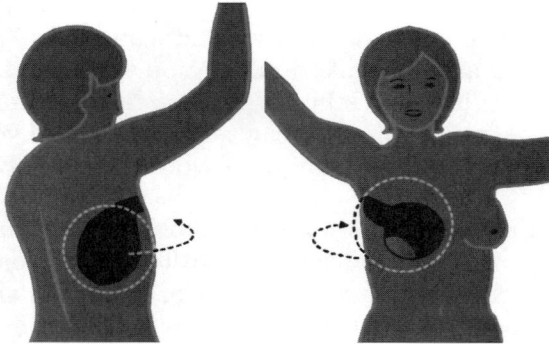

Figure 35.6. Tissue Flap Reconstruction: *This flap of skin, muscle, and fat is moved while still connected to its blood supply. It is then shaped to form a new breast mound.*

What You Should Know

Most women who have breast reconstruction are happy with their decisions. A woman starting this process, however, should know that breast reconstruction requires more than one surgery. Extra steps may include:

- Adding a nipple.
- Changing the shape or size of the reconstructed breast.
- Surgery on the opposite breast to create a good match.

With most of these extra surgeries, you can go home the same day as the operation.

Questions to Ask Your Plastic Surgeon about Breast Reconstruction

- What is the latest information about the safety of breast implants?

- How many breast reconstructions have you done?
- Which type of surgery would give me the best results?
- How long will the surgery take? What kind of anesthesia?
- When do you recommend I begin breast reconstruction?
- How many surgeries will I need?
- What are the risks at the time of surgery? Later?
- Will there be scars? Where? How large?
- Will flap surgery cause any permanent changes where tissue was removed?
- What complications should I report to you?
- How long will my recovery take? When can I return to my normal activities? What activities should I avoid?
- Will I need followup care?
- How much will it cost? Will my health insurance pay for breast reconstruction?

Complementary Therapies

In addition to medical treatment, some cancer patients want to try complementary therapies. Complementary therapies include acupuncture, herbs, biofeedback, visualization, meditation, yoga, nutritional supplements, and vitamins. Some breast cancer patients feel that they benefit from some of these therapies.

Before you try any of these therapies, you should discuss their possible value and side effects with your medical doctors. You should let them know if you are using any such therapies. These therapies should never be used instead of medical treatment. Be aware that these therapies may be expensive and some are not paid for by health insurance. You should consider asking the therapist for evidence of how the therapy has helped others, possibly by giving you references.

Emotional Health

It is normal to have trouble coping with the diagnosis and treatment of breast cancer. Some women feel anger, fear, denial, frustration, loss of control, confusion, or grief. Others feel lonely, isolated, and depressed. Some breast cancer patients may be concerned about self-image, future priorities, sexuality, concerns about family members and medical bills, and possible death. Like other women, you can deal with these issues and your diagnosis of cancer in your own way and at your own pace. You may want to talk with a friend or family member who can listen and let you sort out your feelings without giving any advice. When you reach out, you give loved ones and friends the chance to support you during this difficult time. You may want to talk about your concerns with members of your health care team. You will feel more confident and in control as you become comfortable with your treatment decisions.

Like other cancer survivors, you may experience an emotional letdown once treatment is completed. This could happen because you may feel that you should keep doing something to continue fighting your disease. Concerns and fears about breast cancer are likely to stay with you. A new ache or pain, or the anniversary of your diagnosis, may get you down or worried. Making appointments for followup exams, returning to a treatment location, and waiting for test results may be especially stressful. These feelings are part of being a cancer survivor. Having faced one of life's greatest challenges, you will find relief from these anxieties as you return to routine activities and focus on your future goals.

Many women are helped by talking about their feelings with other women who have had breast cancer. Hospitals often offer support groups or meetings with counselors or psychologists. Ask your doctor if your hospital offers these services. You also may want to look into family or individual therapy. Growing numbers of therapists offer services to individuals, families, and friends affected by cancer.

Followup Care

After your breast cancer treatment is completed, you will need to have regularly scheduled followup care.

Because you have had breast cancer in one breast, you are at increased risk of developing breast cancer again. To be sure that the cancer has not returned, your checkups will include physical exams and mammograms. You also may have blood tests, chest x-rays, bone scans, or other tests. If you find any unusual changes in your treated area or in your other breast, or if you have swollen lymph glands or bone pain, you should call your doctor as soon as possible.

Chapter 36

Understanding Your Pathology Report

This text is designed to give you the tools you need to understand your pathology report. It's not really as difficult as you may think. Contrary to popular belief, the pathology report is actually in English, but it is replete with elements to make it seem more complicated than it is. Some of these elements include the use of multiple words that sound different but actually mean the same thing (example: "invasive" and "infiltrating" are synonyms, as are "intraductal" and "ductal carcinoma *in situ*", and "cancer" and "carcinoma"). Just when you think it begins to sound easy again, be prepared for detailed use of frightening sounding words which seem complicated but which actually have little or no clinical significance ("florid papillomatosis," "sclerosing adenosis," "fibrosis," and "apocrine metaplasia" to name a few). To be fair, we are still collecting data, and the pathologists are not to be faulted for being as detailed as possible as they speak to each other; they are also communicating to each other that they evaluated several areas that may be confused with patterns of cancer. Just don't let the use of these terms deter you from trying to understand your own report.

By law you are entitled to copies of your medical records, though a copying fee can be charged if you ask for a large number of sheets of paper. Most physicians and clinics will not begrudge you a few copies, however, and if there is anything which you should have and always

By Dr. Ellen Mahoney, Understanding Your Pathology Report, Community Breast Health Project, Stanford University, July 1999; reprinted with permission.

keep with your important papers, it is a copy of each of the pathology reports generated on your behalf. In the future, the possession of these records will save you time and trouble. Other reports that you may want to have include the treatment summary for radiation and for chemotherapy.

Check Identifying Data

Your pathology report will begin with some identifying data. Just as the pros always double-check the name on the x-ray label before acting, it is worth taking a moment to check your date of birth and social security number, especially if you have a common name. The date of the procedure and the specimens submitted will be named next, along with a brief clinical history, the operation performed, and the clinical diagnosis. Your doctor should take time to communicate his pre-operative thoughts to the pathologist by filling out this form. If he doesn't, the nurse will often try to glean the information from the chart and fill out the information during a rare, brief idle moment. The pathologist is a consultant as important (or maybe more important) than the doctors you meet face-to-face, and there are many times when the interpretation is aided by physician-to-physician communication.

Gross Description

The next paragraph is the "gross description." This is not an aesthetic judgment. It refers to "obvious" and it is the description of what the pathologist sees before making any slides. There is a statement of the documentation which links the tissue to the identified patient, the measured size (remember that there are 2.5 centimeters and 25 millimeters to the inch), and the description of the markings attached to the specimen. As an aside, most breast experts are providing suture markings on the main biopsy specimens so that different colored inks can be applied to the surface of the tissue before it is cut. That way, if one margin is involved with tumor, the color of the margin is noted, and the surgeon knows which aspect of the biopsy cavity is involved. I use what I call "The Sesame Street Protocol" where the Long suture is Lateral, the Double is Deep and the Short is Superior. With these three sides of the approximately six-sided object noted, the other three aspects are easily defined. The specimen is sometimes x-rayed in the pathology lab so that the pathologist can tell in advance which slice may contain the most suspicious areas. At Stanford, all of the biopsy is processed, but thinner slices may be taken in the block which has calcifications.

Under the Microscope

The next paragraph of the report contains the description of what the pathologist sees under the microscope. If your biopsy is benign, be on the lookout for descriptions which include the words "atypical" or "atypia." If this word is not accompanied by a negative (for example, "no atypia is seen"), you may have a slightly increased risk of breast cancer in the future, and your surveillance program may change, especially if you also have a family history of breast cancer.

A special word about "lobular carcinoma *in situ*": This is not cancer! It too is a benign condition, but one associated with a higher risk of future cancer in either breast.

If you are told that you have "ductal carcinoma *in situ*" (DCIS), you have cells which appear malignant but are trapped inside the walls of the duct. This too is technically not real cancer ("pre-malignant" in Dr. Love's book [NOTE: see Chapter 65 for information about this publication]), but some types are more dangerous than others; the treatment may need to be similar to that for invasive cancer. The more dangerous ones are described as "high-grade with necrosis" or "comedocarcinoma." Less dangerous forms are described as "solid," "cribriform," or "papillary." If you have DCIS, you need to know the type, the size and the approximate margin. The margin is the distance from the DCIS to the edge of the tissue removed. The more dangerous the cell type, the wider the margin should be whether or not radiation is suggested.

Tumor size and margin are also very important in invasive cancer. The margin is not only described in terms of size, but also in terms of any DCIS in the tissue between the cancer and the edge of the tissue removed. The cancer is also "graded" I, II, or III depending on how closely it resembles normal breast tissue. This used to be done subjectively, but the Bloom-Scharf-Richardson is a commonly used scoring system which attempts to objectify the impression. Grade I is best; most tumors are Grade II ("moderately well-differentiated"). Invasive tumors can be ductal or lobular, but the distinction is less important practically than it used to be, and we recognize that many tumors are on a spectrum between the two types. Prognostic measures, such as hormone receptors, DNA index, S-phase, her-2-neu expression and others may be mentioned in the main report, but they are typically included in an addendum since they take longer to do. If lymph nodes were taken, the total number is noted, and the number involved with tumor is described. If an involved lymph node is described as having a "micrometastasis," or if a tumor is seen in the fat outside the lymph node, this is important information that can affect prognosis, and you should ask your doctor to comment on it.

Staging

Important information which is not mentioned explicitly in your pathology report is your "stage." Stages are I-IV, with DCIS being Stage 0. Usually the pathology reports contain the information we need to calculate the stage. Staging is a way of stratifying breast cancer cases for purposes of research and for comparing outcomes in various treatment protocols, and it is therefore important to know not only the number assigned but also the details of how the stage was calculated. The stage is also used in treatment, but as we become more sophisticated, we recognize that nature is a spectrum—not a series of compartments. A case which is Stage II but at the low end of the spectrum may behave more like a Stage I tumor, whereas a Stage II which is almost a III may have a less favorable prognosis. Just remember that stage does not tell the future or the results for people being treated today. There are long-term survivors who began as Stage III cases, and some Stage IV patients who survive for years.

Keep your pathology reports and treatment summaries, know your cell type and stage. With just a little practice, you too can speak "Pathologese."

Community Breast Health Project

For more information about the Community Breast Health Project, contact:

Community Breast Health Project
545 Bryant Street
Palo Alto, CA 94301
Phone: 650-326-6686
Fax: 650-626-6673
Website: http://med.stanford.edu/CBHP

Chapter 37

Preventive Mastectomy

Preventive mastectomy (also called prophylactic mastectomy) is the surgical removal of one or both breasts in an effort to prevent or reduce the risk of breast cancer. The surgeon removes the entire breast and nipple (total mastectomy). In the past, the surgeon may have removed the breast tissue but spared the nipple (subcutaneous mastectomy). This procedure is no longer recommended.

Preventive mastectomy may be considered for several reasons. Women who have already had one breast removed due to cancer may consider this procedure in an effort to avoid developing a new cancer in the other breast. Preventive mastectomy may also be an option for women with a strong family history of breast cancer, especially if several close relatives developed the disease before age 50. Women in families with hereditary breast cancer who test positive for a known cancer-causing gene alteration may also consider this surgery. In addition, preventive mastectomy is sometimes considered for women who have had lobular carcinoma *in situ*, a condition that increases their risk of developing breast cancer in the same and/or in the opposite breast. Infrequently, preventive mastectomy may be considered for women with breast calcifications or for women whose breast tissue is very dense. Dense breast tissue is linked to an elevated risk of breast cancer and also makes diagnosing breast abnormalities difficult. Multiple biopsies, which may be necessary for diagnosing abnormalities in dense breasts, cause scarring and further complicate examination of the breast tissue.

Cancer Facts, National Cancer Institute, March 1999.

Because all women are different and the degree to which preventive mastectomy can protect an individual woman from breast cancer is not known, the procedure should be considered in the context of each woman's unique risk factors and her level of concern.

It is important for a woman to know that having a preventive mastectomy does not guarantee that she will never develop breast cancer. It is impossible for a surgeon to remove all breast tissue, and breast cancer can develop in the small amount of remaining tissue. A woman who is considering preventive mastectomy should talk with a doctor about her risk factors, the mastectomy procedure, potential complications, followup care, her feelings about mastectomy, and alternatives to surgery. She may wish to get a second medical opinion to help with the decision.

Women who choose to have preventive mastectomy may decide to have breast reconstruction (plastic surgery to restore the shape of the breast). Before performing this type of procedure, the plastic surgeon carefully examines the breasts and discusses the appropriate types of reconstruction.

In one type of reconstructive procedure, the surgeon inserts an implant under the skin and the chest muscles. Another procedure to create the shape of a breast uses skin, fat, and muscle from the woman's abdomen or back. After both types of reconstructive surgery, the surgeon will discuss any limitations on exercise or arm motion.

Women who have reconstructive surgery will be followed carefully in the postoperative period to detect and treat complications, such as infection, movement of the implant, or contracture (the formation of a firm, fibrous shell around the implant caused by the body's reaction to it). Routine screening for breast cancer is also part of the postoperative followup because the risk of cancer cannot be completely eliminated. When women with breast implants have mammograms, they should tell the radiology technician about the implant. Special procedures may be necessary to improve the accuracy of the mammogram.

Doctors do not always agree on the most effective way to manage the care of women who have a strong family history of breast cancer and/or have other risk factors for the disease. Some doctors may recommend preventive mastectomy, while others may prescribe tamoxifen, a medication that has recently been shown to decrease the chances of getting breast cancer in women at high risk for the disease. Some doctors may advise very close monitoring (periodic mammograms, regular checkups, and monthly breast self-examination) to increase the chance of detecting breast cancer at an early stage. Although the effects are not proven, doctors may also encourage women at high risk to limit their consumption of alcohol, eat a low-fat diet, engage in regular exercise, and avoid hormone replacement therapy.

For More Information about Breast Implants

The U.S. Food and Drug Administration (FDA) regulates the use of breast implants and can supply detailed information about these devices. Consumers may write to the FDA Center for Devices and Radiological Health (CDRH) at HFZ-210, 5600 Fishers Lane, Rockville, MD 20857; or call the FDA's Office of Consumer Affairs toll-free at 1-888-INFO-FDA (1-888-463-6332) to listen to recorded information or to request free printed material on breast implants. The CDRH Web site is located at http://www.fda.gov/cdrh/ on the Internet.

Chapter 38

Breast Reconstruction

Choices in Reconstructive Procedures

The type of breast reconstruction procedure available to you depends on your medical situation, breast shape and size, general health, lifestyle, and goals. Women with small or medium sized breasts are the best candidates for breast reconstruction.

Breast reconstruction can be accomplished by the use of a breast implant, your own tissues (a tissue flap), or a combination of the two. A tissue flap is a section of skin, fat and/or muscle which is moved from your stomach, back or other area of your body, to the chest area and shaped into a new breast.

Whether or not you have reconstruction with or without breast implants, you will probably undergo additional surgeries to improve symmetry and appearance. For example, after your breast has healed from the original implant surgery, you may want to build a new nipple and darken the areola (skin around the nipple). This procedure can usually be performed on an outpatient basis. Ask your doctor to explain the various ways this can be done, such as using a skin graft from the opposite breast or by tattooing the area.

Ask your doctor about the pros and cons of each implant technique. If you decide to have reconstruction for one breast, you may need to

---

Excerpted from *Breast Implants: An Information Update*, Center for Devices and Radiological Health, U.S. Food and Drug Administration (FDA), September 2000. The complete text of this document may be viewed on FDA's website at http://www.fda.gov/cdhr/breastimplants.

think about surgery on the other breast to achieve a similar appearance.

Special Surgical Concerns for Women with Breast Cancer

The following issues should be considered for women with breast cancer:

- The physical and cosmetic results with breast implants may be affected by chemotherapy, radiation therapy, or any other factor that significantly alters the healing process.

- Skin necrosis (cell death) may occur because circulation to the remaining tissue has been changed by a mastectomy (breast removal). Also, skin necrosis may be increased as a result of radiation treatment.

- It usually takes more than one operation to achieve the desired cosmetic outcome, especially if this procedure includes building a new nipple.

Breast Reconstruction with Breast Implants

Your surgeon will decide whether your health and medical condition makes you an appropriate candidate for breast implant reconstruction. Women with larger breasts may require reconstruction with a combination of a tissue flap and an implant. Your surgeon may recommend breast implantation of the opposite, uninvolved breast in order to make them more alike (maximize symmetry) or he/she may suggest breast reduction (reduction mammoplasty) or a breast lift (mastopexy) to improve symmetry. Mastopexy involves removing a strip of skin from under the breast or around the nipple and using it to lift and tighten the skin over the breast. Reduction mammoplasty involves removal of breast tissue and skin. If it is important to you not to alter the unaffected breast, you should discuss this with your surgeon, as it may affect the breast reconstruction methods considered for your case.

Timing of Breast Implant Reconstruction

The breast reconstruction process may begin at the time of your mastectomy (immediate reconstruction) or weeks to years afterwards (delayed reconstruction). Immediate reconstruction may involve placement of a breast implant, but typically involves placement of a tissue expander, which will eventually be replaced with a breast implant. It is important to know that any type of surgical breast reconstruction may take several steps to complete.

Two potential advantages to immediate reconstruction are that your breast reconstruction starts at the time of your mastectomy and that there may be cost savings in combining the mastectomy procedure with the first stage of the reconstruction. However, there may be a higher risk of complications such as deflation with immediate reconstruction, and your initial operative time and recuperative time may be longer.

A potential advantage to delayed reconstruction is that you can delay your reconstruction decision and surgery until other treatments, such as radiation therapy and chemotherapy, are completed. Delayed reconstruction may be advisable if your surgeon anticipates healing problems with your mastectomy, or if you just need more time to consider your options.

There are medical, financial, and emotional considerations to choosing immediate versus delayed reconstruction. You should discuss with your surgeon, plastic surgeon, and oncologist, the pros and cons with the options available in your individual case.

Breast Implant Reconstruction Procedures

One-Stage Immediate Breast Implant Reconstruction

Immediate one-stage breast reconstruction may be done at the time of your mastectomy. After the general surgeon removes your breast tissue, the plastic surgeon will then implant a breast implant that completes the one-stage reconstruction.

Two-Stage (Immediate or Delayed) Breast Implant Reconstruction

Breast reconstruction usually occurs as a two-stage procedure, starting with the placement of a breast tissue expander, which is replaced several months later with a breast implant. The tissue expander placement may be done immediately, at the time of your mastectomy, or be delayed until months or years later.

Tissue Expansion. During a mastectomy, the general surgeon often removes skin as well as breast tissue, leaving the chest tissues flat and tight. To create a breast shaped space for the breast implant, a tissue expander is placed under the remaining chest tissues.

The tissue expander is a balloon-like device made from elastic silicone rubber. It is inserted unfilled, and over time, sterile saline fluid is added by inserting a small needle through the skin to the filling port of the device. As the tissue expander fills, the tissues over the expander begin to stretch, similar to the gradual expansion of a woman's abdomen during pregnancy. The tissue expander creates a new breast shaped pocket for a breast implant.

Tissue expander placement usually occurs under general anesthesia in an operating room. Operative time is generally one to two hours. The procedure may require a brief hospital stay, or be done on an outpatient basis. Typically, you can resume normal daily activity after two to three weeks.

Because the chest skin is usually numb from the mastectomy surgery, it is possible that you may not experience pain from the placement of the tissue expander. However, you may experience feelings of pressure or discomfort after each filling of the expander, which subsides as the tissue expands. Tissue expansion typically lasts four to six months.

Placing the Breast Implant. After the tissue expander is removed, the breast implant is placed in the pocket. The surgery to replace the

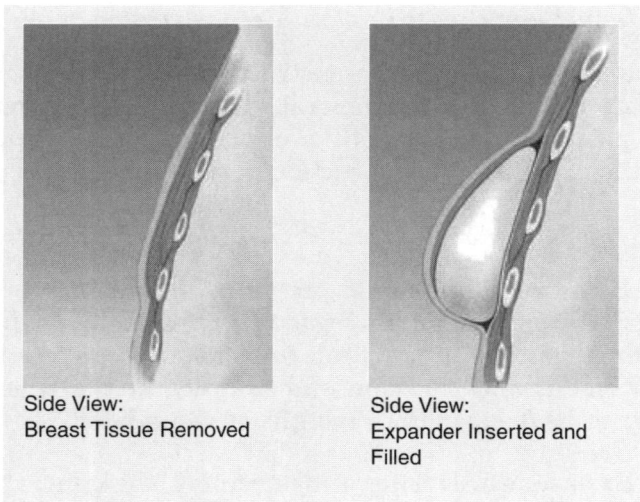

Side View:
Breast Tissue Removed

Side View:
Expander Inserted and Filled

Figure 38.1. Side view of breast with tissue removed and with expander inserted and filled.

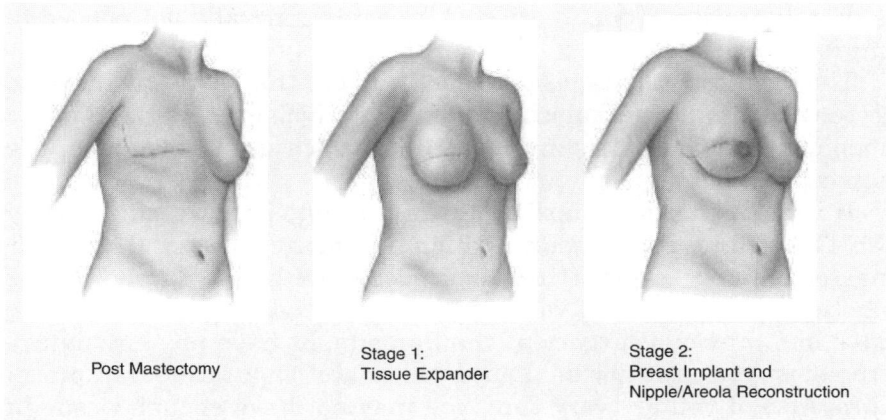

Post Mastectomy

Stage 1:
Tissue Expander

Stage 2:
Breast Implant and
Nipple/Areola Reconstruction

Figure 38.2. Breast reconstruction with implants.

tissue expander with a breast implant (implant exchange) is usually done under general anesthesia in an operating room. It may require a brief hospital stay or be done on an outpatient basis.

Breast Reconstruction without Implants: Tissue Flap Procedures

The breast can be reconstructed by surgically moving a section of skin, fat, and muscle from one area of your body to another. The section of tissue may be taken from such areas as your abdomen, upper back, upper hip, or buttocks.

The tissue flap may be left attached to the blood supply and moved to the breast area through a tunnel under the skin (a pedicled flap), or it may be removed completely and reattached to the breast area by microsurgical techniques (a free flap). Operating time is generally longer with free flaps, because of the microsurgical requirements.

Flap surgery requires a hospital stay of several days and generally a longer recovery time than implant reconstruction. Flap surgery also creates scars at the site where the flap was taken and possibly on the reconstructed breast. However, flap surgery has the advantage of being able to replace tissue in the chest area. This may be useful when the chest tissues have been damaged and are not suitable for tissue expansion. Another advantage of flap procedures over implantation

301

is that alteration of the unaffected breast is generally not needed to improve symmetry.

The most common types of tissue flaps are the TRAM (transverse rectus abdominus musculocutaneous) flap which uses tissue from the abdomen and the Latissimus dorsi flap which uses tissue from the upper back.

It is important for you to be aware that flap surgery, particularly the TRAM flap, is a major operation and more extensive than your mastectomy operation. It requires good general health and strong emotional motivation. If you are very overweight, smoke cigarettes, have had previous surgery at the flap site, or have any circulatory problems, you may not be a good candidate for a tissue flap procedure. Also, if you are very thin, you may not have enough tissue in your abdomen or back to create a breast mound with this method.

The TRAM Flap (Pedicle or Free)

During a TRAM flap procedure, the surgeon removes a section of tissue from your abdomen and moves it to your chest to reconstruct the breast. The TRAM flap is sometimes referred to as a "tummy tuck" reconstruction because it may leave the stomach area flatter.

A pedicle TRAM flap procedure typically takes three to six hours of surgery under general anesthesia; a free TRAM flap procedure generally takes longer. The TRAM procedure may require a blood

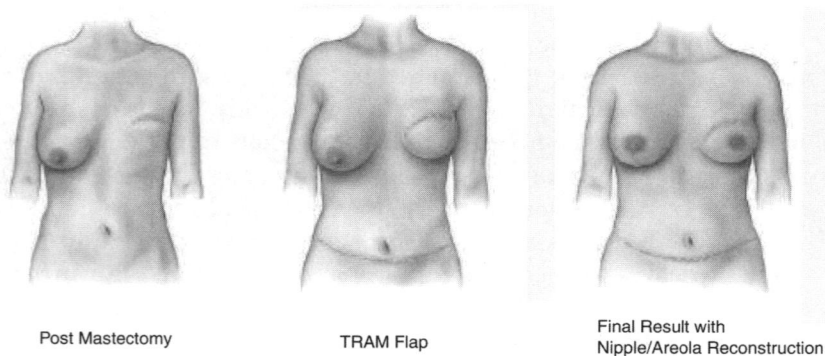

Post Mastectomy   TRAM Flap   Final Result with Nipple/Areola Reconstruction

Figure 38.3. TRAM Flap Procedure.

transfusion. Typically, the hospital stay is two to five days. You can resume normal daily activity after six to eight weeks. Some women, however, report that it takes up to one year to resume a normal lifestyle. You may have temporary or permanent muscle weakness in the abdominal area. If you are considering pregnancy after your reconstruction, you should discuss this with your surgeon. You will have a large scar on your abdomen and may also have additional scars on your reconstructed breast.

The Latissimus Dorsi Flap with or without Breast Implants

During a Latissimus Dorsi flap procedure, the surgeon moves a section of tissue from your back to your chest to reconstruct the breast. Because the Latissimus Dorsi flap is usually thinner and smaller than the TRAM flap, this procedure may be more appropriate for reconstructing a smaller breast.

The Latissimus Dorsi flap procedure typically takes two to four hours of surgery under general anesthesia. Typically, the hospital stay is two to three days. You can resume daily activity after two to three weeks. You may have some temporary or permanent muscle weakness and difficulty with movement in your back and shoulder. You will have a scar on your back, which can usually be hidden in the bra line. You may also have additional scars on your reconstructed breast.

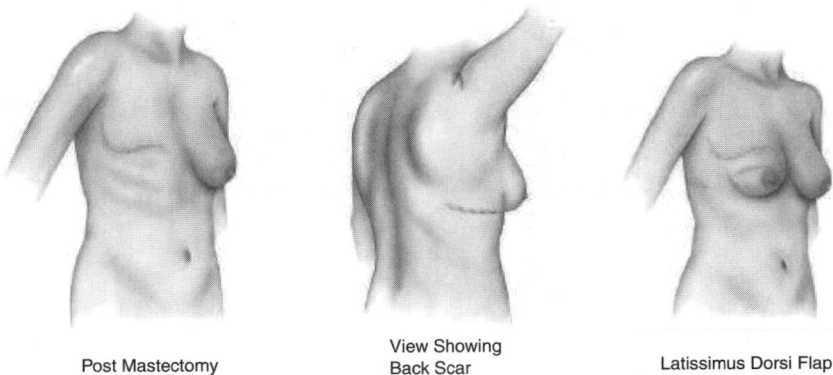

Post Mastectomy

View Showing
Back Scar

Latissimus Dorsi Flap

Figure 38.4. The Latissimus Dorsi flap procedure.

303

General Description of Breast Implant Surgery

Breast implant procedures can be performed on an outpatient (not hospitalized) basis or at a hospital. Breast implant surgery can be done under local anesthesia (only breast area numbed) or under general anesthesia (put to sleep). Breast implant surgery can last from one to several hours depending on whether the implant is inserted behind (submuscular) or in front of (subglandular) the chest muscle and whether surgery is performed on one or both breasts. If the surgery is done in a hospital, the length of the hospital stay will vary according to the type of surgery, the development of any postoperative complications, and your general health. It may also depend on the type of coverage your insurance provides. Before surgery, your doctor should discuss with you the extent of surgery, the estimated time it will take, and the choice of drugs for pain and nausea.

Your Expectations

Your consideration of breast implants should be based on realistic expectations of the outcome. You may also want to talk with women who have had this surgery at least a year ago by the same surgeon. Keep in mind, however, that there is no guarantee that your results will match those of other women.

Your results will depend on many individual factors, such as:

- your overall health
- chest structure and body shape
- healing capabilities (which may be hindered by radiation and chemotherapy, smoking, alcohol, and various medications)
- bleeding tendencies/likelihood.
- prior breast surgery(ies)
- possibility of infection
- the skill and experience of the surgical team
- the type of surgical procedure
- the type and size of implant

You will be given general or local anesthesia, and in most cases, antibiotics. The surgery may last from 1-2 hours for augmentation to several hours for reconstruction or revision.

Scarring is a natural outcome of surgery, and your doctor can describe the location, size, and appearance of the scars you can expect to have. For most women, scars will fade over time to thin lines, although the darker your skin, the more prominent the scars are likely to be. You should ask your doctor about the types of surgical procedures, where your scar will be, and what to expect after surgery.

Postoperative Care

Your doctor should describe the usual postoperative (after surgery) recovery process, the possible complications that can arise, and the expected recovery period. Following the operation, as with any surgery, some pain, swelling, bruising, and tenderness can be expected. These complications may last for a month or longer, but they should disappear with time.

Medications for pain and nausea can be prescribed. Some women may experience bleeding and some may experience fever, warmth, or redness of the breast, or other symptoms of infection. These symptoms should be reported immediately to your doctor. You should be told about wound healing and how to care for your wound. Drains may be used for a few days.

Post-operative care may involve the use of a post-operative bra, compression bandage, or jog bra for extra support and positioning while you heal. At your doctor's recommendation, you will most likely be able to return to work within a few days, although you should avoid any strenuous activities that could raise your pulse and blood pressure for at least a couple of weeks. Your doctor may also recommend breast massage exercises.

Ask your doctor about a schedule of follow-up examinations, limits on your activities, precautions you should take, and when you can return to your normal routine. (If you are enrolled in a clinical study, your doctor should give you a schedule for follow-up examinations set by the study plan.)

Breast Implant Risks

The Institute of Medicine (IOM) completed its independent, unbiased review of all past and ongoing scientific research study of silicone breast implant safety in June 1999.[1] Among the major findings from this study were that local complications with silicone breast implants were the primary safety issue with breast implants, that these have not been well studied, and that information on these complications is crucial for women deciding whether or not they want breast implant surgery. The IOM report said:

"First, reoperations and local and perioperative [right after surgery] complications are frequent enough to be a cause for concern and to justify the conclusion that they are the primary safety issue with silicone breast implants. Complications may have risks themselves, such as pain, disfigurement, and serious infection and they may lead to medical and surgical interventions, such as reoperations, that have risks. Second, risks accumulate over the lifetime of the implant, but quantitative data on this point are lacking for modern implants and deficient historically. Third, information concerning the nature and the relative high frequency of local complications and reoperations is an essential element of adequate informed consent for women undergoing breast implantation."

There are risks or complications associated with any surgical procedure, such as the effects of anesthesia, infection, swelling, redness, bleeding, and there are complications specific to breast implants. These complications are described below.

Capsular Contracture

Capsular contracture is when the scar tissue or capsule that normally forms around the implant tightens and squeezes the implant. It may be more common following infection, hematoma (collection of blood), and seroma (collection of watery portion of blood). There are four grades of capsular contracture—Baker Grades I through IV.

The Baker grading is as follows:

- Grade I the breast is normally soft and looks natural.
- Grade II the breast is a little firm but looks normal.
- Grade III the breast is firm and looks abnormal (visible distortion).
- Grade IV the breast is hard, painful, and looks abnormal (greater distortion).

Additional surgery may be needed to correct the capsular contracture. This surgery ranges from removal of the implant capsule tissue to removal (and possibly replacement) of the implant itself. Capsular contracture may happen again after this additional surgery.

In a prospective clinical study of saline-filled breast implants conducted by Mentor, the cumulative, 3-year, by patient rates of a first occurrence of capsular contracture Grades III and IV were 9% for the 1264 augmentation patients and 30% for the 416 reconstruction patients. In a prospective clinical study of saline-filled breast implants conducted by McGhan, the cumulative, 3-year, by patient rates of a first occurrence of capsular contracture Grades III and IV were 9% for the 901 augmentation patients and 25% for the 237 reconstruction patients.

A randomized controlled study comparing silicone gel-filled and saline-filled implants in women undergoing reconstruction reported a 54% contracture rate of Baker Grades III and IV in the silicone gel group after 6 months.[2]

A retrospective study by Gabriel *et al.* indicated that 131 of 749 (17.5%) women had at least one surgical procedure over an average of 7.8 years because of capsular contracture.[3] This would not include capsular contracture that may have been severe but did not result in surgery. This study included women who had implants for cosmetic and reconstruction purposes, most of whom had silicone gel-filled breast implants.

Deflation/Rupture/Leakage

Breast implants are not lifetime devices and cannot be expected to last forever. Some implants deflate or rupture in the first few months after being implanted and some deflate after several years; others are intact 10 or more years after the surgery.

Silicone Gel-Filled Breast Implants. When silicone gel-filled implants rupture, some women may notice decreased breast size, nodules (hard knots), uneven appearance of the breasts, pain or tenderness, tingling, swelling, numbness, burning, or changes in sensation. Other women may unknowingly experience a rupture without any symptoms (i.e., "silent rupture"). Magnetic resonance imaging (MRI) with equipment specifically designed for imaging the breast may be used for evaluating patients with suspected rupture or leakage of their silicone gel-filled implant.

Silicone gel which escapes the fibrotic capsule surrounding the implant may migrate away from the breast. The free silicone may cause lumps called granulomas to form in the breast or other tissues where the silicone has migrated, such as the chest wall, armpit, arm, or abdomen.

Plastic surgeons usually recommend removal of the implant if it has ruptured, even if the silicone is still enclosed within the scar tissue capsule, because the silicone gel may eventually leak into surrounding tissues. If you are considering the removal of an implant and the implantation of another one, be sure to discuss the benefits and risks with your doctor.

FDA completed a retrospective study on rupture of silicone gel-filled breast implants.[4] This study was performed in Birmingham, Alabama and included women who had their first breast implant before 1988. Women with silicone gel-filled breast implants had a MRI examination of their breasts to determine the status of their current breast implants. The 344 women who received a MRI examination had a total of 687 implants. Of the 687 implants in the study, at least two of the three study radiologists agreed that 378 implants were ruptured (55%). This means that 69% of the 344 women had at least one ruptured breast implant. Of the 344 women, 73 (21%) had extracapsular silicone gel in one or both breasts. Factors that were associated with rupture included increasing age of the implant, the implant manufacturer, and submuscular rather than subglandular location of the implant. (A summary of the findings of this study is also available on FDA's website at http://www.fda.gov/cdrh/breastimplants/studies/biinterview.pdf and http://www.fda.gov/cdrh/breastimplants/studies/birupture.pdf.)

Robinson *et al.* studied 300 women who had their implants for 1 to 25 years and had them removed for a variety of reasons.[5] Visible signs of rupture in 51% of the women studied were found. Severe silicone leakage (silicone outside the implant without visible tears or holes) was seen in another 20%. Robinson *et al.* also noted that the chance of rupture increases as the implant ages.

Other studies indicate that silicone may escape the capsule in 11-23% of rupture cases.[6,7,8,9]

Saline-Filled Breast Implants. Saline-filled breast implants deflate when the saline solution leaks either through an unsealed or damaged valve or through a break in the implant shell. Implant deflation can occur immediately or progressively over a period of days and is noticed by loss of size or shape of the implant. Some implants deflate or rupture in the first few months after being implanted and some deflate after several years. You should also be aware that the breast implant may wear out over time and deflate. Additional surgery is needed to remove deflated implants.

In a prospective clinical study conducted by Mentor, the cumulative, 3-year, by patient rates of a first occurrence of deflation were 3% for 1264 augmentation patients and 9% for 416 reconstruction patients.

In a prospective clinical study conducted by McGhan, the cumulative, 3-year, by patient rates of a first occurrence of deflation were 5% for the 901 augmentation patients and 6% for the 237 reconstruction patients.

A retrospective study of saline breast implants by Gutowski *et al.* indicates that 10.1% of women followed for an average of 6 years had at least one implant deflated.[10]

For silicone gel and saline-filled implants, some causes of rupture or deflation include:

- damage by surgical instruments during surgery
- overfilling or underfilling of the implant with saline solution (specific only to saline-filled breast implants)
- capsular contracture
- closed capsulotomy (described below)
- stresses such as trauma or intense physical manipulation
- excessive compression during mammographic imaging
- placement through umbilical incision site
- injury to the breast
- normal aging of the implant
- unknown/unexplained reasons

Closed capsulotomy is a technique used to relieve capsular contracture. It involves manually squeezing the breast to break the hard capsule. This has been implicated as a possible cause of breast implant rupture. Closed capsulotomy is not recommended by breast implant manufacturers.

Additional Surgeries

You should understand there is a high chance that you will need to have additional surgery at some point to replace or remove your implant(s) due to problems such as deflation, capsular contracture, infection, shifting, and calcium deposits. Many women decide to have the implants replaced, but some women do not. Those who do not have their implants replaced may have cosmetically undesirable dimpling and/or puckering of the breast following removal of the implant.

In a prospective clinical study of saline-filled breast implants conducted by Mentor, the cumulative, 3-year, by patient rates of a first occurrence of additional surgeries were 13% for the 1264 augmentation patients and 40% for the 416 reconstruction patients. In a prospective clinical study of saline-filled breast implants conducted by McGhan, the cumulative, 3-year, by patient rates of a first occurrence of additional surgeries were 21% for the 901 augmentation patients and 39% for the 237 reconstruction patients.

A retrospective study by Gabriel *et al.* shows that 24% of women with breast implants experience adverse events resulting in surgery during the first five years after implantation (silicone and saline implants were studied together).[11] According to this study, about 1 in 3 women getting breast implants for reconstruction may need a second surgery within five years, and about 1 in 8 women getting breast implants for augmentation may need a second surgery within five years. These additional surgeries may result in the loss of breast tissue.

Pain

Women may feel pain of varying severity (degrees) and duration (length of time) following breast implant surgery. In addition, improper size, placement, surgical technique, or capsular contracture may result in pain associated with nerve entrapment or interference with muscle motion. You should tell your doctor if you have pain.

Dissatisfaction with Cosmetic Results

Dissatisfying results such as wrinkling, asymmetry, implant displacement (shifting), incorrect size, unanticipated shape, implant palpability, scar deformity, hypertrophic (irregular, raised scar) scarring, and/or sloshing may occur. Careful surgical planning and technique can minimize, but not always prevent, such results.

Additionally, for saline-filled implants that have a valve, you also might be able to feel the valve of the implant with your hand.

Repeated surgeries to improve the appearance of the breasts and/or to remove ruptured or deflated prostheses may result in an unsatisfactory cosmetic outcome.

Infection

Infection can occur with any surgery. Most infections resulting from surgery appear within a few days to weeks after the operation. However, infection is possible at any time after surgery. Infections with an implant present are harder to treat than infections in normal body tissues. If an infection does not respond to antibiotics, the implant may have to be removed, and another implant may be placed after the infection has cleared up.

In rare instances, Toxic Shock Syndrome has been noted in women after breast implant surgery, and it is a life-threatening condition. Symptoms include sudden fever, vomiting, diarrhea, fainting, dizziness, and/or sunburn-like rash. A doctor should be seen immediately for diagnosis and treatment.

Hematoma/Seroma

Hematoma is a collection of blood inside a body cavity, and seroma is a collection of the watery portion of the blood around the implant or around the incision. Postoperative hematoma and seroma may contribute to infection and/or capsular contracture. Swelling, pain, and bruising may result. If a hematoma occurs, it will usually be soon after surgery; however, this can also occur at any time after injury to the breast. While the body absorbs small hematomas and seromas, large ones will require the placement of surgical drains for proper healing. A small scar can result from surgical draining. Implant deflation/rupture can occur from surgical draining if damage to the implant occurs during the draining procedure.

Changes in Nipple and Breast Sensation

Feeling in the nipple and breast can increase or decrease after implant surgery. The range of changes varies from intense sensitivity to no feeling in the nipple or breast following surgery. Changes in feeling can be temporary or permanent and may affect sexual response or the ability to nurse a baby.

Calcium Deposits in the Tissue Around the Implant

Deposits of calcium can be seen on mammograms and can be mistaken for possible cancer, resulting in additional surgery to biopsy and/ or remove the implant to distinguish these deposits from cancer. Calcium deposits may be felt as nodules (hard knots) under the skin around the implant.

Delayed Wound Healing

In some cases, the incision site fails to heal normally or takes longer to heal.

311

Extrusion

An unstable or compromised tissue covering and/or interruption of wound healing may result in extrusion of the implant, which is when the breast implant comes through the skin. The additional surgery needed to correct this complication can result in unacceptable scarring or loss of breast tissue.

Necrosis

Necrosis is the formation of dead tissue around the implant. This may prevent wound healing and require surgical correction and/or implant removal. Permanent scar and/or deformity may occur following necrosis. Factors associated with increased necrosis include infection, use of steroids in the surgical pocket, smoking, chemotherapy/radiation, and excessive heat or cold therapy.

Breast Tissue Atrophy/Chest Wall Deformity

The pressure of the breast implant may cause the breast tissue to thin and shrink. This can occur while implants are still in place or following implant removal without replacement.

Interference with Mammography

Interference with mammography due to breast implants may delay or hinder the early detection of breast cancer either by hiding suspicious lesions (wounds or injuries or tumors) or by making it more difficult to include them in the image. Implants increase the difficulty of both taking and reading mammograms. Some women who undergo reconstruction will have some breast tissue remaining, and some have all of their breast tissue removed. It is important that a woman with breast tissue remaining continue to have mammography of that breast, as well as of the other breast, to detect breast cancer.

Mammography requires breast compression (hard pressure) that could contribute to implant rupture. In addition to special care taken by the technologist to reduce the risk of implant rupture during this compression, other techniques are used to maximize what is seen of the breast tissue during mammography. These techniques are called breast implant displacement views, Eklund displacement views, or Eklund views, after the radiologist who developed them. These special implant displacement views are done in addition to those views done during routine mammograms.

Because of the extra views and time needed, women with implants should always inform the receptionist or scheduler that they have breast implants when making an appointment for mammography. They should also tell the radiology technologist about the presence of implants before mammography is performed. This is to make sure that the technologist uses these special displacement techniques and takes extra care when compressing the breasts to avoid rupturing the implant.

The displacement procedure involves pushing the implant back and gently pulling the breast tissue into view. Several factors affect the success of this special technique in imaging the breast tissue in women with breast implants. The location of the implant, the hardness of the capsular contracture, the size of the breast tissue compared to the implant, and other factors may affect how well the breast tissue can be imaged. Also, a radiologist may find it difficult to distinguish calcium deposits in the scar tissue around the implant from a breast tumor when he or she is interpreting the mammogram. Occasionally, it is necessary to remove and examine a small amount of tissue (biopsy) to see whether or not it is cancerous. This can frequently be done without removing the implant.

Galactorrhea

Sometimes after breast implant surgery, you may begin producing breast milk. In some cases, the milk production stops spontaneously or when medication is given to suppress milk production. In other cases, removal of the implant(s) may be needed.

Questions to Ask Your Surgeon about Breast Reconstruction

The following list of questions may help to remind you of topics to discuss with your doctor. You may have additional questions as well.

1. What are all my options for breast reconstruction?

2. What are the risks and complications of each type of breast reconstruction surgery and how common are they?

3. What if my cancer recurs or occurs in the other breast?

4. Will reconstruction interfere with my cancer treatment?

5. How many steps are there in each procedure, and what are they?

6. How long will it take to complete my reconstruction?

7. How much experience do you have with each procedure?

8. Do you have before and after photos I can look at for each procedure and what results are reasonable for me?

9. What will my scars look like?

10. What kind of changes in my implanted breast can I expect over time?

11. What kind of changes in my implanted breast can I expect with pregnancy?

12. What are my options if I am dissatisfied with the cosmetic outcome of my implanted breast?

13. Would you suggest other patients I could talk to about their experiences?

14. What is the estimated total cost of each procedure?

15. How much pain or discomfort will I feel, and for how long?

16. How long will I be in the hospital?

17. Will I need blood transfusions, and can I donate my own blood?

18. When will I be able to resume my normal activity (or sexual activity, or athletic activity)?

Notes

1. *Safety of Silicone Breast Implants*. IOM Report, Institute of Medicine National Academy Press, Washington, D.C. 2000.

2. Asplund, O. Capsular contracture in silicone gel and saline-filled breast implants after reconstruction. *Plast Reconstru Surg* 1984;73:270-5.

3. Gabriel SE, Woods JE, O'Fallon WM, Beard CM, Kurland LT, Melton LJ. Complications leading to surgery after breast implantation. *New Engl J Med* 1997; 336:679-682.

4. Brown SL, Middleton MS, Berg WA, Soo MS, Pennello G. Prevalence of rupture of silicone gel breast implants in a

population of women in Birmingham, Alabama. *American Journal of Roentgenology* 2000;175:1-8.

5. Robinson OG, Bradley EL, Wilson DS. Analysis of explanted silicone implants: a report of 300 patients. *Ann Plast Surg* 1995; 34:1-7.

6. Vinnik CA. Migratory silicon—clinical aspects. Silicone in Medical Devices—Conference Proceedings. 1991 February 1-2; Baltimore, MD: U.S. Department of Health and Human Services, FDA Publication No. 92-4249 (p.59-67).

7. Duffy MJ, Woods JE. Health risks of failed silicone gel breast implants: a 30-year clinical experience. *Plast Reconstr Surg* 1994;94:295-299.

8. Berg WA, Caskey CI, Hamper UM, Kuhlman JE, Anderson ND, Chang BW, Sheth S, Zerhouni EA. Single- and double-lumen silicone breast implant integrity: Prospective evaluation of MR and US criteria. *Radiology* 1995;197:45-52.

9. Gorczyca DP, Schneider E, DeBruhl ND, Foo TKF, Ahn CY, Sayre JW, Shaw WW, Bassett LW. Silicone breast implant rupture: Comparison between three-point Dixon and fast spin-echo MR imaging. *AJR* 1994;162:305-310.

10. Gutowski KA, Mesna GT, Cunningham BL. Saline-filled Breast Implants: A Plastic Surgery Educational Foundation Multicenter Outcomes Study. *Plastic Reconstructive Surgery*. 1997 (100): 1019-27.

11. Gabriel SE, Woods JE, O'Fallon WM, Beard CM, Kurland LT, Melton LJ. Complications leading to surgery after breast implantatation. *New Engl J Med* 1997; 336:679-682.

Chapter 39

Questions and Answers about Adjuvant Therapy for Breast Cancer

Researchers have been studying breast cancer for many years to learn how best to treat this disease. They have given special attention to ways to prevent breast cancer from recurring (returning) after primary treatment.

Scientists once thought that breast cancer metastasizes (spreads) first to nearby tissue and underarm lymph nodes before spreading to other parts of the body. They now believe that cancer cells may break away from the primary tumor in the breast and begin to metastasize even when the disease is in an early stage.

Adjuvant therapy is treatment given in addition to the primary therapy to kill any cancer cells that may have spread, even if the spread cannot be detected by radiologic or laboratory tests. Studies have shown that adjuvant therapy for breast cancer may increase the chance of long-term survival by preventing a recurrence.

What types of primary therapy are used for breast cancer?

Primary therapy for breast cancer generally involves lumpectomy and radiation therapy or modified radical mastectomy. A lumpectomy is the removal of the primary breast tumor and a small amount of

This chapter contains text from "Questions and Answers about Adjuvant Therapy for Breast Cancer," Cancer Facts, National Cancer Institute (NCI), April 7, 2000, and "NIH Consensus Panel Recommends a Range of Adjuvant Therapies for Women with Breast Cancer," National Institutes of Health (NIH) News Release, November 3, 2000.

surrounding tissue. Usually, most of the underarm lymph nodes are also removed. A lumpectomy is followed by radiation treatment to the breast. A modified radical mastectomy is the removal of the whole breast, most of the lymph nodes under the arm, and often the lining over the chest muscles. The smaller of the two chest muscles is sometimes taken out to help in removing the lymph nodes.

Doctors are evaluating a new procedure, called sentinel lymph node biopsy or sentinel node biopsy, in which only a single lymph node is removed and tested to determine if the breast cancer has spread to lymph nodes under the arm. Clinical trials (research studies with humans) are in progress to determine the role of this procedure in the treatment of breast cancer.

What types of adjuvant therapy are used for breast cancer?

Because the principal purpose of adjuvant therapy is to kill any cancer cells that may have spread, treatment is usually systemic (uses substances that travel through the bloodstream, reaching and affecting cancer cells all over the body). Adjuvant therapy for breast cancer involves chemotherapy or hormone therapy, either alone or in combination:

- Adjuvant chemotherapy is the use of drugs to kill cancer cells. Research has shown that using chemotherapy as adjuvant therapy for early stage breast cancer helps to prevent the original cancer from returning. Adjuvant chemotherapy is usually a combination of anticancer drugs, which has been shown to be more effective than a single anticancer drug.

- Adjuvant hormone therapy deprives cancer cells of the female hormone estrogen, which some breast cancer cells need to grow. Most often, adjuvant hormone therapy is treatment with the drug tamoxifen. Research has shown that when tamoxifen is used as adjuvant therapy for early stage breast cancer, it helps to prevent the original cancer from returning and also helps to prevent the development of new cancers in the other breast.

The ovaries are the main source of estrogen prior to menopause. For premenopausal women with breast cancer, adjuvant hormone therapy may involve tamoxifen to deprive the cancer cells of estrogen. Drugs to suppress the production of estrogen by the ovaries are under investigation. Alternatively, surgery may be performed to remove the ovaries.

Although this chapter sheet focuses on systemic adjuvant therapy, radiation therapy is sometimes used as a local adjuvant treatment. Radiation therapy is considered adjuvant treatment when it is given before or after a mastectomy. Such treatment is intended to destroy breast cancer cells that have spread to nearby parts of the body, such as the chest wall or lymph nodes. Radiation therapy is part of primary therapy, not adjuvant therapy, when it follows breast-sparing surgery.

What are prognostic factors, and what do they have to do with adjuvant therapy?

Prognostic factors are characteristics of breast tumors that help predict whether the disease is likely to recur. Doctors consider these factors when they are deciding which patients might benefit from adjuvant therapy.

Several prognostic factors are commonly used to plan breast cancer treatment:

- *Tumor size.* Prognosis (probable outcome of the disease) is closely linked to tumor size. In general, patients with small tumors (2 centimeters [a little more than three-quarters of an inch] or less in diameter) have a better prognosis than do patients with larger tumors (especially those that are more than 5 centimeters [2 inches] in diameter).

- *Lymph node involvement.* Lymph nodes in the underarm are a common site of breast cancer spread. Doctors usually remove some of the underarm lymph nodes to determine whether they contain cancer cells. If cancer is found, the nodes are said to be "positive." If the lymph nodes are free of cancer, the nodes are said to be "negative." Breast cancer that is node-positive is more likely to recur than cancer that is node-negative because, if cancer cells have spread to the lymph nodes, it is more likely that they have also spread elsewhere in the body.

- *Hormone receptor status.* Cells in the breast contain receptors for the female hormones estrogen and progesterone. These receptors allow the breast tissue to grow or change in response to changing hormone levels.

Research has shown that about two-thirds of all breast cancers contain significant levels of estrogen receptors. These tumors are said to be estrogen receptor positive (ER+). About 40 percent

319

to 50 percent of all breast cancers have progesterone receptors. These tumors are said to be progesterone receptor positive (PR+).

ER+ tumors tend to grow less aggressively than ER- tumors. The result is a better prognosis for patients with ER+ tumors.

- *Histologic grade.* This term refers to how much the tumor cells resemble normal cells when viewed under the microscope. Tumors composed of cells that closely resemble normal breast cells and structures are called well-differentiated. Tumors with cells that bear little or no resemblance to normal breast cells are called poorly differentiated. Tumors that have "in between" cells are called moderately differentiated. For most types of invasive breast cancer, patients who have tumors with cells that are well-differentiated tend to have a better prognosis.

- *Proliferative capacity of a tumor.* This factor refers to the rate at which the cancer cells divide to form more cells. Cells that have a high proliferative capacity divide more often and are more aggressive (fast growing) than those with a low proliferative capacity. Patients who have tumors with cells that have a low proliferative capacity (that is, divide less often and grow more slowly) tend to have a better prognosis.

  Scientists estimate the proliferative capacity of the tumor using such tests as flow cytometry, which includes the S-phase fraction measurement. The S-phase fraction is the percentage of tumor cells that are dividing. Tumors with a high S-phase fraction tend to have an increased risk of recurrence.

- *Oncogene activation.* The activation of an oncogene (a gene that causes or promotes unrestrained cell growth) can make normal cells become abnormal or convert a normal cell into a tumor cell. Patients whose tumor cells contain an oncogene called HER-2/neu, also called erb B-2, may be more likely to have a recurrence. Some research studies suggest that HER-2/neu may be associated with resistance to certain anticancer drugs; however, more research is needed.

Who is given adjuvant therapy?

Although prognostic factors provide important information about the risk of recurrence, they do not enable doctors to predict exactly who will be cured by primary therapy and who may benefit from adjuvant therapy. Decisions about adjuvant therapy for breast cancer must be made on an individual basis, taking into account the prognostic factors described above, the woman's menopausal status (whether she has gone through menopause), her general health, and her personal preference. This complicated decision-making process is best carried out by consulting an oncologist, a doctor who specializes in cancer treatment.

Clinical trials are in progress to learn how to identify women most likely to benefit from adjuvant therapy and those who do not require this treatment.

When is adjuvant therapy started?

Adjuvant therapy usually begins within 6 weeks after surgery, based on the results of clinical trials in which the therapy was started within that time period. Doctors do not know how effective adjuvant therapy is in reducing the chance of recurrence when treatment is started at a later time.

How is adjuvant therapy given, and how long does it last?

Chemotherapy is given by mouth or by injection into a blood vessel. Either way, the drugs enter the bloodstream and travel throughout the body. Chemotherapy is given in cycles: a treatment period followed by a recovery period, then another treatment period, and so on. Most patients receive treatment in an outpatient part of the hospital or at the doctor's office. Adjuvant chemotherapy usually lasts for 3 to 6 months.

In adjuvant hormone therapy, tamoxifen is taken orally. Tamoxifen enters the bloodstream and travels throughout the body. Most women take tamoxifen every day for 5 years. Studies have indicated that taking tamoxifen for longer than 5 years is not any more effective than taking it for 5 years. Premenopausal women may receive hormones by injection to suppress ovarian function. Alternatively, surgery can be performed to remove the ovaries.

What are some of the side effects of adjuvant therapy, and what can be done to help manage them?

The side effects of chemotherapy depend mainly on the drugs the patient receives. As with other types of treatment, side effects vary from person to person. In general, anticancer drugs affect rapidly dividing cells. These include blood cells, which fight infection, cause the blood to clot, and carry oxygen to all parts of the body. When blood cells are affected by anticancer drugs, patients are more likely to get infections, bruise or bleed easily, and may have less energy during treatment and for some time afterward. Cells in hair follicles and cells that line the digestive tract also divide rapidly. As a result of chemotherapy, patients may lose their hair and may have other side effects, such as loss of appetite, nausea, vomiting, diarrhea, or mouth sores.

Doctors can prescribe medications to help control nausea and vomiting caused by chemotherapy. They also monitor patients for any signs of other problems and may adjust the dose or schedule of treatment if problems arise. In addition, doctors advise women who have a lowered resistance to infection because of low blood cell counts to avoid crowds and people who are sick or have colds. The side effects of chemotherapy are generally short-term problems. They gradually go away during the recovery part of the chemotherapy cycle or after the treatment is over.

In general, the side effects of tamoxifen are similar to some of the symptoms of menopause. The most common side effects are hot flashes, vaginal discharge, and nausea. As is the case with menopause, not all women who take tamoxifen have these symptoms. Most of these side effects do not require medical attention.

Doctors carefully monitor women taking tamoxifen for any signs of more serious side effects. Women taking tamoxifen, particularly those who are receiving chemotherapy along with tamoxifen, have a greater risk of developing a blood clot. The risk of having a blood clot due to tamoxifen is similar to the risk of a blood clot when taking estrogen replacement therapy. Women who are taking tamoxifen also have an increased risk of developing cancer of the uterus. They should talk with their doctor about having regular pelvic exams and should be examined promptly if they have any abnormal vaginal bleeding.

Careful studies have shown that the risks of adjuvant therapy for breast cancer are outweighed by the benefit of the treatment—increasing the chance of survival. Still, it is important for women to share any concerns they may have about their treatment or side effects with their doctor or other health care provider.

More information and printed materials about the side effects of chemotherapy and tamoxifen can be obtained from the National Cancer Institute's Cancer Information Service.

How are doctors and scientists trying to answer questions about adjuvant therapy for breast cancer?

Doctors and scientists are conducting research studies called clinical trials to learn how to treat breast cancer more effectively. In these studies, researchers compare two or more groups of patients who receive different treatments. Such studies can show whether new treatments are more or less effective than standard ones and how the side effects compare. People who participate in clinical trials have the first opportunity to benefit from new treatments while helping to increase medical knowledge.

Women with breast cancer who are interested in taking part in a clinical trial can ask their doctor whether this would be appropriate for them. Information about current clinical trials can be obtained from the National Cancer Institute (NCI)-supported Cancer Information Service (1-800-422-6237) or from the NCI's cancerTrials™ Web site at http://cancertrials.nci.nih.gov on the Internet.

NIH Consensus Panel Recommends a Range of Adjuvant Therapies for Women with Breast Cancer

Treatment with a combination of chemotherapy drugs improves survival and should be recommended for most women with localized breast cancer, according to a consensus panel convened by the National Institutes of Health. The panel also recommended hormonal therapy for women whose tumors have estrogen receptors, and radiation therapy for women who have had mastectomies and who are at high risk for recurrence of cancer.

These and other recommendations emerged from a 3-day NIH Consensus Development Conference on Adjuvant Therapy for Breast Cancer held November 1-3, 2000 at the NIH in Bethesda, Maryland. Adjuvant therapy—treatments used in addition to surgery to kill cancer cells that may have begun to spread to other organs—includes chemotherapy and hormonal therapy, typically tamoxifen. In addition to these systemic therapies, radiation therapy is sometimes used as a local adjuvant treatment to help destroy breast cancer cells that have spread to nearby tissues.

"Clinical trials over the past ten years have contributed an enormous amount of new information about adjuvant therapies," said panel chair Patricia Eifel, M.D., Professor of Radiation Oncology at M.D. Anderson Cancer Center in Houston. "Women with breast cancer have more treatment options and a better chance of surviving their disease than ever before. At the same time, making treatment decisions has become a more complex process for them and their physicians due to a growing list of effective options."

The conference brought together national and international experts to clarify, for clinicians, patients, and the general public, key questions regarding the selection of treatments, quality of life, and new research directions in adjuvant therapy.

Dr. Eifel and her colleagues noted that decisions about the choice of adjuvant therapy should be based on age, tumor size, presence or absence of hormone receptors, presence or absence of cancerous lymph nodes, and other generally accepted factors. New technologies and molecular markers hold potential but require further study.

Hormonal therapy was recommended by the panel for women whose breast tumors contain estrogen receptors, regardless of age, menopausal status, tumor size, or whether the cancer has spread to nearby lymph nodes. Five years of tamoxifen is currently the standard adjuvant hormonal therapy.

The panel noted that no data support the use of tamoxifen for longer than five years outside of a clinical trial but that this is an important area for investigation. The panel emphasized that hormonal therapy is not indicated for women whose tumors do not have hormone receptors. The panel recommended chemotherapy with a combination of drugs for most pre- and post-menopausal women regardless of lymph node involvement or estrogen receptor status. Including anthracycline drugs as part of chemotherapy regimens produces a small but statistically significant survival advantage over regimens that do not contain anthracyclines. However, there are not enough data to support the routine use of taxanes or dose-intensive chemotherapy.

Women who have undergone mastectomy and who have four or more cancerous lymph nodes or an advanced primary tumor benefit from post-surgical radiation, the panel concluded. The panel added that it is unclear whether women with one to three cancerous lymph nodes benefit from radiation therapy and that this question should be tested in a randomized clinical trial.

Adjuvant treatments often involve serious short- and long-term side effects such as premature menopause, weight gain, mild memory loss, and fatigue. The panel recommended that selected trials of adjuvant therapy include quality-of-life measures. It emphasized that long term follow-up of women in these trials is important to fully understand the effects of adjuvant therapies. It also endorsed continued development of decision-making tools to help patients and their physicians weigh the risks and benefits of adjuvant treatments.

Among its other recommendations for future research, the panel called for carefully designed studies of:

• combined hormonal therapy

- hormonal therapy versus chemotherapy in premenopausal women whose tumors have estrogen receptors

- high dose chemotherapy

- taxanes

- factors that predict the effectiveness of treatments in individual patients

- new drugs, including trastuzumab and bisphosphonates

- radiation techniques that reduce the dose to normal tissue such as the heart and lungs

- the effectiveness and side effects of adjuvant therapies in women older than 70

The National Cancer Institute and the NIH Office of Medical Applications of Research sponsored the conference. Cosponsors included the National Institute of Nursing Research and the NIH Office of Research on Women's Health.

The full NIH Consensus Statement on Adjuvant Therapy for Breast Cancer is available by calling 1-888-NIH-CONSENSUS (1-888-644-2667) or by visiting the NIH Consensus Development Program Web site at http://consensus.nih.gov.

The consensus statement is the report of an independent panel and is not a policy statement of the NIH or the Federal Government. The NIH Consensus Development Program was established in 1977 to resolve in an unbiased manner controversial topics in medicine. To date, NIH has conducted 113 such conferences addressing a wide range of controversial medical issues important to health care providers, patients, and the general public.

Chapter 40

Herceptin (Trastuzumab)

Questions and Answers about Herceptin-R (Trastuzumab)

What is Herceptin? How does it work?

Herceptin (trastuzumab) is a monoclonal antibody. It belongs to a group of drugs made in the laboratory that are designed to attack specific cancer cells. Herceptin is given intravenously (by injection into a blood vessel) to treat some breast cancers. Genentech Inc., located in South San Francisco, manufactures Herceptin.

Herceptin targets cancer cells that "overexpress," or make too much of, a protein called HER-2 or erb B2, which is found on the surface of cancer cells. Herceptin slows or stops the growth of these cells. Herceptin is used only to treat cancers that overexpress the HER-2 protein.

Approximately 25 percent of breast cancers overexpress HER-2. These tumors tend to grow faster and are generally more likely to recur (come back) than tumors that do not overproduce HER-2.

The amount of HER-2 protein in the tumor is measured in the laboratory using a scale from 0 (negative) to 3+ (strongly positive). The result helps the doctor determine whether a patient might benefit from treatment with Herceptin. Patients whose tumors are strongly positive for HER-2 protein overexpression (a score of 3+ on the laboratory

"Questions and Answers about Herceptin (Trastuzumab)," Cancer Facts, National Cancer Institute, August 2000.

test) are more likely to benefit. There is no evidence of benefit in patients whose tumors do not overexpress HER-2 (a score of 0 or 1+ on the laboratory test).

How is Herceptin currently used in the treatment of cancer?

Herceptin is approved by the U.S. Food and Drug Administration (FDA) for the treatment of metastatic breast cancer (breast cancer that has spread to other parts of the body). Herceptin can be given by itself or along with chemotherapy.

Researchers continue to study Herceptin in clinical trials (research studies with people). These studies can show whether new treatments are more or less effective than standard ones and how the side effects compare.

What are some of the common side effects of Herceptin?

Side effects that most commonly occur during the first treatment with Herceptin include fever and/or chills. Other possible side effects include pain, weakness, nausea, vomiting, diarrhea, headaches, difficulty breathing, and rashes. These side effects generally become less severe after the first treatment with Herceptin.

Patients who receive Herceptin along with chemotherapy may experience side effects that are different from those of patients who take Herceptin by itself. Patients should discuss any concerns about the side effects of treatment with their doctor. The doctor may be able to make suggestions for managing side effects.

Can Herceptin cause any serious side effects?

Herceptin can cause damage to the heart muscle that can lead to heart failure. Symptoms of heart failure include shortness of breath, difficulty breathing, a fast or irregular heartbeat, increased cough, and swelling of the feet or lower legs.

Herceptin can also affect the lungs, causing severe or life-threatening breathing problems that require immediate medical attention.

Herceptin may also cause allergic reactions that can be severe or life-threatening. These reactions can involve a drop in blood pressure, shortness of breath, rashes, and wheezing. These reactions may be more common in patients who already have breathing difficulties or lung disease.

Because of these potentially life-threatening side effects, patients are evaluated carefully for any heart or lung problems before starting treatment and are monitored closely during treatment. Patients who develop any problems during or after treatment should call the doctor immediately or go to the nearest emergency care facility.

How do scientists know whether Herceptin is effective?

The safety and effectiveness of Herceptin were studied in two clinical trials with women whose metastatic breast cancers produced excess amounts of HER-2. In one clinical trial, women received either Herceptin and chemotherapy or chemotherapy alone. The women who received Herceptin and chemotherapy had slower tumor growth, greater reduction in tumor size, and longer survival than the women who received chemotherapy alone. In another trial, women received Herceptin alone. In 15 percent of these women, the tumor got smaller or disappeared.

Is Herceptin being studied to treat nonmetastatic breast cancer?

Yes. The National Cancer Institute (NCI) is sponsoring two large, multicenter phase III clinical trials of Herceptin as adjuvant therapy to treat node-positive breast cancer; this is breast cancer that has spread to the lymph nodes under the arm (regional lymph nodes), but not to other parts of the body. These trials will take place in hospitals and cancer centers around the country. Adjuvant therapy is treatment given in addition to the primary therapy to kill any cancer cells that may have spread, even if the spread cannot be detected by radiologic or laboratory tests.

- The National Surgical Adjuvant Breast and Bowel Project (NSABP) is comparing chemotherapy to chemotherapy plus Herceptin for patients with node-positive breast cancer. Patients will be divided randomly into two groups. One group will receive doxorubicin (Adriamycin-R) and cyclophosphamide (Cytoxan-R) followed by paclitaxel (Taxol-R). The second group will receive doxorubicin and cyclophosphamide followed by paclitaxel and Herceptin. This trial will enroll 2,700 patients.

- The North Central Cancer Treatment Group (NCCTG) is leading an Intergroup study to compare three different treatments in patients with node-positive breast cancer. The three regimens are as follows: 1) doxorubicin and cyclophosphamide followed by weekly paclitaxel treatments; 2) doxorubicin and cyclophosphamide followed by weekly paclitaxel and Herceptin treatments; or 3) doxorubicin and cyclophosphamide, followed by weekly paclitaxel treatments, followed by Herceptin. This trial will enroll 3,000 patients.

Patients who are interested in receiving Herceptin as adjuvant therapy for breast cancer should consider participating in a clinical trial. For more information about these and other clinical trials, patients and doctors may call the Cancer Information Service (CIS) or visit the NCI's cancerTrials-R Web site on the Internet.

Cancer Information Service (CIS)
Telephone: 1-800-422-6237
TTY: 1-800-332-8615
Internet: http://cancertrials.nci.nih.gov

Is Herceptin under study for cancers other than breast cancer?

Yes. Herceptin is also being studied in clinical trials for other types of cancer, including cancers of the lung, pancreas, salivary gland, colon, prostate, and ovaries. About 30 to 40 percent of patients with these types of cancer have tumors that overexpress the HER-2 protein and will be possible candidates for clinical trials with Herceptin.

Researchers are exploring the use of Herceptin by itself and in combination with anticancer drugs. They are also investigating the use of Herceptin with other types of cancer treatment.

Is the NCI supporting studies of other anti-HER-2 antibodies?

Yes. The NCI is involved in early trials of other monoclonal antibodies directed against the HER-2 protein. For example, several phase I studies sponsored by NCI are testing an HER-2 antibody, designated 520C9xH22 or MDXH-210, produced by the Medarex Corporation in Annandale, New Jersey. Another NCI-sponsored study is evaluating a different HER-2 antibody, 2B1, from Chiron Corporation in Emeryville, California.

Chapter 41

Tamoxifen

Questions and Answers about Tamoxifen

What is tamoxifen?

Tamoxifen is a medication in pill form that interferes with the activity of estrogen (a female hormone). Tamoxifen has been used for more than 20 years to treat patients with advanced breast cancer. It has also been used as adjuvant, or additional, therapy following surgery or radiation therapy for early stage breast cancer. Tamoxifen has recently been found to reduce the incidence of breast cancer in women at high risk of developing this disease. Tamoxifen continues to be studied for the prevention of breast cancer. It is also being studied in the treatment of several other types of cancer.

How does tamoxifen work on breast cancer?

Estrogen promotes the growth of breast cancer cells. Tamoxifen works against the effects of estrogen on these cells. It is often called an "anti-estrogen." As a treatment for breast cancer, the drug slows or stops the growth of cancer cells that are already present in the body. As adjuvant therapy, tamoxifen has been shown to help prevent the original breast cancer from returning and also prevent the development of new cancers in the opposite breast.

This chapter includes text from "Questions and Answers about Tamoxifen," Cancer Facts, National Cancer Institute (NCI), June 1999; and "Tamoxifen Approved for DCIS: More Trials On the Way," Cancer Trials, National Cancer Institute, August 2000.

Are there other beneficial effects of tamoxifen?

While tamoxifen acts against the effects of estrogen in breast tissue, it acts like estrogen in other body systems. This means that women who take tamoxifen may derive many of the beneficial effects of menopausal estrogen replacement therapy, such as a lowering of blood cholesterol and a slowing of bone loss (osteoporosis).

Can tamoxifen prevent breast cancer?

Research has shown that when tamoxifen is used as adjuvant therapy for early stage breast cancer, it not only prevents the recurrence of the original cancer but also prevents the development of new cancers in the opposite breast. Based on these findings, the National Cancer Institute (NCI) funded a large research study, the Breast Cancer Prevention Trial (BCPT) conducted by the National Surgical Adjuvant Breast and Bowel Project (NSABP), to determine the usefulness of tamoxifen in preventing breast cancer in women who have an increased risk of developing the disease. Results from this study showed a 49 percent reduction in diagnoses of invasive breast cancer among women who took tamoxifen. Women who took tamoxifen also had 50 percent fewer diagnoses of noninvasive breast tumors, such as ductal or lobular carcinoma in situ. However, there are some risks associated with tamoxifen, some even life threatening. The decision to take tamoxifen is an individual one in which the woman and her doctor must carefully consider the benefits and risks of therapy.

Women with an increased risk of developing breast cancer have the option to consider taking tamoxifen to reduce their chance of developing this disease. They may also consider participating in the Study of Tamoxifen and Raloxifene that will compare tamoxifen with the osteoporosis prevention drug raloxifene, which could have similar breast cancer risk reduction properties, but might be associated with fewer adverse effects.

At this time, there is no evidence that tamoxifen is beneficial for women who do not have an increased risk of breast cancer.

What is the Study of Tamoxifen and Raloxifene (STAR), and how can a woman learn more about it?

The National Surgical Adjuvant Breast and Bowel Project (NSABP), a component of NCI's Clinical Trials Cooperative Group Program, has launched a new breast cancer study. The new trial, known as STAR, began recruiting participants in June 1999. It will involve about 22,000 postmenopausal women who are at least 35 years old and are at increased risk for developing breast cancer. The study is designed to determine whether raloxifene, a drug similar to tamoxifen, is also effective in reducing the chance of developing breast cancer in women who have not had the disease, and whether the drug has benefits over tamoxifen, such as fewer side effects.

Women can learn more about the STAR trial in several ways. They can call NCI's Cancer Information Service at 1-800-4-CANCER (1-800-422-6237). The number for deaf and hard of hearing callers with TTY equipment is 1-800-332-8615. Information is also available on NSABP'S Web site at http://www.nsabp.pitt.edu or NCI's clinical trials Web site at http://cancertrials.nci.nih.gov on the Internet.

Does tamoxifen cause blood clots?

Data from large treatment studies suggest that there is a small increase in the number of blood clots in women taking tamoxifen, particularly in women who are receiving anticancer drugs (chemotherapy) along with tamoxifen. The total number of women who have experienced this side effect is small. Women in the BCPT who took tamoxifen also had an increased chance of developing blood clots. The risk of having a blood clot due to tamoxifen is similar to the risk of blood clots for women on single-agent estrogen replacement therapy.

Does tamoxifen cause uterine cancer?

The BCPT found that women taking tamoxifen had more than twice the chance of developing uterine cancer compared with women on placebo (an inactive substance that looks the same as, and is administered in the same way as, tamoxifen). The risk of uterine cancer in women taking tamoxifen was in the same range as (or less than) the risk in postmenopausal women taking single-agent estrogen replacement therapy. Additional studies are under way to define more clearly the role of other risk factors for uterine cancer, such as prior hormone use, in women receiving tamoxifen.

Like many cancers, uterine cancer is potentially life threatening. Most of the uterine cancers that have occurred during studies of women taking tamoxifen have been found in the early stages, and treatment was usually effective. However, breast cancer patients who developed uterine cancer while taking tamoxifen have died from the disease. Abnormal vaginal bleeding and lower abdominal (pelvic) pain are two symptoms of the disease. Women on tamoxifen should see their doctor if they experience these symptoms.

Does tamoxifen cause eye problems?

As women age, they are more likely to develop cataracts (a clouding of the lens inside the eye). Women taking tamoxifen appear to be at increased risk for developing cataracts. Other eye problems, such as corneal scarring or retinal changes, have been reported in a few patients.

Does tamoxifen cause other types of cancer?

There have been a few reports of liver cancer and reports of other liver toxicities that have occurred in women taking tamoxifen. Although tamoxifen can cause liver cancer in particular strains of rats, it is not known to cause liver cancer in humans. Tamoxifen did not cause liver cancer in the BCPT. It is clear that tamoxifen can sometimes cause other liver toxicities in women, which rarely can be severe or life threatening. Doctors may order blood tests from time to time to check liver function.

Although one study suggested a possible increase in cancers of the digestive tract among women receiving tamoxifen for breast cancer, other trials, including the BCPT, have not shown an association between tamoxifen and these cancers.

Studies such as the BCPT show no increase in cancers other than uterine cancer. This potential risk is being evaluated.

Should women taking tamoxifen avoid pregnancy?

Yes. Tamoxifen may make premenopausal women more fertile, but doctors advise women on tamoxifen to avoid pregnancy because animal studies have suggested that the use of tamoxifen in pregnancy can cause fetal harm. Women who have questions about fertility, birth control, or pregnancy should discuss their concerns with their doctor.

What are some of the more common side effects of taking tamoxifen?

In general, the side effects of tamoxifen are similar to some of the symptoms of menopause. The most common side effects are hot flashes and vaginal discharge. Some women experience irregular menstrual periods, dizziness, headaches, fatigue, loss of appetite, nausea and/ or vomiting, vaginal dryness or bleeding, and irritation of the skin around the vagina. As is the case with menopause, not all women who take tamoxifen have these symptoms.

Does tamoxifen cause a woman to begin menopause?

Tamoxifen does not cause a woman to begin menopause, although it can cause some symptoms that are similar to those that may occur during menopause. In most premenopausal women taking tamoxifen, the ovaries continue to act normally and produce female hormones (estrogens) in the same or slightly increased amounts.

Do the benefits of tamoxifen in treating breast cancer outweigh its risks?

The benefits of tamoxifen as a treatment for breast cancer are firmly established and far outweigh the potential risks. Women concerned about the risks and benefits of medications they are taking are encouraged to discuss these concerns with their doctor.

How long should a woman take tamoxifen for the treatment of breast cancer?

Women with advanced breast cancer may take tamoxifen for varying lengths of time depending on their response to prior treatment and other factors. When used as adjuvant therapy for early stage breast cancer, tamoxifen is generally prescribed for 5 years. However, the ideal length of treatment with tamoxifen is not known.

Two studies have confirmed the benefit of taking tamoxifen daily for 5 years. These studies compared 5 years of treatment with tamoxifen with 10 years of treatment. When taken for 5 years, the drug prevents the recurrence of the original breast cancer and also prevents the development of a second primary cancer in the opposite breast. Taking tamoxifen for longer than 5 years is not more effective than 5 years of therapy.

Tamoxifen Approved for DCIS; More Trials On the Way

The drug tamoxifen reached another milestone in June 2000 with its approval by the Food and Drug Administration for ductal carconoma in situ, or DCIS. Women who have had DCIS—a small, non-invasive group of abnormal cells—are at high risk of developing invasive breast cancer. Tamoxifen reduces that risk substantially, accordi ng to the clinical trial that led to FDA approval.

In this 1,804-patient trial, women first received lumpectomy and radiation therapy, a standard treatment for DCIS, and then were randomly divided into two groups to receive either tamoxifen or a placebo.

After five years, the tamoxifen group had 43% percent fewer cases of invasive breast cancer.

The study is the latest, but by no means last, in a series of findings from clinical trials exploring the uses of tamoxifen. First studied as a treatment for advanced breast cancer, the drug later moved into studies to treat early breast cancer, and then into primary prevention trials.

But even with FDA approval in these three settings, the tamoxifen story is not yet over. Researchers continue to ask questions about the drug. For instance, when used for prevention of breast cancer, will it reduce overall death rates from that disease? The landmark Breast Cancer Prevention Trial in the United States showed that tamoxifen reduced incidence (number of new cases) of breast cancer in postmenopausal women at increased risk who had been taking the drug for about four years. The study was not designed to show whether the tamoxifen would reduce breast cancer death rates, however.

Some information on mortality may come from the International Breast Cancer Intervention Study, which is comparing tamoxifen to a placebo in 7,000 women at increased risk of the disease. The primary aim of this trial is to compare the incidence of breast cancer in the two groups, but it will also assess mortality, other cancers, cardiovascular disease, and fractures according to Jack Cuzick, Ph.D., of the Imperial Cancer Research Fund, London.

Cuzick spoke at a workshop at the National Institutes of Health, Bethesda, Maryland, in April, 2000, when enrollment had passed the 6000 mark. He projected all 7000 participants needed would be enrolled by the end of the year.

New Combinations

For some investigators, tamoxifen's success in both prevention and treatment studies has set the stage for its use in combination with other agents that may also span these two uses. "It helps to think of breast cancer as a continuum," said JoAnne Zujewski, M.D., who leads several breast cancer clinical trials at the National Cancer Institute in Bethesda. "I'm interested in compounds that may be useful from prevention to in situ disease to invasive cancer."

Such compounds include a class of drugs known as retinoids—4HPR or Fenretidine is one of most-studied—and another group known as farnesyl transferase inhibitors. In a pilot prevention trial, Zujewski and colleagues have shown that Fenretidine combined with tamoxifen is safe and, they concluded, warrants further study as a preventive agent.

Treatment studies have also combined tamoxifen and Fenretidine. In metastatic disease, these include a phase I/II study by Melody Cobleigh, M.D., and colleagues at the University of Chicago and a phase II trial by Zujewski and colleagues at NCI. In early breast cancer, studies of the combination are under way in Chicago and in Italy, at the National Institute for Cancer Research, where A. Decenzi, M.D. has been working with the two drugs.

Another retinoid, 9-cis-retinoic acid, has also been studied in combination with tamoxifen to treat metatastic breast cancer. Zujewski said that a phase I trial showed the combination is safe and holds some promise and that phase II trials of tamoxifen in combination with 9-cis or similar retinoids are under consideration.

Comparisons

In other studies, tamoxifen now serves as the benchmark against which newer therapies are measured. Perhaps the most widely watched of the current tamoxifen trials is the one comparing it to raloxifene for the primary prevention of breast cancer in women at increased risk. The Study of Tamoxifen and Raloxifene (STAR), launched in July 1999, has enrolled about 6,000 of the 22,000 women needed for the study.

Raloxifene is also an estrogen-like drug—both it and tamoxifen are called selective estrogen receptor modulators or SERMS—and was originally developed to prevent osteoporosis. Other novel SERMs are in development, including one known as LY353381, which is now being tested against tamoxifen in a small phase I study.

Treatment studies have compared tamoxifen to Arimidex, an aromatase inhibitor, and a randomized trial of the two drugs has been under way for several years. This trial has completed enrolling patients and preliminary results could be available next year, according to a spokesperson for AstraZeneca Pharmaceuticals, maker of both drugs and sponsor of the trial.

Another DCIS Trial

Also under way is more tamoxifen research in DCIS. Approved by the FDA for use with radiotherapy, the drug will now be tested without radiotherapy in a large trial conducted by the Radiation Therapy Oncology Group and the Cancer and Leukemia Group B, both NCI-sponsored Cooperative Clinical Trials Groups. Patients in this trial will be randomized, after lumpectomy, to receive either tamoxifen with radiation therapy—the combination that was just approved by the FDA—or tamoxifen alone.

This trial is one of the first to be open to members of all NCI-sponsored Groups through the new Cancer Trial Support Unit (CTSU). One aim of the CTSU is to speed and facilitate the completion of trials, so enrollment in this trial may proceed rapidly.

Chapter 42

Paclitaxel (Taxol) and Related Anticancer Drugs

Paclitaxel (Taxol-R) is a compound originally isolated from the bark of the Pacific yew tree (Taxus brevifolia). It has been approved by the U.S. Food and Drug Administration (FDA) to treat breast, ovarian, and lung cancers as well as AIDS-related Kaposi's sarcoma.

Paclitaxel has a unique way of preventing the growth of cancer cells: it affects cell structures called microtubules, which play an important role in cell functions. In normal cell growth, microtubules are formed when a cell starts dividing. Once the cell stops dividing, the microtubules are broken down or destroyed. Paclitaxel stops the microtubules from breaking down. With paclitaxel, cancer cells become so clogged with microtubules that they cannot grow and divide.

Early Research

In 1984, NCI began clinical trials (research studies with people) that looked at paclitaxel's safety and how well it worked to treat certain cancers. In 1989, NCI-supported researchers at The Johns Hopkins Oncology Center reported that tumors shrank or disappeared in 30 percent of patients who were being given paclitaxel for the treatment of advanced ovarian cancer. Although the responses to paclitaxel were not permanent (they lasted an average of 5 months, some up to 9 months), it was clear that advanced ovarian cancer patients could benefit from the treatment. In December 1992, FDA approved the use of paclitaxel for ovarian cancer that was resistant to treatment (refractory).

CancerNet, National Cancer Institute, February 2000.

Other clinical trials using paclitaxel have shown that the drug is effective in the treatment of advanced breast cancer. In April 1994, FDA approved paclitaxel for treating breast cancers that recur within 6 months after adjuvant chemotherapy (chemotherapy that is given after the primary treatment to enhance the effectiveness of the primary treatment). At that time, it was also approved for breast cancer that has spread (metastasized) and has not responded to combination chemotherapy.

In August 1997, paclitaxel was also approved by the FDA as a treatment for the AIDS-related cancer called Kaposi's sarcoma. In April 1998, it was approved for first-line therapy for the treatment of ovarian cancer in combination with cisplatin. Most recently, in June 1998, the FDA approved paclitaxel, in combination with other anticancer drugs, to treat common forms of advanced lung cancer.

Like most cancer drugs, paclitaxel has side effects that can be serious. It is important for patients to talk with their doctor about possible side effects from paclitaxel. For example, it can cause temporary damage to the bone marrow. The bone marrow is the soft, sponge-like tissue in the center of large bones that produces cells that fight infection, carry oxygen, and help prevent bleeding by causing blood clots to form. This damage can cause a person to bruise or bleed easily and be more susceptible to infection. However, the benefits for many patients with advanced cancer outweigh the risks associated with this drug.

Current Clinical Trials

Researchers continue to look for new and better ways to use paclitaxel to treat cancer. For example, they are studying paclitaxel for treatment of early breast, ovarian, and lung cancer. Preliminary findings from ongoing clinical trials suggest that combining paclitaxel with other anticancer drugs may be an effective treatment for patients with lymph node-positive breast cancer. Other studies are looking at paclitaxel as a treatment for lymphomas, and stomach, head and neck, and bladder cancers. In addition, researchers are studying ways to overcome some cancers' resistance to paclitaxel.

Paclitaxel Supplies: Old Problems and New Approaches

Early research using paclitaxel was limited due to difficulties in obtaining the drug. The amount of paclitaxel in yew bark is low, and extracting it is a complicated and expensive process. In addition, bark collection is restricted because the Pacific yew is a limited resource located in forests that are home to the endangered spotted owl.

As demand for paclitaxel grew, NCI, in collaboration with other Government agencies and Bristol-Myers Squibb, worked to increase the availability of paclitaxel. Bark collection and processing expanded to increase the short-term supply of the drug while NCI encouraged research to find other sources of paclitaxel and related compounds.

One option is to synthesize paclitaxel. Currently, a semi-synthetic form of the drug is being studied. To produce the semi-synthetic drug, a substance from the needles of yew trees grown for this purpose is chemically changed to produce paclitaxel.

Another alternative is docetaxel (Taxotere-R), a substance that is similar to paclitaxel. Docetaxel, like the semi-synthetic paclitaxel, comes from the needles of the yew tree. Docetaxel has been approved by the FDA to treat advanced breast and nonsmall cell lung cancers that have not responded to other anticancer drugs. The side effects of docetaxel are similar to those related to paclitaxel. The NCI is sponsoring clinical trials to test the effectiveness of docetaxel alone or in combination with other anticancer drugs for several types of cancer, including cancers of the head and neck, prostate, breast, lung, and uterus.

Chapter 43

Complementary and Alternative Medicine Sometimes Used in Breast Cancer Treatment

hapter Contents

Section 43.1

Questions and Answers about Complementary and Alternative Medicine in Cancer Treatment

National Cancer Institute, available at http://cancernet.nci.nih.gov; last modified July 7, 1999.

What is complementary and alternative medicine?

Complementary and alternative medicine (CAM)—also referred to as integrative medicine—includes a broad range of healing philosophies, approaches, and therapies. A therapy is generally called complementary when it is used in addition to conventional treatments; it is often called alternative when it is used instead of conventional treatment. (Conventional treatments are those that are widely accepted and practiced by the mainstream medical community.) Depending on how they are used, some therapies can be considered either complementary or alternative.

Complementary and alternative therapies are used in an effort to prevent illness, reduce stress, prevent or reduce side effects and symptoms, or control or cure disease. Some commonly used methods of complementary or alternative therapy include mind/body control interventions such as visualization or relaxation, manual healing including acupressure and massage, homeopathy, vitamins or herbal products, and acupuncture.

Are complementary and alternative cancer therapies widely used?

Although there are few studies on the use of complementary and alternative therapies for cancer, one large-scale study found that the percentage of cancer patients in the United States using these therapies was nine percent overall (Lerner and Kennedy, 1992).

Can complementary and alternative medicine be evaluated using the same methods used in conventional medicine?

Scientific evaluation is important in understanding if and when complementary and alternative therapies work. A number of medical centers are evaluating complementary and alternative therapies by developing scientific studies to test them.

Conventional approaches to cancer treatment have generally been studied for safety and effectiveness through a rigorous scientific process, including clinical trials with large numbers of patients. Often, less is known about the safety and effectiveness of complementary and alternative methods. Some of these complementary and alternative therapies have not undergone rigorous evaluation. Others, once considered unorthodox, are finding a place in cancer treatment—not as cures, but as complementary therapies that may help patients feel better and recover faster. One example is acupuncture. According to a panel of experts at a National Institutes of Health Consensus Conference in November 1997, acupuncture has been found to be effective in the management of chemotherapy-associated nausea and vomiting and in controlling pain associated with surgery. Some approaches, such as laetrile, have been studied and found ineffective or potentially harmful.

What should patients do when considering complementary and alternative therapies?

Cancer patients considering complementary and alternative medicine should discuss this decision with their doctor or nurse, as they would any therapeutic approach, because some complementary and alternative therapies may interfere with their standard treatment or may be harmful when used with conventional treatment.

When considering complementary and alternative therapies, what questions should patients ask their health care provider?

- What benefits can be expected from this therapy?
- What are the risks associated with this therapy?
- Do the known benefits outweigh the risks?
- What side effects can be expected?
- Will the therapy interfere with conventional treatment?
- Will the therapy be covered by health insurance?

What government agencies can provide patients and their health care providers more information about complementary and alternative therapies?

The NIH National Center for Complementary and Alternative Medicine (NCCAM) facilitates research and evaluation of complementary and alternative practices and has information about a variety of methods.

345

NCCAM Clearinghouse
Post Office Box 8218
Silver Spring, MD 20907-8218
Toll free: 1-888-644-6226
TTY/TDY (for deaf and hard of hearing callers): 1-888-644-6226 (toll free)
Website: http://nccam.nih.gov

The Food and Drug Administration (FDA) regulates drugs and medical devices to ensure that they are safe and effective.

Food and Drug Administration
5600 Fishers Lane
Rockville, MD 20857
Toll free: 1-888-463-6332
Website: http://www.fda.gov

The Federal Trade Commission (FTC) enforces consumer protection laws. Publications available from the FTC include:

- "Who Cares: Sources of Information about Health Care Products and Services"

- "Fraudulent Health Claims: Don't Be Fooled"

Consumer Response Center
Federal Trade Commission
Room 130
600 Pennsylvania Avenue, NW
Washington, DC 20580
Phone: 1-877-382-4357 (toll free)
TTY (for deaf and hard of hearing callers): 202-326-2502
Web site: http://www.ftc.gov

References for This Section

Cassileth B, Chapman C. Alternative and Complementary Cancer Therapies. *Cancer* 1996; 77(6):1026-1033.

Jacobs J. Unproven Alternative Methods of Cancer Treatment. In: DeVita, Hellman, Rosenberg, editors. *Cancer: Principles and Practice of Oncology. 5th edition.* Philadelphia: Lippincott-Raven Publishers; 1997. 2993-3001.

Lerner IJ, Kennedy BJ. The Prevalence of Questionable Methods of Cancer Treatment in the United States. *CA-A Cancer Journal* 1992;42:181-191.

Nelson W. Alternative Cancer Treatments. *Highlights in Oncology Practice* 1998; 15(4):85-93.

Section 43.2

714-X

Excerpted from "714-X," National Cancer Institute, full text available at http://cancernet.nci.nih.gov/cam/714X.htm; last modified November 2000.

General Information

714-X was developed over 30 years ago in a privately funded laboratory in Quebec, Canada, where it continues to be produced. The primary component of 714-X is naturally-derived camphor that has been chemically altered by the addition of an extra nitrogen atom and then combined with ammonium salts, sodium chloride, and ethanol.

The laboratory currently makes 714-X available through physicians in Canada (where it is available on compassionate grounds only, but not approved for general therapeutic use), Mexico, and some western European countries. The U.S. Food and Drug Administration (FDA) has not approved 714-X for use in the United States.

714-X is usually administered by injection into lymph nodes in the groin, but it can be administered nasally, using a nebulizer, for patients with lung or oral cancers. The producers of 714-X do not recommend intravenous or oral administration. A usual treatment cycle consists of daily injection for 21 days followed by a 3-day rest period. Between three and 12 treatment cycles are recommended, depending on the stage of the cancer. It has been suggested that 714-X is more effective if administered early in the disease process and before chemotherapy or radiation therapy, but that it can also be used in conjunction with conventional treatments. It has been recommended that vitamin B_{12} supplements, vitamin E supplements, and alcohol be avoided during 714-X therapy.

It has been proposed that 714-X works by protecting, stabilizing, and reactivating the patient's immune system, so the body can defend itself against tumor growth and metastasis. The camphor component of 714-X is purportedly attracted to cancer cells, where the added nitrogen is released, thus preventing tumor cells from depleting the nitrogen required by normal cells, including immune system cells, for proper metabolism and function.

Laboratory/Animal/Preclinical Studies

There have been no laboratory or animal studies published in peer-reviewed, scientific journals in which the safety or the efficacy of 714-X was evaluated. Results of studies using tumor models in rats, dogs, and cows were presented at a scientific conference in 1982, and no benefit of 714-X could be demonstrated.

A few laboratory and animal studies have suggested that camphor (a component of 714-X) may be able to enhance the immune response observed after vaccine administration and increase the sensitivity of tumor cells to radiation therapy. In one series of studies, investigators used camphor vapors as a "conditioned stimulus" to promote an immune response. These studies demonstrated that mice exposed to camphor vapors at the same time they received an antitumor vaccine showed decreased growth of transplanted lymphoma cells and increased survival when they were re-exposed to camphor vapors plus the vaccine or to camphor vapors alone, in comparison with mice re-exposed to only the vaccine. These investigators also demonstrated that exposure to camphor vapors led to an increase in natural killer cells and in tumor-specific cytotoxic T cells. Another study reported that breast adenocarcinoma cells transplanted under the skin of mice responded better to local radiation therapy when small doses of camphor were given by intraperitoneal injection before irradiation. Finally, researchers examined nine compounds, including a camphor-containing compound, for their ability to inhibit the activity of estrone sulfatase, an enzyme involved in the production of estrone, which is a precursor of the various forms of estrogen. Estrogens are thought to promote the growth of hormone-dependent breast cancer cells. The camphor-containing compound showed only modest inhibition of estrone sulfatase activity in human breast cancer cells grown in the laboratory.

Human/Clinical Studies

No clinical trials, clinical series, or case reports have been published in peer-reviewed, scientific journals to support the efficacy or safety of 714-X. A number of anecdotal reports and testimonials have been published in newspapers and other non-medical literature. The producers of 714-X state that they have tried to document the long-term experience of patients treated with 714-X, but they have encountered difficulty in obtaining information from patients and their health-care providers.

Adverse Effects

714-X is reported to be nontoxic, with the only side effects of treatment being local redness, tenderness, and swelling at injection sites.

Levels of Evidence for Human Studies of Cancer Complementary and Alternative Medicine

To assist readers in evaluating the results of human studies of CAM treatments for cancer, the strength of the evidence associated with each type of treatment is provided whenever possible. To qualify for a levels of evidence analysis, a study must 1) be published in a peer-reviewed, scientific journal; 2) report on a therapeutic outcome(s), such as tumor response, improvement in survival, or measured improvement in quality of life; and 3) describe clinical findings in sufficient detail that a meaningful evaluation can be made. No levels of evidence analysis could be performed for 714-X because no study of its use in humans has been published in a peer-reviewed, scientific journal.

Section 43.3

Cartilage

Excerpted from "Cartilage" National Cancer Institute, full text available at http://cancernet.nci.nih.gov/cam/cartilage.htm; last modified July 1999.

General Information

Cartilage products are widely used in the United States for the treatment of medical conditions such as cancer, arthritis, and psoriasis. It is estimated that more than 50,000 Americans used shark cartilage in 1992, and with media attention increasing, this number is likely to have grown substantially. In 1995 more than 40 brand names of shark cartilage products were being sold in the United States. Most purchases are made over the counter. Use of these products is not limited to humans. Products containing shark and bovine (cattle) cartilage for both human and veterinary use have been marketed and sold throughout the world.

Cartilage compounds are marketed as dietary supplements that do not require Food and Drug Administration (FDA) pre-marketing evaluation or approval. Before researchers can conduct clinical drug research in the United States, they must file an Investigational New Drug (IND) application; the FDA so far has granted IND status to 3 groups of investigators studying the use of cartilage as a cancer treatment.

The major components of shark cartilage are proteins (approximately 40%), glycosaminoglycans (GAGs, approximately 5%-20%), and calcium salts. Chondroitin sulfate, one of the most plentiful glycosaminoglycans found in cartilage, is under investigation to determine if it is one of the active ingredients. Cartilage reportedly has been sold in many forms and is given in many ways. It can be taken orally as a pill, powder, or liquid extract; given as a topical agent, an enema, or an intravenous (i.v.) infusion; or administered as a subcutaneous (under the skin), intraperitoneal (into the lining of the abdomen), or intramuscular (into the muscle) injection. Administration schedules and the length of treatment in animal models and in humans vary widely.

The use of shark cartilage as a cancer treatment has drawn attention because of the popular belief that the incidence of cancer in cartilaginous fish (sharks, skates, and rays) is very rare or nonexistent. However, literature on cancer in fish shows this may not be true. Comprehensive lists of literature compiled in 1933, 1948, and 1969 document that a sampling of cartilaginous fish captured over the years were found to have cancer. Although there is no way to establish the prevalence of cancer among all sharks, various types of tumors have been found in cartilaginous fish. The majority of these cancers are melanomas and soft-tissue sarcomas.

Mechanisms of action proposed to explain why cartilage compounds might be useful as a cancer therapy are based on information derived from experiments using animal models and human cell cultures. The most frequently cited is antiangiogenesis, a process that slows or stops the growth of blood vessels that supply nutrients and oxygen to the tumor. Other mechanisms of action include blocking the formation of certain enzymes (metalloproteinases) that tumors use to invade tissue surrounding the tumor and stimulating the immune system. Some researchers have hypothesized that bovine and shark cartilage have different mechanisms of action.

Human/Clinical Studies

Studies using bovine and shark cartilage on human subjects with cancer have been ongoing since the early 1980s. However, little information exists on how treatment was administered and how patients were monitored during the study, and the long-term outcome of treatment is limited. Most reports on tumor response and survival after cartilage treatment consist of anecdotal information that provides few details. Very little scientifically based data have been published on this subject. Two clinical series, one using shark cartilage with 32 breast and prostate patients and another utilizing bovine cartilage with 35 renal cell carcinoma patients, and a phase II trial of oral shark cartilage powder with 60 advanced cancer patients have been presented as abstracts at national oncology meetings. Only 2 bovine cartilage case series and 1 phase I/II shark cartilage case series have been published in peer-reviewed, scientific journals. The majority of studies have used bovine or shark cartilage as a treatment for advanced cancer patients, but the response rate to cartilage therapy for these patients has not been impressive. Randomized clinical trials to test whether cartilage may be effective for patients with limited disease have not been conducted.

351

The results of a clinical series that used intensive i.v. and oral bovine cartilage therapies for patients with advanced cancer were reported in 1985. Although the study claimed to have induced a 90% initial response rate (complete and partial responses) in a group of 31 patients, confounding factors such as concomitant treatment with chemotherapy, radiation, or surgery may be the reason for many of the positive responses. The ability to generalize these data to other groups of patients is difficult. No standard dosing schedule or route of administration was used for the entire group of patients or within groups of patients with a particular type of cancer. In addition, prior treatment among patients varied widely, ranging from no prior therapy at all to heavy pretreatment. In one clinical series, a less intensive dose of bovine cartilage was administered subcutaneously to 9 patients with advanced disease who had received no chemotherapy for a month. Strict entry criteria were used and baseline staging and follow-up were performed during the study. A complete response was achieved by a patient with renal cell carcinoma, but no other patients responded to therapy. Another study used oral and injectable forms of bovine cartilage with 4 different schedules of administration to treat patients with metastatic renal cell carcinoma. Of the 22 patients who could be evaluated, 3 had durable partial responses and 1 had stable disease.

Two phase II clinical trials for cancer patients using shark and bovine tracheal cartilage (sponsored by Cancer Treatment Centers of America (CTCA)) and a clinical trial using shark cartilage in AIDS patients with Kaposi's sarcoma (sponsored by Lane Labs) have been conducted and are listed in the closed clinical trial section of PDQ. Results from the phase II CTCA shark cartilage study, published in November 1998, concluded that oral shark cartilage given as a single agent was ineffective in 47 patients with advanced breast, colon, lung, and prostate cancer. For more information on clinical trials, call the National Cancer Institute's Cancer Information Service at 1-800-4-CANCER (1-800-422-6237); TTY at 1-800-332-8615.

Adverse Effects

Information on side effects associated with taking cartilage preparations is limited, but cartilage therapy apparently has few side effects regardless of route of administration. Reported side effects include dysgeusia (bad taste in the mouth), fatigue, dyspepsia (problems with digestion), nausea, fever, dizziness, hypercalcemia, scrotal edema (swelling of the scrotum), and discomfort at the injection site.

Section 43.4

Coenzyme Q10

Excerpted from "Coenzyme Q10" National Cancer Institute, full text available at http://cancernet.nci.nih.gov/cam/Q10.htm; last modified July 1999.

General Information

Coenzyme Q10 (also known as Co Q10, Q10, vitamin Q10, ubiquinone, or ubidecarenone) is a benzoquinone compound synthesized naturally in the human body. The "Q" and the "10" in the name refer to the quinone chemical group and the 10 isoprenyl chemical subunits, respectively, that are part of this compound's structure. Coenzyme Q10 is used by cells of the body in a process known variously as aerobic respiration, aerobic metabolism, oxidative metabolism, or cell respiration. Through this process, energy for cell growth and maintenance is created inside cells in compartments called mitochondria. Coenzyme Q10 is also used by the body as an endogenous antioxidant. An antioxidant is a substance that protects cells from free radicals, which are highly reactive chemicals, often containing oxygen atoms, capable of damaging important cellular components such as DNA and lipids. In addition, the plasma level of coenzyme Q10 has been used, in studies, as a measure of oxidative stress (a situation in which normal antioxidant levels are reduced).

Coenzyme Q10 is present in most tissues, but the highest concentrations are found in the heart, liver, kidneys, and pancreas. The lowest concentration is found in the lungs. Tissue levels of this compound decrease as people age, due to increased requirements, decreased production, or insufficient intake of the chemical precursors needed for synthesis.

Given the importance of coenzyme Q10 to optimal cellular energy production, use of this compound as a treatment for diseases other than cancer has been investigated. Most of these investigations have focused on coenzyme Q10 as a treatment for cardiovascular disease. In patients with cancer, coenzyme Q10 has been shown to protect the heart from anthracycline-induced cardiotoxicity (anthracyclines are a family of chemotherapy drugs, including doxorubicin, that have the potential to damage the heart) and to stimulate the immune system. Stimulation of the immune system by this compound has also been observed in animal studies and in humans without cancer. In part because of its immunostimulatory potential, coenzyme Q10 has been used as an adjuvant therapy in patients with various types of cancer.

While coenzyme Q10 may show indirect anticancer activity through its effect(s) on the immune system, there is evidence to suggest that analogs of this compound are able to suppress cancer growth directly. Analogs of coenzyme Q10 have been shown to inhibit the proliferation of cancer cells in vitro and the growth of cancer cells transplanted into rats and mice. In view of these findings, it has been proposed that analogs of coenzyme Q10 may function as antimetabolites to disrupt normal biochemical reactions that are required for cell growth and/or survival and, thus, that they may be useful for short periods of time as chemotherapeutic agents.

Several companies distribute coenzyme Q10 as a dietary supplement. In the United States, dietary supplements are regulated as foods not drugs. Therefore, premarket evaluation and approval by the Food and Drug Administration (FDA) are not required unless specific disease prevention or treatment claims are made. Because dietary supplements are not formally reviewed for manufacturing consistency, there may be considerable variation from lot to lot.

To conduct clinical drug research in the United States, researchers must file an Investigational New Drug (IND) application with the FDA. The IND application process is highly confidential, and IND information can only be disclosed by the applicants. To date, no investigators have announced that they have applied for an IND to study coenzyme Q10 as a treatment for cancer.

Human/Clinical Studies

The use of coenzyme Q10 as a treatment for cancer in humans has been investigated in only a limited fashion. With the exception of a single randomized trial, which involved 20 patients and tested the ability of coenzyme Q10 to reduce anthracycline-induced cardiotoxicity, the studies that have been published consist of anecdotal reports, case reports, case series, and uncontrolled clinical studies.

In view of the promising results from animal studies, coenzyme Q10 was tested as a protective agent against the cardiac toxicity observed in cancer patients treated with the anthracycline drug doxorubicin. It has been postulated that doxorubicin interferes with energy generating biochemical reactions involving coenzyme Q10 in heart muscle mitochondria and that this interference can be overcome by coenzyme Q10 supplementation. Studies with adults and children, including the aforementioned randomized trial, have confirmed the decrease in cardiac toxicity observed in animal studies.

The potential of coenzyme Q10 as an adjuvant therapy for cancer has also been explored. In view of observations that blood levels of coenzyme Q10 are frequently reduced in cancer patients, supplementation with this compound has been tested in patients undergoing conventional treatment. An open-label (nonblinded), uncontrolled clinical study in Denmark followed 32 breast cancer patients for 18 months. The disease in these patients had spread to the axillary lymph nodes, and an unreported number had distant metastases. The patients received antioxidant supplementation (vitamin C, vitamin E, and beta-carotene), other vitamins and trace minerals, essential fatty acids, and coenzyme Q10 (at a dose of 90 milligrams per day), in addition to standard therapy (surgery, radiation therapy, and chemotherapy, with or without tamoxifen). The patients were seen every 3 months to monitor disease status (progressive disease or recurrence), and, if there was a suspicion of recurrence, mammography, bone scan, x-ray, or biopsy was performed. The survival rate for the study period was one hundred percent (four deaths were expected). Six patients were reported to show some evidence of remission; however, incomplete clinical data were provided, and information suggestive of remission was presented for only three of the six patients. None of the six patients had evidence of further metastases. For all 32 patients, decreased use of painkillers, improved quality of life, and an absence of weight loss were reported. Whether painkiller use and quality of life were measured objectively (e.g., from pharmacy records and validated questionnaires, respectively) or subjectively (from patient self-reports) was not specified.

In a follow-up study, one of the six patients with a reported remission and a new patient were treated for several months with higher doses of coenzyme Q10 (390 and 300 milligrams per day, respectively). Surgical removal of the primary breast tumor in both patients had been incomplete. After 3 to 4 months of high-level coenzyme Q10 supplementation, both patients appeared to experience complete regression of their residual breast tumors (assessed by clinical examination and mammography). It should be noted that a different patient identifier was used in the follow-up study for the patient who had participated in the original study. Therefore, it is impossible to determine which of the six patients with a reported remission took part in the follow-up study. In the follow-up study report, the researchers noted that all 32 patients from the original study remained alive at 24 months of observation, whereas six deaths had been expected.

The above-mentioned human studies had important design flaws that could have influenced their outcome. Study weaknesses include the absence of a control group (i.e., all patients received coenzyme Q10), possible selection bias in the follow-up investigations, and multiple confounding variables (i.e., the patients received a variety of supplements in addition to coenzyme Q10, and they received standard therapy either during or immediately before supplementation with coenzyme Q10). Thus, it is impossible to determine whether any of the beneficial results was directly related to coenzyme Q10 therapy.

Adverse Effects

No serious toxicity associated with the use of coenzyme Q10 has been reported. Doses of 100 milligrams per day or higher have caused mild insomnia in some individuals. Liver enzyme elevation has been detected in patients taking doses of 300 milligrams per day for extended periods of time, but no liver toxicity has been reported. Researchers in one cardiovascular study reported that coenzyme Q10 caused rashes, nausea, and epigastric (upper abdominal) pain that required withdrawal of a small number of patients from the study. Other reported side effects have included dizziness, photophobia (abnormal visual sensitivity to light), irritability, headache, heartburn, and fatigue.

Certain lipid-lowering drugs, such as the "statins" (lovastatin, pravastatin, and simvastatin) and gemfibrozil, as well as oral agents that lower blood sugar, such as glyburide and tolazamide, cause a decrease in serum levels of coenzyme Q10 and reduce the effects of coenzyme Q10 supplementation. Beta-blockers (drugs that slow the heart rate and lower blood pressure) can inhibit coenzyme Q10-dependent enzyme reactions. The contractile force of the heart in patients with high blood pressure can be increased by coenzyme Q10 administration. Coenzyme Q10 can reduce the body's response to the anticoagulant drug warfarin. Finally, coenzyme Q10 can decrease insulin requirements in individuals with diabetes.

Section 43.5

Mistletoe

Excerpted from "Mistletoe," National Cancer Institute, full text available at http://cancernet.nci.nih.gov/cam/mistletoe.htm; last modified June 2000.

General Information

Mistletoe, a parasitic plant, holds interest as a possible anticancer agent because extracts derived from it have been shown to kill cancer cells *in vitro* and to stimulate immune system cells both *in vitro* and *in vivo*. Several components of mistletoe, namely alkaloids, viscotoxins, and lectins, may be responsible for these effects. Alkaloids comprise a large group of nitrogen-containing chemicals produced by plants, and some alkaloids, from other types of plants, are widely used as cancer chemotherapy agents. Limited experimental evidence indicates that mistletoe alkaloids may also have anticancer activity. Viscotoxins are small proteins that exhibit cell-killing activity and possible immune system stimulating activity. Lectins are complex molecules that contain both protein and sugars and are capable of binding to the outside of cells (for example, immune system cells) and inducing biochemical changes in them. In view of mistletoe's ability to stimulate the immune system, it has been classified as a type of biological response modifier. Biological response modifiers constitute a complex group of biologic substances that have been used individually, or in combination with other agents, to treat cancer or to lessen the adverse effects of anticancer drugs.

Mistletoe is used mainly in Europe and Asia, where commercially available products are marketed under the brand names Iscador, Eurixor, Helixor, Isorel, Vysorel, and ABNOBAviscum. These products are not sold commercially in the United States. Mistletoe products have not been tested and found by the U.S. Food and Drug Administration (FDA) to be safe and effective in treating cancer in humans. Before researchers can conduct clinical drug research in the United States, they must file an Investigational New Drug (IND) application with the FDA. Since the existence of an IND application is often highly confidential, it is not known whether one has been submitted or approved for the study of mistletoe as a treatment for cancer.

357

Mistletoe grows on various trees such as apple, oak, maple, elm, pine, and birch. Each mistletoe species (for example., *Viscum album Loranthacea* [*Viscum album L.* or "European mistletoe"] and *Viscum album coloratum* ["Korean mistletoe"]) is capable of growing on a variety of trees. The chemical composition of commercial mistletoe products varies greatly depending on the species of the host tree, the time of year harvested, the species of mistletoe, how it is prepared for use, and the commercial producer. This summary discusses research using primarily *Viscum album L.*

In modern studies, mistletoe extracts have been administered by intramuscular injection, subcutaneous injection (sometimes in the vicinity of a tumor), or intravenous infusion.

Human/Clinical Studies

Mistletoe has been used for centuries to treat a number of ailments in humans, but scientific data from controlled or uncontrolled studies of cancer are limited and often of poor quality. To a great extent, research in this area has concentrated on immune system effects. Relatively few studies have used tumor response or survival as study endpoints, and conflicting results have been obtained. Furthermore, the use of different mistletoe products, or combinations of mistletoe products, from one study to the next makes comparison of the findings difficult, and, in some studies, patients have required different doses of the same product to achieve comparable effects on immune system function. Although there is substantial evidence of mistletoe's ability to modulate the human immune system, there is no evidence that this enhanced immunity leads to improved cancer destruction.

It has been suggested that mistletoe may fail to inhibit tumor growth in humans because 1) antibodies can be produced against the active component(s), 2) plasma proteins may break down or interfere with the active component(s), or 3) the plant lectins in mistletoe extracts may not be able to bind to certain types of human cells.

Several studies involving patients with breast cancer have demonstrated that extracts of *Viscum album L.*, or the lectin ML-I purified from them, can stimulate increases in a variety of white blood cell types and may be able to induce cells to repair damaged DNA.

Adverse Effects

Although numerous formulations of mistletoe have been used in animal and human studies, the associated side effects have been minimal and non-life threatening. Common side effects found with mistletoe-product injection include soreness and inflammation at the injection site, headache, fever, and chills. Seizures, slowing of the heart rate, abnormally high blood pressure, abnormally low blood pressure, vomiting, and death have been observed after ingestion of mistletoe plants and berries. The severity of the toxic effects associated with mistletoe ingestion may depend on the amount consumed and the type of mistletoe plant.

Section 43.6

Hydrazine Sulfate

Excerpted from "National Cancer Institute Studies of Hydrazine Sulfate," National Cancer Institute, reviewed July 24, 1998; full text available at http://cis.nci.nih.gov/fact/7_39.htm.

In the 1980s and early 1990s, the National Cancer Institute (NCI) sponsored studies of hydrazine sulfate to evaluate whether the compound might improve patient survival or help reverse cancer cachexia, a wasting syndrome that occurs in many patients who have advanced cancer. This syndrome profoundly affects patients' quality of life as well as their health, causing weight loss, fatigue, weakness, and loss of appetite.

After hydrazine sulfate showed promising results in a small pilot study, three large-scale, randomized clinical trials of the compound were conducted in patients with advanced cancers. (Clinical trials are carried out to determine whether new treatments are safe and effective in people.) These three clinical trials did not show any improvement in cancer patient survival, weight loss, or quality of life from hydrazine sulfate.

In two of the three clinical trials, patients were permitted to take tranquilizers, alcohol, and barbiturates. Some people believed these compounds may have interfered with hydrazine sulfate, based on animal and laboratory studies. At the request of Congress, the General Accounting Office (GAO) examined this issue beginning in July 1994 and ending in April 1995. The GAO concluded that, although

359

tranquilizers, alcohol, and barbiturates were permitted, the use of these substances did not affect the findings of the studies. The GAO published its conclusions in the 1995 report, "Cancer Drug Research: Contrary to Allegation, NIH Hydrazine Sulfate Studies Were Not Flawed." Copies of the GAO report are available from the U.S. General Accounting Office, Post Office Box 6015, Gaithersburg, MD 20884–6015, or call 202–512–6000. The first copy of the report is free; additional copies are $2.00 each.

Although the Food and Drug Administration (FDA) has not approved hydrazine sulfate for marketing in the United States, a number of drugs that help fight cancer cachexia have been approved by the FDA and are available to cancer patients. No new NCI–supported studies of hydrazine sulfate are planned, but studies of other compounds that may reverse cachexia and other treatments to fight advanced cancers are under way.

Section 43.7

Guided Imagery and Hypnosis

by Jeanne Fournier, Medical Hypnotherapist, Community Breast Health Project, Stanford University, July 1997; reprinted with permission.

Guided imagery and hypnotherapy are examples of what is known as mind/body medicine, or more accurately, mind/body therapy. These are therapies which use the power of the mind to help heal the body. The idea that our thoughts and emotions can contribute to illness is not a new one, but the belief that they can also contribute to our health and sense of well-being is something that is often minimized due to lack of scientific proofs. Even though the American Medical Association approved the use of hypnosis as a valid medical treatment in 1958, there has been little funding to do the type of studies being done for drug therapies. With the establishment of the new field of Psychoneuroimmunology (PNI)—a rather long word for a study that seems to establish a link between our thoughts and the function of our immune cells—and the establishment of the National Institutes of

Health's Office of Alternative Medicine, the value of these and other mind/body techniques is finally becoming better understood.

Guided imagery and hypnosis are both ways of focusing the mind's attention. This is usually done by first relaxing the body, and then, shifting the attention away from the external environment toward a narrow range of ideas or images suggested by the hypnotherapist. The idea is that once the patient's conscious mind is quieted, the unconscious mind is more accessible. The unconscious mind, which is basically non-critical, then allows healing suggestions and images to have a better chance of being effective than they would if given during a normal waking state. While in this state of advanced relaxation, the patient has complete control of his participation while the hypnotherapist is the facilitator of the process.

Imagery and Hypnosis

In the last couple of years as I've begun to focus more in my practice on working with people with serious illness, I've noticed that these people are basically in a kind of trance state, with their thoughts, emotions, and actions pretty narrowly focused on the facts, the treatment, the helplessness, the limitations, and the fears associated with their disease. They are in an almost constant state of stress and anxiety; they are angry and frightened—all conditions which are known to contribute to illness and impede the body's natural ability to heal. My believe has been that if we could change the focus of this near-trance state from one that is disease-based to one that is healing-focused, then it would allow a sense of well-being, empowerment, hope of recovery, and an enhancement of the immune system to occur.

At Community Breast Health Project (CBHP), I've been facilitating group healing guided imagery sessions. I believe that healing is much broader than curing, which is the worthy goal of most medical treatments; it is about wholeness, about bringing into balance all the aspects of who we are, our body, our mind, our emotions, and our spirit. Healing involves looking within to discover meaning, looking to others to establish connections, and looking beyond to face the future with hope and joy.

In addition, in my practice, I've created a protocol to support people through various stages of their healing journey. Imagery and hypnosis is used to create relaxation and relieve stress, to allow for a shift in consciousness from disease to healing, to prepare patients for surgery and other medical treatments, to enhance recovery, and to focus powerful life energy on returning to health and well-being. This may include support for lifestyle changes such as weight control or smoking cessation. The result has been that people have been able to move through their experience with more calm and hope, developing a strong sense of who they really are beyond the disease and how they want to live their lives. Many even use this experience as an opportunity to recreate their lives in a more healthy, meaningful way.

For more information about the Community Breast Health Project, contact:

Community Breast Health Project
545 Bryant Street
Palo Alto, CA 94301
Phone: 650-326-6686
Fax: 650-626-6673
Website: http://med.stanford.edu/CBHP

Section 43.8

Halted Studies and Banned Products

Antineoplastons

Information in this section is taken from "National Cancer Institute–Sponsored Clinical Trials of Antineoplastons," National Cancer Institute, reviewed February 1999; full text available at http://cis.nci.nih.gov/fact/7_43.htm.

Antineoplastons are a group of synthetic compounds that were originally isolated from human blood and urine by Stanislaw Burzynski, M.D., Ph.D., in Houston, Texas. Dr. Burzynski has used antineoplastons to treat patients with a variety of cancers. In 1991, the National Cancer Institute (NCI) conducted a review to evaluate the clinical responses in a group of patients treated with antineoplastons at the Burzynski Research Institute in Houston.

The medical records of seven brain tumor patients who were thought to have benefited from treatment with antineoplastons were reviewed by NCI. This did not constitute a clinical trial but, rather, was a retrospective review of medical records, called a "best case series." The reviewers of this series found evidence of antitumor activity, and NCI proposed that formal clinical trials be conducted to further evaluate the response rate and toxicity of antineoplastons in adults with advanced brain tumors.

Investigators at several cancer centers developed protocols for two phase II clinical trials with review and input from NCI and Dr. Burzynski. These NCI-sponsored studies began in 1993 at the Memorial Sloan-Kettering Cancer Center, the Mayo Clinic, and the Warren Grant Magnussen Clinical Center at the National Institutes of Health. Patient enrollment in these studies was slow, and by August 1995 only nine patients had entered the trials. Attempts to reach a consensus on proposed changes to increase accrual could not be reached by Dr. Burzynski, NCI staff, and investigators, and on August 18, 1995, the studies were closed prior to completion. A paper describing this research, "Phase II Study of Antineoplastons A10 (NSC 648539) and AS2-1 (NSC 620261) in Patients With Recurrent Glioma," appears in *Mayo Clinic Proceedings* 1999, 74:137-145. Because of the small number of patients in these trials, no definitive conclusions can be drawn about the effectiveness of treatment with antineoplastons.

Cancell

Information in this section is excerpted from "Cancell," National Cancer Institute, reviewed November 2000; full text available at http://cis.nci.nih.gov/fact/9_13.htm.

Cancell is also known as Entelev, Sheridan's Formula, Jim's Juice, Crocinic Acid, JS-114, JS-101, 126-F, and Cantron. It has been promoted as a therapy for cancer and a wide range of other diseases. The U.S. Food and Drug Administration has listed the components of Cancell as inositol, nitric acid, sodium sulfite, potassium hydroxide, sulfuric acid, and catechol. Cancell can be administered orally or rectally. It can also be applied to the skin of the wrist or the ball of the foot.

Cancell was developed by James V. Sheridan, a former researcher at the Michigan Cancer Center, in the 1930s. Mr. Sheridan and his associate, Edward J. Sopcak, offered the mixture free of charge to any seriously ill patient who requested it.

The principal manufacturers of Cancell state that they have performed numerous animal experiments with the mixture, and that it has been used by many cancer patients. However, these findings have not been published in peer-reviewed, scientific journals, and no clinical trials (research studies with patients) of Cancell have been conducted. The National Cancer Institute (NCI) has evaluated Cancell in the laboratory and in animal studies and found that it had no effect on cancer cells.

Because studies of Cancell have not shown it to be effective in treating cancer, it has not been approved by the U.S. Food and Drug Administration (FDA). In 1989, the FDA obtained a permanent injunction against the manufacturers of Cancell. The injunction prohibited the manufacture or distribution of the product. The Cancell mixture is reportedly being sold under various names as a dietary supplement in health food stores.

Immuno-Augmentative Therapy

Information in this section is from " Immuno-Augmentative Therapy," National Cancer Institute, reviewed October 1999; text available at http:/ / cis.nci.nih.gov / fact / 9_15.htm.

Immuno-augmentative therapy (IAT) consists of daily injections of processed human blood products that are designed to stimulate the patient's immune system to attack cancer cells. IAT was developed by Dr. Lawrence Burton, Ph.D. In the mid-1970s, Dr. Burton established the Immunological Researching Foundation in Great Neck, New York, and filed an investigational new drug application for IAT with the Food and Drug Administration (FDA). However, because Dr. Burton did not provide the experimental evidence for IAT that the FDA requested, the application was not approved. In 1977, Dr. Burton relocated to the Commonwealth of the Bahamas, established The Immunology Researching Centre, and began using IAT to treat persons with cancer.

In the mid-1980s, the safety of all products derived from human blood, including IAT, came under questioning as the scientific community learned about the human immunodeficiency virus (HIV), which causes acquired immunodeficiency syndrome (AIDS). In 1985, at the request of the families of two patients who had returned to the United States from Dr. Burton's clinic, a Washington state blood bank examined 18 sealed IAT specimens. All of the samples tested positive for hepatitis B; some of the samples were positive for HIV. These findings were confirmed by subsequent analyses by the Centers for Disease Control and Prevention (CDC), the National Cancer Institute (NCI), and independent laboratories.

In July 1985, at the request of the Bahamian Ministry of Health, representatives from the CDC and the Pan American Health Organization (PAHO) visited the Immunology Researching Centre to investigate the manufacturing process used for IAT. The CDC and PAHO concluded that the manufacture of IAT represented a serious health hazard, and the Bahamian Government closed the clinic. The clinic reopened in March 1986 after Dr. Burton agreed to follow certain quality control procedures, including screening blood sources for HIV and hepatitis B and conducting standard blood donor screening and collection practices. In July 1986, the FDA issued an import ban prohibiting anyone from bringing IAT into the United States. This ban is still in effect.

A sample of IAT frozen in a block of ice was offered to and analyzed by the FDA during the summer of 1987. Although the sample was not sterile (free from contamination), there was no evidence of HIV or hepatitis B.

Although Dr. Burton described his success in treating cancer patients in newspaper, magazine, and television interviews, several attempts to plan a clinical trial (research study with humans) in collaboration with Dr. Burton were unsuccessful. Dr. Burton died in 1993. The Immunology Researching Centre remains open under the direction of Dr. R. J. Clement.

Laetrile

Information in this section is from "Laetrile," National Cancer Institute, reviewed September 1999; available at http://cis.nci.nih.gov/fact/9_3.htm.

Laetrile, also called amygdalin or vitamin B_{17}, is derived primarily from apricot pits and almonds. It has been proposed by some as an alternative to the standard treatment for cancer.

In the 1970s, the National Cancer Institute (NCI) tested Laetrile in laboratory animals and did not find significant evidence that it was effective against animal cancers. In 1978, because of public interest in the use of Laetrile, the NCI sponsored an independent review of this substance. The review involved an evaluation of the records of people with cancer who had previously been treated with Laetrile. Letters were mailed to 385,000 physicians and 70,000 other health professionals to request information on whether patients treated with Laetrile had shown benefit. Advocacy groups were also contacted. Although an estimated 70,000 Americans had used Laetrile, only 67 cases were available for review. (The records of 93 patients treated with Laetrile were submitted for evaluation; however, 26 of the patient records lacked enough information to evaluate.) A panel of 12 oncologists, who did not know what treatments were given, reviewed the records and identified a response to Laetrile in 6 of the 67 patient records. No definite conclusions could be drawn about the anticancer effects of Laetrile because of the small number of patient responses.

In 1981, NCI sponsored a clinical trial (research study) of Laetrile in 178 people with cancer. Most of the patients were in overall good condition before treatment; one-third had not received any prior chemotherapy. The patients were treated with Laetrile plus a metabolic therapy program that included diet, enzymes, and vitamins. The Laetrile dosage and treatment schedule were consistent with that in use by practitioners who prescribed Laetrile in the community. The results of the study indicated no significant patient benefit in terms of a decrease in the size of the tumor, a decrease in or relief of cancer-related symptoms, or a longer lifespan. Several patients displayed symptoms of cyanide poisoning, including muscle weakness and impaired reflexes, or had life-threatening levels of cyanide in their blood. (Laetrile can release cyanide, which is a highly toxic chemical.) The researchers concluded that Laetrile is not effective as a cancer treatment and is harmful in some cases. A detailed report on this study was published in *The New England Journal of Medicine*, January 28, 1982, volume 306, number 4.

On March 24, 1987, a Federal judge signed an order making it illegal to import Laetrile into the United States. Previously, importation had been allowed for the treatment of patients with very advanced cancer or for the treatment of cancer pain. Laetrile is not approved by the Food and Drug Administration.

Gerson Therapy

Information in this section is from "Gerson Therapy," National Cancer Institute, reviewed December 1999; available at http://cis.nci.nih.gov/fact/9_7.htm.

Gerson therapy, a dietary approach that has been used by some to treat cancer and other diseases, focuses on the role of minerals, enzymes, hormones, and other dietary factors in restoring health and well-being. The daily regimen calls for drinking 13 glasses of juice prepared from fresh, organic fruits and vegetables, and eating vegetarian meals prepared from organically grown fruits, vegetables, and whole grains. Various supplements are given, including an iodine solution called Lugol, Vitamin B_{12}, potassium, thyroid hormone, an injectable crude liver extract, and pancreatic enzymes. Enemas, including coffee or chamomile enemas, are recommended on a regular basis to detoxify the body. Salt, spices, and aluminum cookware or utensils are not used when preparing food. Gerson therapy was named after Dr. Max B. Gerson, who initially developed this approach to treat his migraine headaches.

Dr. Gerson's therapy first came to public attention in the 1930s as a treatment for a type of tuberculosis. Gerson therapy was later used to treat other conditions, including cancer. In a presentation before a Congressional subcommittee in 1946, Dr. Gerson estimated that about 30 percent of cancer patients treated with his therapy had a favorable response. In 1947, the National Cancer Institute (NCI) reviewed 10 cases submitted by Dr. Gerson. However, because the patients were also receiving other anticancer treatments, the NCI could not determine whether the patients' condition was due to the Gerson therapy or another treatment. The NCI has not conducted any further evaluation of Dr. Gerson's therapy.

For most cancer patients, nutrition recommendations stress a well-balanced diet that includes a generous amount of fruits, vegetables, and whole-grain products. However, general guidelines such as these may have to be modified to meet the specific needs of an individual patient. Patients should talk with their doctor about an appropriate diet to follow.

Part Six

Clinical Trials and Other Research

Chapter 44

Breast Cancer Research Highlights

Introduction

Each year, about 185,000 U.S. women are newly diagnosed with breast cancer, and nearly 45,000 women die from this disease. The risk of breast cancer rises with age. Other risk factors include a history of prior breast cancer, two or more first degree relatives with premenopausal and/or bilateral breast cancer, atypical hyperplasia on previous breast biopsy, and ethnic origins in Northern Europe. Obesity, first full-term pregnancy after age 30, childlessness, and a history of ovarian or endometrial cancer also may increase a woman's risk of breast cancer.

Although substantial progress has been made in diagnosing and treating breast cancer, it continues to take a heavy toll, particularly among black women. Breast cancer survival rates rose slightly among white women over the past two decades, but they declined for black women during the same period. There are several reasons for this disparity: (1) black women are more likely than white women to be diagnosed at a later stage when the cancer has spread, (2) they may lack access to the most up-to-date treatments, and (3) they may be biologically at greater risk for more aggressive tumors.

Below are examples of current and completed breast cancer research projects sponsored by the Agency for Health Care Policy and Research (AHCPR).

Agency for Health Care Policy and Research (AHCPR), Publication No. 97-R087, October 1999.

Extramural Research

Breast cancer treatment for older women. This 5-year study is surveying older women with localized breast cancer about their treatment decisions and preferences and how they assess their quality of life. These considerations will be factored into a cost-effectiveness analysis of alternative therapies for treating breast cancer. Participating centers include the Lombardi Cancer Center at Georgetown University, Howard University, and the Washington Hospital Center, in Washington DC; the Dana Farber Cancer Institute/Harvard; the M.D. Anderson Cancer Center/University of Texas; and the Roswell Park Cancer Institute, Buffalo, NY. Jack Hadley, Principal Investigator, Georgetown University; project period September 1994 to October 1999; grant HS08395.

Effectiveness of methods for recruiting low-income women into breast and cervical cancer screening. The researchers will examine the effectiveness of methods used to increase scheduling of appointments for breast and cervical cancer screening in low-income women ages 18 to 64. They also will study the effectiveness and interaction of interventions by race and ethnicity among Mexican-American, black, and white women. Mari Jibaja, principal investigator, Baylor College of Medicine; project period September 1994 to October 1999; grant HS08581.

Breast and colon cancer screening evaluated by cancer mortality. This study will evaluate the effectiveness of screening for breast and colon cancers over time. Graham Colditz, Principal Investigator, Brigham and Women's Hospital; March 1992 to summer 1997; grant HS07038.

Prophylactic mastectomy may provide substantial gains in life expectancy for women with cancer-disposing genes. Technology now permits women to be tested for genetic mutations that markedly increase the risk of breast and ovarian cancer. The cumulative breast cancer risk for women with mutations in the BRCA1 and BRCA2 genes ranges from 40 to 85 percent, compared with 12 percent among the general population. Their risk of ovarian cancer ranges from 5 to 60 percent (vs. 1.5 percent for other women). According to this study, 30-year-old women who carry BRCA1 or BRCA2 mutations may gain from 2.9 to 5.3 years of life expectancy from preventive mastectomy and from 0.3 to 1.7 years from preventive removal of the ovaries (oophorectomy), depending on individual risk factors. The gains in life expectancy for 35-year-old women carrying mutations that place them at intermediate risk who undergo both surgeries are similar to the benefits expected for women of the same age who have very high cholesterol levels and reduce them to normal. *New Engl J Med* 336:1465-1471, May 1997. (Grant HS00020)

Statistical variation in screening mammography diagnosis. The researchers studied the variability in interpretation of screening mammograms in a large random sample of U.S. radiologists. Craig Beam, Principal Investigator, Marshfield Medical Research and Education Foundation; project period February 1992 to September 1994; grant HS07845. Selected significant findings include:

- Wide variation in interpretation of mammograms.

  Diagnostic accuracy varies substantially among radiologists specializing in the interpretation of mammograms, which may limit the effectiveness of mammography screening. *Arch Intern Med* 156:209-213, 1996.

- Effects on diagnostic accuracy of double reading of mammograms.

  By pairing with another radiologist, the average radiologist can expect an 8 to 14 percent gain in the true-positive rate (that is, diagnosis of cancer that is proven to be cancer). However, this gain comes at the expense of a 4 to 10 percent increase in the false-positive rate (a diagnosis of cancer that is proven not to be cancer). *Acad Radiol* 3(11):891-897, 1996.

Evaluation of practice variations and costs for cancer care. The objective of this study was to evaluate the choice of initial treatment for cancer in elderly women; assess the effects of choice of therapy, patient characteristics, tumor characteristics, comorbidity, and geographic location on outcomes; and estimate the costs associated with cancer care. Sheldon Retchin, Principal Investigator, People to People Health Foundations, Inc.; project period August 1991 to July 1994; grant HS06589. Selected significant findings include:

- Variations by age in receipt of adjuvant therapy following breast cancer surgery.

  As women age the likelihood decreases that they will receive chemotherapy or radiation treatment (adjuvant therapy) following surgery to prevent breast cancer recurrence. They also are less apt to have their axillary lymph nodes assessed to determine how far the cancer has spread. *Breast Cancer Res Treat* 40:75-86, 1996.

Cancer prevention for minority women in a Medicaid HMO. The purpose of this study was to investigate the impact of feedback and financial incentives on physician compliance with cancer screening guidelines for women 50 years of age and over in a mandatory Medicaid HMO. Alan Hillman, Principal Investigator, University of Pennsylvania; project period September 1993 to September 1996; grant HS07720. Selected significant findings include:

• Feedback and financial incentives do not improve physician screening compliance.

This randomized controlled trial was carried out in 54 primary care sites and involved semiannual reports to providers and a financial bonus (ranging from $570 to $1,260) when compliance criteria were met. Compliance with guidelines for mammography, clinical breast exam, colorectal screening, and Papanicolaou testing was evaluated through semiannual chart reviews in 1994 and 1995. The intervention did not improve physician compliance with the screening guidelines over an 18-month period during which cancer screening rates were improving in general. Grant final report available from the National Technical Information Service, NTIS accession no. PB97-13449.

Intramural Research

Treatment for Early-Stage Breast Cancer.

• Women treated in urban hospitals for early-stage breast cancer are much more likely to have breast-conserving surgery than women treated in rural hospitals.

The 1981 to 1987 discharge data from the Hospital Cost and Utilization Project show that patients treated in urban hospitals are nearly twice as likely to have a breast-conserving procedure and 40 percent less likely to have a radical mastectomy than rural patients. *Am J Public Health* 85(10):1432-1434, 1995. Reprints (AHCPR Publication Number 96-R028) are available free from AHRQ's Publications Clearinghouse.

- Women treated in teaching hospitals for early-stage breast cancer are nearly three times more likely to have breast-conserving surgery than women treated in non-teaching hospitals.

  This study of the surgical treatment of early-stage breast cancer in Colorado found that women treated in hospitals with an intern or resident program are almost three times as likely to have breast-conserving surgery as women treated in hospitals that do not have teaching programs. Other factors that significantly increase the odds of a breast-conserving procedure include having surgery during the fall months, treatment in a high- or medium-occupancy hospital, and treatment in a hospital located in a metropolitan area. *Dissertation Abstracts International*. May 21, 1997. (Johantgen ME, Doctoral dissertation, Virginia Commonwealth University, 1994.)

Breast and Cervical Cancer Screening.

- Female physicians are more likely to provide their patients with Pap tests and mammograms than male doctors.

  These findings take into account differences in age, race, education, lifestyle, and other factors. Med Care 31(3):213-218, 1993. Reprints (AHCPR Publication No. 97-R048) are available free from the Publications Clearinghouse.

AHCPR-Sponsored Clinical Practice Guideline on Mammography. Quality Determinants of Mammography is an evidence-based *Clinical Practice Guideline* on the quality and delivery of mammography services. The guideline was issued by AHCPR in October 1994. It was developed by a multidisciplinary panel of experts and consumers led by Lawrence W. Bassett, M.D., and R. Edward Hendrick, Ph.D. The guideline begins with the point at which a woman or her provider calls to schedule mammography and continues through the tracking, monitoring, and followup of the screened patient. Companion documents include a *Quick Reference Guide for Clinicians* (AHCPR Publication No. 95-0633), which provides information for providers who refer women for screening or diagnostic mammography, and a *Woman's Guide* (AHCPR Publication Nos. 95-0634, English; 95-0635, Spanish; 95-0636, Vietnamese; 95-0637, Tagalog; 95-0638, Korean; 95-0639, Chinese; 96-G001, Laotian; and 96-G002, Creole), which outlines seven steps to breast health. Print copies of the *Quick Reference Guide* and *Consumer Guide* (English and translations indicated) are available free from the AHRQ Clearing-house.

Call the FDA Los Angeles District Office at (714) 798-7609 for print copies or electronic access to the consumer guide in Samoan (FDA 96-8291), Thai (FDA 96-8292), or Cambodian (FDA 96-8290).

Print copies of the *Clinical Practice Guideline* are available from the U.S. Government Printing Office (stock number 017-026-00137-9; $6.50 per copy); call the GPO order desk at 202-512-1800.

For More Information

For more information on AHRQ's initiatives concerning breast cancer or other women's health topics, contact:

Agency for Healthcare Research and Quality
6010 Executive Boulevard, Room 332
Rockville, MD 20852
Telephone: (301) 594-2429
Fax: (301) 594-3211

To obtain print copies of grant announcements or an application kit, contact:

AHRQ Publications Clearinghouse
P.O. Box 8547
Silver Spring, MD 20907-8547
Telephone: 800-358-9295
TDD service: 888-586-6340
E-mail: info@ahrq.gov

To order free print copies of items from the AHRQ Publications Clearinghouse, call (800) 358-9295 or write to:

AHRQ Publications Clearinghouse
P.O. Box 8547
Silver Spring, MD 20907

Please use the AHCPR publication number when ordering.

Chapter 45

What Cancer Patients Need to Know about Taking Part in Clinical Trials

Introduction

This chapter is for people with cancer, their families, and others who care about them. It is divided into three sections. Each section answers questions many people have about clinical trials:

1. What are clinical trials?

2. What happens in a clinical trial?

3. Should I take part in a clinical trial?

The first two sections provide background information on the important role clinical trials play in improving cancer care. They also explain some of the technical terms you may hear from your doctor or nurse.

The third section of the chapter is designed to help you answer question three for yourself. It raises issues to think about as you decide whether a clinical trial is right for you. For example, what are the pros and cons of being in a clinical trial from the patient's point of view? This section also lists some questions to ask the doctor or nurse about any study you are considering. The resources section at the end of the chapter lists other sources of information about cancer and treatment studies.

National Cancer Institute, NIH Pub. No. 98-4270, June 1998. Support for this publication was provided by Novartis Oncology.

This chapter is a part of the patient education program of the National Cancer Institute (NCI). The NCI sponsors, conducts, and oversees clinical trials and other cancer research, and provides research-based information to health professionals, patients, and the public.

What Are Clinical Trials?

Clinical trials, also called cancer treatment or research studies, test new treatments in people with cancer. The goal of this research is to find better ways to treat cancer and help cancer patients. Clinical trials test many types of treatment such as new drugs, new approaches to surgery or radiation therapy, new combinations of treatments, or new methods such as gene therapy.

A clinical trial is one of the final stages of a long and careful cancer research process. The search for new treatments begins in the laboratory, where scientists first develop and test new ideas. If an approach seems promising, the next step may be testing a treatment in animals to see how it affects cancer in a living being and whether it has harmful effects. Of course, treatments that work well in the lab or in animals do not always work well in people. Studies are done with cancer patients to find out whether promising treatments are safe and effective.

Why Are Clinical Trials Important?

Clinical trials are important in two ways.

First, cancer affects us all, whether we have it, care about someone who does, or worry about getting it in the future. Clinical trials contribute to knowledge and progress against cancer. If a new treatment proves effective in a study, it may become a new standard treatment that can help many patients. Many of today's most effective standard treatments are based on previous study results. Examples include treatments for breast, colon, rectal, and childhood cancers. Clinical trials may also answer important scientific questions and suggest future research directions. Because of progress made through clinical trials, many people treated for cancer are now living longer.

Second, the patients who take part may be helped personally by the treatment(s) they receive. They get up-to-date care from cancer experts, and they receive either a new treatment being tested or the best available standard treatment for their cancer. Of course, there is no guarantee that a new treatment being tested or a standard treatment will produce good results. New treatments also may have unknown risks. But if a new treatment proves effective or more effective than standard treatment, study patients who receive it may be among the first to benefit. Some patients receive only standard treatment and benefit from it.

In the past, clinical trials were sometimes seen as a last resort for people who had no other treatment choices. Today, patients with common cancers often choose to receive their first treatment in a clinical trial.

What Happens in a Clinical Trial?

In a clinical trial, patients receive treatment and doctors carry out research on how the treatment affects the patients. While clinical trials have risks for the people who take part, each study also takes steps to protect patients.

What Is It Like to Receive Treatment in a Study?

When you take part in a clinical trial, you receive your treatment in a cancer center, hospital, clinic, and/or doctor's office. Doctors, nurses, social workers, and other health professionals may be part of your treatment team. They will follow your progress closely. You may have more tests and doctor visits than you would if you were not taking part in a study. You will follow a treatment plan your doctor prescribes, and you may also have other responsibilities such as keeping a log or filling out forms about your health. Some studies continue to check on patients even after their treatment is over.

How Is the Research Carried Out? How Are Patients Protected?

In clinical trials, both research concerns and patient well-being are important. To help protect patients and produce sound results, research with people is carried out according to strict scientific and ethical principles. These include:

1. Each clinical trial has an action plan (protocol) that explains how it will work.

The study's investigator, usually a doctor, prepares an action plan for the study. Known as a protocol, this plan explains what will be done in the study and why. It outlines how many people will take part in the study, what medical tests they will receive and how often, and the treatment plan. The same protocol is used by each doctor that takes part.

For patient safety, each protocol must be approved by the organization that sponsors the study (such as the National Cancer Institute)

379

and the Institutional Review Board (IRB) at each hospital or other study site. This board, which includes consumers, clergy, and health professionals, reviews the protocol to try to be sure that the research will not expose patients to extreme or unethical risks.

2. Each study enrolls people who are alike in key ways.

Each study's protocol describes the characteristics that all patients in the study must have. Called eligibility criteria, these guidelines differ from study to study, depending on the research purpose. They may include age, gender, the type and stage of cancer, and whether cancer patients who have had prior cancer treatment or who have other health problems can take part.

Using eligibility criteria is an important principle of medical research that helps produce reliable results. During a study, they help protect patient safety, so that people who are likely to be harmed by study drugs or other treatments are not exposed to the risk. After results are in, they also help doctors know which patient groups will benefit if the new treatment being studied is proven to work. For instance, a new treatment may work for one type of cancer but not for another, or it may be more effective for men than women.

3. Cancer clinical trials include research at three different phases.

Each phase answers different questions about the new treatment.

- Phase I trials are the first step in testing a new treatment in humans. In these studies, researchers look for the best way to give a new treatment (e.g., by mouth, IV drip, or injection? how many times a day?). They also try to find out if and how the treatment can be given safely (e.g., best dose?); and they watch for any harmful side effects. Because less is known about the possible risks and benefits in Phase I, these studies usually include only a limited number of patients who would not be helped by other known treatments.

- Phase II trials focus on learning whether the new treatment has an anticancer effect (e.g., Does it shrink a tumor? improve blood test results?). As in Phase I, only a small number of people take part because of the risks and unknowns involved.

- Phase III trials compare the results of people taking the new treatment with results of people taking standard treatment (e.g., Which group has better survival rates? fewer side effects?). In most cases, studies move into Phase III testing only after a treatment shows promise in Phases I and II. Phase III trials may include hundreds of people around the country.

4. In Phase III trials, people are assigned at random to receive either the new treatment or standard treatment.

Researchers assign patients by chance either to a group taking the new treatment (called the treatment group) or to a group taking standard treatment (called the control group). This method, called randomization, helps avoid bias: having the study's results affected by human choices or other factors not related to the treatments being tested.

In some studies, researchers do not tell the patient whether he or she is in the treatment or control group (called a single blind study). This approach is another way to avoid bias, because when people know what drug they are taking, it might change the way they react. For instance, patients who knew they were taking the new treatment might expect it to work better and report hopeful signs because they want to believe they are getting well. This could bias the study by making results look better than they really were.

Why Do Phase III Clinical Trials Compare Treatment Groups?

Comparing similar groups of people taking different treatments for the same type of cancer is another way to make sure that study results are real and caused by the treatment rather than by chance or other factors. Comparing treatments with each other often shows clearly which one is more effective or has fewer side effects.

Another reason Phase III trials compare the new treatment with standard treatment is so that no one in a study is left without any treatment when standard treatment is available, which would be unethical. When no standard treatment exists for a cancer, some studies compare a new treatment with a placebo (a look-alike pill that contains no active drug). However, you will be told if this is a possibility before you decide whether to take part in a study.

Your Doctor Can Tell You More

If you have any questions about how clinical trials work, ask your doctor, nurse, or other health professional. It may be helpful to bring this chapter and discuss points you want to understand better.

Should I Take Part in a Clinical Trial?

This is a question only you, those close to you, and your health professionals can answer together. Learning you have cancer and deciding what to do about it is often overwhelming. This section has information you can use in thinking about your choices and making your decision.

Clinical Trials: Weighing the Pros and Cons

While a clinical trial is a good choice for some people, this treatment option has possible benefits and drawbacks. Here are some factors to consider. You may want to discuss them with your doctor and the people close to you.

Possible Benefits

- Clinical trials offer high-quality cancer care. If you are in a study and do not receive the new treatment being tested, you will receive the best standard treatment. This may be as good as, or better than, the new approach.

- If a new treatment approach is proven to work and you are taking it, you may be among the first to benefit.

- By looking at the pros and cons of clinical trials and your other treatment choices, you are taking an active role in a decision that affects your life.

- You have the chance to help others and improve cancer treatment.

Possible Drawbacks

- New treatments under study are not always better than, or even as good as, standard care. They may have side effects that doctors do not expect or that are worse than those of standard treatment.

- Even if a new treatment has benefits, it may not work for you. Even standard treatments, proven effective for many people, do not help everyone.

- If you receive standard treatment instead of the new treatment being tested, it may not be as effective as the new approach.

- Health insurance and managed care providers do not always cover all patient care costs in a study. What they cover varies by plan and by study. To find out in advance what costs are likely to be paid in your case, talk to a doctor, nurse or social worker from the study.

Your Rights, Your Protections

Before and during a cancer treatment study, you have a number of rights. Knowing these can help protect you from harm.

- Taking part in a treatment study is up to you. It may be only one of your treatment choices. Talk with your doctor. Together, you can make the best choice for you.

- If you do enter a study, doctors and nurses will follow your response to treatment carefully throughout the research.

- If researchers learn that a treatment harms you, you will be taken off the study right away. You may then receive other treatment from your own doctor.

- You have the right to leave a study at any time.

One of your key rights is the right to informed consent. Informed consent means that you must be given all the facts about a study before you decide whether to take part. This includes details about the treatments and tests you may receive and the possible benefits and risks they may have. The doctor or nurse will give you an informed consent form that goes over key facts. If you agree to take part in the study, you will be asked to sign this informed consent form.

The informed consent process continues throughout the study. For instance, you will be told of any new findings regarding your clinical trial, such as new risks. You may be asked to sign a new consent form if you want to stay in the study.

Signing a consent form does not mean you must stay in the study. In fact, you can leave at any time. If you choose to leave the study, you will have the chance to discuss other treatments and care with your own doctor or a doctor from the study.

Questions You Should Ask

Finding answers and making choices may be hard for people with cancer and those who care about them. It is important to discuss your treatment choices with your doctor, a cancer specialist (an oncologist) to whom your doctor may refer you, and the staff of any clinical trial you consider entering.

Ask questions about the information you receive during the informed consent process and about any other issues that concern you. Getting answers can help you work better with the doctor. You may want to take a friend or relative along when you talk to the doctor. It also may help to write down your questions and the answers you receive, or bring a tape recorder to record what is said. No question about your care is foolish. It is very important to understand your choices.

Here are some questions you may want to ask:

The Study

- What is the purpose of the study? In what phase is this study?
- Why do researchers believe the new treatment being tested may be effective? Has it been tested before?
- Who sponsors the study, and who has reviewed and approved it?
- How are the study data and patient safety being checked?
- When and where will study results and information go?

Possible Risks and Benefits

- What are the possible short- and long-term risks; side effects, and benefits to me?
- Are there standard treatments for my type of cancer?
- How do the possible risks, side effects, and benefits in the study compare with standard treatment?

Your Care

- What kinds of treatments, medical tests, or procedures will I have during the study? Will they be painful? How do they compare with what I would receive outside the study?
- How often and for how long will I receive the treatment, and how long will I need to remain in the study? Will there be follow-up after the study?
- Where will my treatment take place? Will I have to be in the hospital? If so, how often and for how long?
- How will I know if the treatment is working?
- Will I be able to see my own doctor? Who will be in charge of my care?

Personal Issues

- How could the study affect my daily life?
- Can you put me in touch with other people who are in this study?
- What support is there for me and my family in the community?

Cost Issues

- Will I have to pay for any treatment, tests, or other charges?
- What is my health insurance likely to cover?
- Who can help answer any questions from my insurance company or managed care plan?

Other Questions

Write down other questions you have.

Others Can Help

As you make your treatment decisions, remember that you are not alone. Doctors, nurses, social workers, other people with cancer, clergy, family, and those who care about you can help and support you. The resources in the next section also can provide more information and links to other contacts in your community.

National Cancer Institute Information Resources

You may want more information for yourself, your family, and your doctor. The following National Cancer Institute (NCI) services are available to help you.

Telephone

Cancer Information Service (CIS)
Provides accurate, up-to-date information on cancer to patients and their families, health professionals, and the general public. Information specialists translate the latest scientific information into understandable language and respond in English, Spanish, or on TTY equipment.
Toll-free: 1-800-4-CANCER (1-800-422-6237)
TTY: 1-800-332-8615

Internet... these web sites may be useful

http://www.nci.nih.gov
NCI's primary web site; contains information about the Institute and its programs.

http://cancerTrials.nci.nih.gov
cancerTrials; NCI's comprehensive clinical trials information center for patients, health professionals, and the public. Includes information on understanding trials, deciding whether to participate in trials, finding specific trials, plus research news and other resources.

http://cancernet.nci.nih.gov
CancerNet™; contains material for health professionals, patients, and the public, including information from PDQ® about cancer treatment, screening, prevention, supportive care, and clinical trials, and CANCERLIT ®, a bibliographic database.

http://rex.nci.nih.gov
Includes news, upcoming events, educational materials, and publications for patients, the public, and the mass media.

http://chid.nih.gov/ncichid/
Cancer Patient Education Database; provides information on cancer patient education resources for cancer patients, their family members, and health professionals.

E-Mail

CancerMail
Includes NCI information about cancer treatment, screening, prevention, and supportive care. To obtain a contents list, send e-mail to cancermail@icicc.nci.nih.gov with the word "help" in the body of the message.

Fax

CancerFax®
Includes NCI information about cancer treatment, screening, prevention, and supportive care. To obtain a contents list, dial 301-402-5874 from a fax machine hand set and follow the recorded instructions.

Glossary

This glossary contains a list of words used in the chapter and their definitions. It also explains some other terms related to treatment studies that you may hear from your doctor or nurse.

Bias: Human choices or any other factors beside the treatments being tested that affect a study's results. Clinical trials use many methods to avoid bias, because biased results may not be correct.

Clinical trials: Research studies that involve people. Each study tries to answer scientific questions and to find better ways to prevent or treat cancer.

Control group: In a clinical trial, the group of people that receives standard treatment for their cancer. (See Treatment group.)

Informed consent: The process in which a person learns key facts about a clinical trial or research study and then agrees voluntarily to take part or decides against it. This process includes signing a form that describes the benefits and risks that may occur if the person decides to take part.

Institutional Review Board (IRB): Groups of scientists, doctors, clergy, and consumers at each health care facility at which a clinical trial takes place. Designed to protect patients who take part in studies, IRBs review and must approve the protocols for all clinical trials funded by the Federal Government. They check to see that the study is well-designed, does not involve undue risks, and includes safeguards for patients.

Investigator: A researcher in a treatment study.

Oncologist: A doctor who specializes in treating cancer.

Placebo: A tablet, capsule, or injection that looks like the drug or other substance being tested but contains no drug.

Protocol: An action plan for a clinical trial. The plan states what will be done in the study and why. It outlines how many people will take part in the study, what types of patients may take part, what tests they will receive and how often, and the treatment plan.

Randomization: A method used to prevent bias in research. People are assigned by chance to either the treatment or control group.

Remission: When the signs and symptoms of cancer go away, the disease is said to be "in remission." A remission can be temporary or permanent.

Side effects: Problems that occur when treatment affects healthy cells. Common side effects of standard cancer treatments are fatigue, nausea, vomiting, decreased blood cell counts, hair loss, and mouth sores. New treatments being tested may have these or other unknown side effects.

Single blind study: A method used to prevent bias in treatment studies. In a single blind study, the patient is not told whether he/she is taking the standard treatment or the new treatment being tested. Only the doctors know.

Stage: The extent of a cancer and whether the disease has spread from the original site to other parts of the body. Numbers with or without letters are used to define cancer stages (e.g., Stage IIb).

Standard treatment: The best treatment currently known for a cancer, based on results of past research.

Treatment group: The group that receives the new treatment being tested during a study. (See Control group.)

Chapter 46

Participating in Cancer Prevention Studies

Cancer affects us all whether we have the disease, have had it, care about someone with it, or worry about getting it. Cancer prevention studies add to knowledge and progress against cancer.

Introduction

You may have a higher risk for a certain type of cancer than most people, or you may want to learn about ways to prevent cancer. There are two types of prevention clinical trials that study ways to reduce the risk of getting cancer:

- Action studies (doing something)—These focus on finding out whether actions people take, such as getting more exercise or quitting smoking, can prevent cancer.

- Agent studies (taking something)—These studies (also called chemoprevention studies) focus on learning whether taking certain medicines, vitamins, minerals, or food supplements can prevent cancer.

This information is for people who want to learn more about agent studies designed to prevent cancer. When "cancer prevention trials or studies" are mentioned in this chapter, they refer only to *agent studies*.

Taking Part in Clinical Trials: Cancer Prevention Studies: What Participants Need to Know, National Cancer Institute, NIH Pub. No. 98-4250, December 1998.

If you want to learn more about other types of clinical trials, including other types of prevention studies, the resources listed at the end of the chapter can help you.

The chapter explains what prevention clinical trials are, how they work, and why they're done. This can help readers decide whether taking part in a cancer prevention clinical trial is right for them.

What Is Cancer?

Cancer occurs when, for unknown reasons, cells divide without control or order. All parts of the body are made up of cells that normally divide to produce more cells only when the body needs them. When cancer occurs, cells keep dividing even when new cells are not needed. The change from normal to cancerous cells requires several separate, different gene alterations. Eventually uncontrolled growth from altered genes may produce a tumor that can be benign (not cancer) or malignant (cancer). Malignant tumors can invade, damage, and destroy nearby tissues and spread to other parts of the body. A benign tumor won't spread to other parts of the body, but local tissue may be damaged and the growth may need to be removed.

What Are Cancer Risk Factors?

A cancer risk factor may mean you have an increased chance to develop cancer. It *doesn't* mean that you will develop cancer. Some people have a greater than average chance to get a certain cancer because they have one or more risk factors.

Doctors are still learning the role of risk factors in different cancers. Some risk factors make it very likely that a person will develop cancer; others seem to increase a person's risk only slightly.

Risk factors fall into four broad groups and can overlap. For some cancers, different types of risk factors can work together to increase cancer risk.

1. Lifestyle or behavioral risk factors.

These are things people do that make it more likely that they will develop cancer. For example, smoking is strongly linked to lung cancer and a type of sunlight rays (ultraviolet, or U.V., rays) are linked to melanoma, a form of skin cancer.

Lifestyle factors can also reduce cancer risk, such as eating plenty of fruits, vegetables, and fiber to lower the risk for cancer of the colon and rectum.

390

2. Hereditary risk factors.

There are altered or changed genes that are passed on from parent to child, making a person more likely to get cancer. For example, changes in two genes—BRCA1 and BRCA2—can make a person more likely to get breast cancer.

If you know that one type of cancer seems to run in your family, you may wish to speak with a trained genetic counselor. The counselor can answer many of your questions about cancer risk. You also may be able to get a test to see if you were born with a higher risk for getting cancer. Some people worry about how they'll feel if they learn they have a higher risk for cancer, especially if there's no method available to reduce their risk. Other people want to know, no matter what.

3. Environmental risk factors.

There are agents such as asbestos and radon that are linked with a higher cancer risk (an increased risk for cancer). People are sometimes exposed to cancer-causing agents in their workplace.

4. Medical risk factors.

Certain health conditions may increase a person's risk for some cancers, for example:

- colon polyps—abnormal growth of tissue in the lining of the bowel.
- previous cancer—having had radiation or chemotherapy treatment for illness, such as breast cancer, may put you at higher risk for the same type of cancer to return or to get a different type of cancer.

If a person has one or more of these risk factors, he or she may want to know more about cancer prevention trials. If you think you may be at risk for getting cancer, you can find out whether or not you are eligible to join a cancer prevention study. (See the section "Who Can Participate?")

What Is a Cancer Prevention Clinical Trial?

What Is a Clinical Trial?

Clinical trials, also known as clinical studies, are research studies in which people help doctors find ways to improve health and health care. Many of today's treatments for cancer are based on the results of past clinical trials. Examples include clinical studies to treat or prevent breast and childhood cancers. Because of progress made through clinical trials, many people treated for cancer are now living longer.

In cancer prevention trials, people take medicines, vitamins, minerals or other supplements that doctors believe may lower the risk of a certain type of cancer. Scientists who conduct these studies want to learn:

- Does the medicine or supplement (often called a study agent) prevent cancer?
- How safe is it to take the study agent?

How Are Cancer Prevention Clinical Trials Different from Other Cancer Studies?

There are different types of cancer clinical trials or studies. They include:

- chemoprevention trials designed to help people who have not previously had cancer;
- chemoprevention trials designed to prevent a new type of cancer from developing in people who have had cancer;
- early detection trials to find cancer, especially in its early stages;
- treatment trials to test new treatments in people who have cancer; and
- quality of life studies to improve comfort and quality of life for people who have cancer.

Some studies, such as treatment clinical trials and quality-of-life studies, are for people who already have cancer. Certain chemoprevention trials are for people who are cancer survivors who want to lower their risk for getting another cancer. This chapter describes cancer prevention trials or studies for people who haven't had cancer. People in these trials are usually healthy people who want to lower their risk for the disease.

How Do Researchers Design Cancer Prevention Clinical Trials?

A cancer prevention clinical trial that involves people results from a long and careful research process. As with other types of trials, each step, or phase, answers different questions about the study agent which can be a medicine, vitamin, mineral, food supplement, or a combination of these.

Phase I trials are the first step in testing a prevention agent in people. Doctors try to find the best way to give the study agent (for example, by mouth), the best dose, and if there are any harmful side effects.

Phase II trials focus on learning whether the agent has a biologic effect in preventing cancer.

Phase III trials compare a promising new agent to the standard one or to no agent, using two groups of people:

- The intervention group—This is the group taking the study agent.
- The control group—This group takes either:
  1. a standard agent that's being compared with the study agent;
  2. a look-alike pill that contains no active ingredient, called a placebo.

Because less is known about possible risks and benefits in Phase I and II, these trials usually include only a small number of participants. In most cases, studies move into Phase III testing only after an agent shows promise in Phases I and II. Phase III trials may include hundreds of research centers around the country and hundreds or thousands of people.

Clinical trials follow strict guidelines for science and ethics. These guidelines deal with many areas, including the study's design and who can be in the study. Every trial has a chief investigator, who is usually a doctor. The investigator prepares a study action plan, called a protocol. This plan explains what the trial will do, how, and why. For example, it states:

- How many people will be in the study.
- Who is able to be in the study.
- What study agents people will take.
- What medical tests they will have and how often.
- What information will be gathered.

Every research center that takes part in the trial uses the same protocol. This ensures that information from all centers can be combined.

How Do Review Groups Protect Participants?

Clinical trials have several procedures to protect the safety of the people who join the study. Several groups have to approve the protocol for every study. Two of those groups are the sponsor of the study (for example, the National Cancer Institute) and the Institutional Review Board (IRB).

Every study center has an IRB, which includes doctors, other health care providers, consumers, and sometimes members of the clergy who do not have any personal interest in the results of the study which would bias them. They serve as neutral reviewers and ensure that the study is managed fairly and that no one is likely to be harmed who may decide to join. Each Phase III cancer prevention study also has a special group called a Data Safety and Monitoring Committee that looks at the test results and monitors the safety of the participants, and decides whether the study should go forward as originally planned.

What Happens in a Phase III Cancer Prevention Clinical Trial?

If you decide to join a Phase III cancer prevention trial, you'll work with a research team. Team members may include doctors, nurses, social workers, and other health care providers. They will give you clear instructions. You may be asked to take a medication. You also may be asked to keep a diary or answer questions about how you're feeling.

During the study, a research team will review your health carefully. (This means that you may have more tests and doctor visits than you would if you weren't in the study.) Team members also may check on you for a while after the trial ends (followup). To make the trial results as reliable as possible, it is important for you to follow the research team's instructions. That means having all doctor visits and tests, taking medicines on time, and filling out logs or answering questions. Careful review and followup help you and scientists find out quickly what agent is best for reducing cancer risk.

Who Can Participate?

Clinical trials try to enroll people who are alike in certain ways, depending on the study's purpose. Every protocol tells who can join that study and spells out the characteristics that people should have.

These are called eligibility criteria. They may include age, gender, general health, and cancer risk factors.

Eligibility criteria are a key part of medical research. They help produce results we can trust. And after those results are known, the information can help doctors find out who will be helped by the approach being studied if it's shown to work. For example, a new drug may work for people with one type of risk factor but not for another, or it may work better for men than for women.

Eligibility criteria also help protect you. They help make sure that if you are likely to be harmed by something in the study design, you are not exposed to that risk.

How Are Participants Assigned to Groups?

Doctors use a process called randomization (chance) using a computer to assign you to either the intervention group or the control group in Phase III studies. This method ensures that certain factors and human choices don't affect study results, making them less reliable. When groups are compared with each other, it is clear whether the study agent works or has bad side effects. This also helps ensure that the findings really result from the study agent, and not from something else.

Most Phase III cancer prevention studies use a double-blind research design. This means that neither you nor the doctors know which people are taking the study agent or the control agent. Only the researchers at a central office know. Sometimes a doctor needs to find out if a participant has taken the study agent. A doctor can find this out, if needed, by talking with the central office staff.

No one knows whether it is better to be in the intervention or control group until the study is over and the results are ready. If that were known, there would be no need for the study. Either group may have good results or problems. The results help doctors decide whether to advise people to take the study agent for cancer prevention.

What Is Informed Consent?

Informed consent is a process during which you learn key facts about a clinical study before you decide whether or not to join. These facts include details about the study approach and tests you may have, and the benefits and risks that could result. (See the section "Should I Take Part in a Cancer Prevention Study?")

The doctor or nurse will give you a form that goes over key facts. It's called a consent form. If you decide to take part in the study, you'll be asked to sign this form. You can take the form home and discuss it with your family, friends, or others before you make your decision. If you do decide to join the study, be sure to ask for a copy of the consent form so you can look it over at any time.

Don't be afraid to ask questions until you get all the facts you need to decide. This is an important decision, and you should feel at ease with the choice you make. In fact, you should feel free to ask the research team questions at any time.

Informed consent is more than a piece of paper; it's a process that lasts throughout a study. For example, you may be told about new risks or other findings from the study, and asked to sign a new consent form. As always, the choice to join or to continue is yours.

You Can Leave the Study at Any Time

Informed consent lasts as long as you're in the study. You can change your mind and leave the study any time you want—before the study starts or at any time during the study or follow-up period. If you decide to leave, you'll have a chance to talk about other prevention options with your own doctor or with a doctor from the study.

What Protections Do You Have?

Before and during a cancer prevention trial, you have several important rights:

- Informed consent—the right to know all you need to make a thoughtful decision about joining a study.

- Changing your mind—the right to leave the study at any time.

- Medical monitoring—the right to have your health watched throughout the study.

- Removal from harm—the right to be taken off the study if doctors learn that an agent may harm you.

Should I Take Part in a Cancer Prevention Clinical Trial?

People decide to be part of a cancer prevention clinical trial for many reasons. For example:

- Some people who have a higher cancer risk join a cancer prevention trial because they want to take a more active role in their health care. Also, because study participants get regular and careful medical attention, some health problems may be found early.

- Some people feel good about helping medical knowledge advance. If the study agent turns out to work against cancer, it may help others. For example, prevention trials showed that aspirin helps prevent heart attacks, and now many people take aspirin daily on their doctor's advice.

Even when they don't lead to new therapies, clinical trials often answer important questions and help move research forward.

You need to weigh the benefits and risks for yourself. The list in the next section may help you do that. You also may find it useful to talk with family members or friends, your health care providers, and anyone you know who has been in a clinical trial.

Remember: You are the only person who can make this decision, and if you join a clinical trial, you can change your mind *at any time* — even after the study starts.

Prevention Clinical Trials: Weighing the Pros and Cons

Possible Benefits

- If the agent being studied is found to be helpful, you may be among the first to benefit.
- In a cancer prevention clinical trial, your health is reviewed with care.
- A cancer prevention clinical trial gives you a chance to help doctors learn more about cancer prevention and help others.

Possible Drawbacks

- New agents may have side effects or risks unknown to the doctors.
- The side effects, and results, of the agent may be worse than what's now recommended.
- Even if a new agent is helpful, it may not work for you.
- Health insurance and managed care providers don't always cover all costs in a clinical trial. (To find out what costs are likely to be covered for you, talk to a member of the research team or a social worker.)

Questions You Should Ask

Finding answers, and making choices, may be hard for people who are at risk for cancer—and for those who care about them. It's important for you to discuss your concerns and your choices with your doctor and with the staff of any clinical study that you're thinking of joining.

Ask questions about any issues that concern you. You need to review your choices.

Tips for Getting Information

When you talk with your doctor or members of the research team:

- Take a family member or friend along for support and for help in asking questions or recording answers.

- Plan ahead what to ask—but don't be afraid to ask any new questions you think of while you're there.

- Write down your questions in advance, to make sure you remember to ask them all.

- Write down the answers so you can review them when you want.

- Bring a tape recorder to make a record of what's said (even if you write down answers).

Here are some questions you may want to ask about:

The Study

- What's the purpose of the study?

- Why do doctors think the approach may work? (For example, how has it been studied before?)

- Who will sponsor the study?

- Who has reviewed and approved it?

- How are the study results and safety of participants being checked?

- How long will the study last?

- What will I have to do if I join?

- Will I ever know if I'm taking the study agent that's being studied?

Possible Risks and Benefits

- What are the short-term benefits for me?
- What are the long-term benefits for me?
- What are the short-term risks, such as side effects, for me?
- What are the long-term risks for me?
- What other prevention options do people with my risk for cancer have?
- How do the risks and benefits of this trial compare with those options?

Your Participation and Care

- What kinds of therapies, tests, or procedures will I have during the trial?
- Will they hurt, and if so, for how long?
- How do they compare with the care I'd have outside the trial?
- How often, and for how long, will I take the study agent that is being studied?
- Will I be able to take my regular medications?
- Where will I have my medical exams?
- Will I be able to see my own doctor?
- Who will be in charge of my care?

Personal Issues

- How could being in the study affect my daily life?
- Can I talk with other people who are in the study?

Cost Issues

- Will I have to pay for any part of the trial, such as tests or the study agent?
- If I will, what are the charges likely to be?
- What is my health insurance likely to cover?
- Who can help answer any questions from my insurance company or health plan?

Other Questions

• Write down other questions you have.

Others Can Help

• As you make your decisions, remember that there are resources for people who have a higher risk for cancer. The resources below can give you more information and put you in touch with contacts in your community.

National Cancer Institute Information Resources

You may want more information for yourself, your family, and your doctor. The following National Cancer Institute (NCI) services are available to help you.

Telephone: Cancer Information Service (CIS) provides accurate, up-to-date information on cancer to patients and their families, health professionals, and the general public. Information specialists translate the latest scientific information into understandable language and respond in English, Spanish, or on TTY equipment.

Telephone 1-800-4-CANCER (1-800-422-6237)
TTY: 1-800-332-8615 (for deaf and hard of hearing callers)

Internet: These web sites may be useful:

NCI's primary web site; contains information about the Institute and its programs. http://www.nci.nih.gov/

CancerNet; contains material for health professionals, patients, and the public, including information from PDQ about cancer treatment, screening, prevention, genetics, supportive care, and clinical trials, and CANCERLIT, a bibliographic database. http://cancernet.nci.nih. gov/

cancerTrials; NCI's comprehensive clinical trials information center for patients, health professionals, and the public. Includes information on understanding trials, deciding whether to participate in trials, finding specific trials, plus research news and other resources. http://cancertrials.nci.nih.gov/

This site includes news, upcoming events, educational materials, and publications for patients, the public, and the mass media. http://rex. nci.nih.gov

Cancer Patient Education Database; provides information on cancer patient education resources for patients, their families, and health professionals. http://chid.nih.gov/ncichid/

E-mail: CancerMail includes NCI information about cancer treatment, screening, prevention, genetics, and supportive care. To obtain a contents list, send e-mail to cancermail@icicc.nci.nih.gov with the word "help" in the body of the message.

Fax: CancerFax includes NCI information about cancer treatment, screening, prevention, genetics, and supportive care. To obtain a contents list, dial 301-402-5874 or 1-800-624-2511 from a touch-tone telephone or fax machine hand set and follow the recorded instructions.

Glossary

Action studies: In cancer prevention clinical trials, studies that focus on finding out whether actions people take can prevent cancer.

Agent studies: In cancer prevention clinical trials, studies that focus on examining whether taking certain medicines, vitamins, minerals, or food supplements can prevent cancer.

Benign: Not cancerous; cannot invade neighboring tissues or spread to other parts of the body.

Bias: Having an idea about what the study results will show before the clinical trial is conducted.

Chemoprevention studies: Also called "cancer prevention agent studies." Cancer prevention studies that test whether the study agent—usually medicines, vitamins, minerals, food supplements, or a combination of them—can reduce a person's chances of getting cancer.

Clinical trials: Also called "clinical studies." Research studies with people. Each trial tries to answer specific scientific questions and to find better ways to prevent, detect, or treat diseases or to improve care.

Colon polyps: Abnormal growths of tissue on the lining of the bowel. Polyps are a risk factor for cancer of the bowel.

Consent form: A document that provides key facts about a clinical trial. This includes information about the study agent, tests that study participants may have, and possible benefits and risks. Although all participants in a clinical trial must sign a consent form, they can leave the study at any time. As a trial proceeds, there may be new consent forms.

Control group: In a Phase III cancer prevention clinical trial of a study agent, the group that receives either a placebo or a standard agent that is being compared to a new agent.

Data Safety and Monitoring Committee: An impartial group that provides oversight of a clinical trial and reviews the results to see if they are acceptable. This group determines if the trial should be altered or closed.

Double-blind: A method used to prevent bias in a clinical trial. Neither the participants nor the doctor knows who is taking the study agent and who is not. Only researchers at a central office know.

Environmental risk factor: A hazardous agent that is known to cause cancer or increase risk when people are exposed to it, for example asbestos, radon, and second-hand smoke.

Followup: Keeping track of the health of people who participate in a clinical study for a period of time during the study and after the study ends.

Gene alterations: Changes in the cells' unit of inheritance that may be good or bad for the body.

Hereditary risk factor: Altered or mutated genes that make it more likely that a person will develop cancer. Also called an "inherited" risk factor, but this does not necessarily have to be inherited from a parent. It can be acquired in a germline cell through lifestyle behaviors or through exposure to hazards in the environment. Once this cell is altered, the mutated gene can pass to the next generation.

Informed consent: A process in which a person learns key facts about a clinical trial, including potential risks and benefits, before deciding whether or not to participate in a study. Informed consent continues throughout the trial.

Institutional Review Board (IRB): A group of scientists, doctors, clergy, and consumers at each health care facility that participates in a clinical trial. IRBs are designed to protect study participants. They review and must approve the action plan for every clinical trial.

They check to see that the trial is well designed, does not involve undue risks, and includes safeguards for patients.

Intervention group: The group receiving the study agent that's being tested in a clinical trial or clinical study.

Investigator: A researcher in a clinical trial or clinical study.

Lifestyle risk factor: Personal behavior, such as smoking, that may increase a person's risk for cancer. Also called "behavioral risk factor."

Malignant: Cancerous. Malignant tumors can invade surrounding tissues and spread to other parts of the body.

Medical risk factor: Health conditions that may lead to cancer. See colon polyps.

Placebo: A tablet or capsule that looks like the study agent but doesn't contain any active ingredient. Some people call a placebo a "sugar pill."

Protocol: An action plan for a clinical trial. The plan states what the study will do, how, and why. It explains how many people will be in it, who's eligible to participate, what study agents they'll take, what tests they'll receive and how often, and what information is gathered.

Randomization: A method used to prevent bias in research. People are assigned by chance, often by a computer, either to receive the study agent (intervention group) or not (control group).

Risk factor: A condition that increases a person's chance of developing a particular disease. Cancer risk factors include age, lifestyle (including exposure to cancer-causing substances), family history of cancer, or medical conditions that can lead to cancer.

Side effects: Problems that occur when a study agent causes expected but unpleasant conditions, like dry skin or headaches.

Sponsor: The agency or firm responsible for financing the clinical trial.

Study agent: A medicine, vitamin, mineral, food supplement, or a combination of them that's being tested in a cancer prevention trial. A study agent is usually something that's taken by mouth (eaten or swallowed).

Tissue: Specialized cells arranged in a precise pattern in the body.

Tumor: An abnormal growth of tissue. Tumors may be either benign or cancerous.

Ultraviolet: Invisible rays that are part of the energy that comes from the sun which can burn the skin and cause skin cancer.

Chapter 47

The Breast Cancer Prevention Trial

What is the Breast Cancer Prevention Trial?

The Breast Cancer Prevention Trial (BCPT) is a clinical trial (a research study conducted with people) designed to see whether taking the drug tamoxifen (Nolvadex®) can prevent breast cancer in women who are at an increased risk of developing the disease. The BCPT is also looking at whether taking tamoxifen decreases the number of heart attacks and reduces the number of bone fractures in these women. The study began recruiting participants in April 1992 and closed enrollment in September 1997; 13,388 women ages 35 and older are enrolled. Researchers with the National Surgical Adjuvant Breast and Bowel Project (NSABP) are conducting the study in more than 300 centers across the United States and Canada. The study is funded by the National Cancer Institute (NCI), the United States' primary agency for cancer research.

What is tamoxifen?

Tamoxifen is a drug, taken by mouth as a pill. It has been used for 25 years to treat patients with breast cancer. Tamoxifen works against breast cancer, in part, by interfering with the activity of estrogen, a female hormone that promotes the growth of breast cancer cells. For this reason, tamoxifen is often called an "anti-estrogen." In treatment, the drug slows or stops the growth of these cancer cells.

Cancer Trials, National Cancer Institute, October 1999.

Why was tamoxifen tested to prevent breast cancer?

Research had shown that taking tamoxifen as adjuvant therapy for breast cancer not only helps prevent the original breast cancer from returning but also helps to prevent the development of new cancers in the opposite breast. Researchers believed that tamoxifen might have a similar beneficial effect for women at increased risk of breast cancer. While tamoxifen acts against the effects of estrogen in breast tissue, it acts like estrogen in other organs. Tamoxifen's estrogen-like effects include the lowering of blood cholesterol and the slowing of bone loss.

Who participated in the BCPT?

Women at increased risk for developing breast cancer participated in the study. These included women 60 years of age and older who qualified to participate based on age alone, and women between the ages of 35 and 59 with an increased risk of breast cancer equivalent to or greater than that of a 60-year-old woman. At age 60, about 17 of every 1,000 women are expected to develop breast cancer within five years.

About 40 percent of the women on the trial were ages 35 to 49, about 30 percent were ages 50 to 59, and about 30 percent were age 60 or older. Almost 4 percent of the participants were minorities, including Black American, Asian American, Hispanic, and other groups.

Did every woman in the study receive tamoxifen?

No. Participants in the BCPT were randomized (selected by chance) to receive either tamoxifen or a placebo (an inactive pill that looked like tamoxifen). In a process known as "double blinding," neither the participant nor her physician knew which pill she was receiving. Setting up a study in this way allowed the researchers to clearly see the true benefits and side effects of tamoxifen without the influence of other factors. According to the design, all women in the study were to take two pills a day for five years, either a 20-mg dose of tamoxifen (two 10-mg pills) or placebo pills.

Why were women 60 years of age or older eligible for the BCPT based on age alone?

Many diseases, including breast cancer, occur more often in older persons. The risk of developing breast cancer increases with age, so breast cancer occurs more commonly in women over 60 years of age. The risk of developing heart disease or osteoporosis also increases with age, and those diseases are also being studied in the BCPT.

What factors were used to determine increased risk of breast cancer for the participants aged 35 to 59?

To enroll in the study, women between 35 and 59 years of age needed to have a risk of developing breast cancer within the next five years that was equal to or greater than the average risk for 60-year-old women. This increased risk was determined in one of two ways. Women diagnosed as having lobular carcinoma *in situ*, a condition that is not cancer but indicates an increased chance of developing invasive breast cancer, were eligible based on that diagnosis alone. The risk for other women was determined by a computer calculation based on the following factors:

- Number of first-degree relatives (mother, daughters, or sisters) who had been diagnosed as having breast cancer;

- Whether a woman had any children and her age at her first delivery;

- The number of times a woman had breast lumps biopsied, especially if the tissue showed a condition known as atypical hyperplasia; and

- The woman's age at her first menstrual period.

What proportion of women in the United States are estimated to be at the level of risk required for participation in the BCPT?

- At age 35, about three women in 1,000 or .3 percent, would have qualified for the study based on their estimated breast cancer risk.

- At age 40, the proportion is about 27 women in 1,000, or 2.7 percent.

- At age 45, the proportion is about 71 women in 1,000, or 7.1 percent.

- At age 50, the proportion is about 93 women in 1,000, or 9.3 percent.

- At age 55, the proportion is about 125 women in 1,000, or 12.5 percent.

- At age 60 and beyond, all women would have met the breast cancer risk criteria.

Did other factors affect eligibility for the study?

Certain health conditions affected eligibility for the study. For example, women at increased risk for blood clots could not participate. Also, women taking hormone replacements and women using oral contraceptives ("the pill") could not take part in the trial unless they stopped taking these medications. Those who stopped taking these hormones were eligible for the study three months after they discontinued the drugs.

Women who were pregnant or who planned to become pregnant were not eligible to participate. Animal studies have suggested that the use of tamoxifen during pregnancy might harm the fetus. Premenopausal women participating in the BCPT were required to use some method of birth control other than oral contraceptives. Oral contraceptives may change the effects of tamoxifen and may also affect the risk of breast cancer.

What are the results of the BCPT?

At this point (data to March 31, 1998), women on the trial have been followed on the study for about four years (47.7 months). Results show 49 percent fewer diagnoses of invasive breast cancer in women who were randomized to take tamoxifen compared to women who were randomized to take the placebo (89 cases in the tamoxifen group vs. 175 cases in the placebo group). Women on tamoxifen also had 50 percent fewer diagnoses of noninvasive breast cancer, such as ductal or lobular carcinoma *in situ* (35 cases in the tamoxifen group vs. 69 cases in the placebo group). Nine women have died of breast cancer, three women in the tamoxifen group and six women in the placebo group.

Women in the tamoxifen group had almost 20 percent fewer bone fractures of the hip, wrist, and spine than women in the placebo group (111 cases in the tamoxifen group vs. 137 cases in the placebo group), a result that nearly reached statistical significance. There was no difference in the number of heart attacks between the two groups.

Tamoxifen did increase the women's chances of three rare but serious health problems: endometrial cancer (cancer of the lining of the uterus) 36 cases in the tamoxifen group vs. 15 cases in the placebo group; pulmonary embolism (blood clot in the lung) 18 cases in the tamoxifen group vs. six cases in the placebo group; and deep vein thrombosis (blood clots in major veins) 35 cases in the tamoxifen group vs. 22 cases in the placebo group.

What were the participants' chances of developing endometrial cancer?

BCPT participants who were randomized to the tamoxifen group had more than twice the chance of developing endometrial cancer compared with women on placebo (based on 36 cases in the tamoxifen group vs. 15 cases in the placebo group). The increased risk of endometrial cancer was equal to the risk that was expected and is in the same range as (or less than) the endometrial cancer risk for postmenopausal women taking single-agent estrogen replacement therapy. Estrogens and agents that act like estrogens are known to increase the risk of endometrial cancer.

All the participants were informed about the possibility of increased risk of endometrial cancer before they entered the study. Like all cancers, endometrial cancer is potentially life-threatening. All but one (in the placebo group) of the endometrial cancers that occurred during the study were found at an early stage, when treatment is very effective. However, one participant (also in the placebo group) died of endometrial cancer. About 38 percent of BCPT participants in both groups had a hysterectomy (surgery to remove the uterus) for a variety of health reasons before joining the study. Therefore, these women were not at any known risk for endometrial cancer.

What was done to help diagnose endometrial cancer early?

Pap smears are very effective at detecting cancer in the cervix but are not useful for detecting endometrial cancer. Therefore, a screening endometrial sampling—removal of cells in the lining of the uterus for examination under a microscope—was used in the BCPT to check for abnormalities in the endometrium. Women who joined the study after October 1994 were required to have a screening endometrial sampling before entering the study if their uterus had not been removed. All women in the study were strongly urged to have screening endometrial sampling done annually throughout the study (at no cost to them), but could decline if they chose. In addition to these annual tests, women in the BCPT were told to see their physicians if they experienced abnormal vaginal bleeding or pain. The vast majority of the endometrial cancers that were diagnosed in the BCPT caused such symptoms.

What were the participants' chances of getting blood clots?

Women taking tamoxifen had three times the chance of developing a pulmonary embolism (blood clot in the lung) as women on placebo (based on 18 cases in the tamoxifen group vs. six cases in the placebo group). Three women died from these embolisms, all in the tamoxifen group. Women in the tamoxifen group were also more likely to have deep vein thrombosis (a blood clot in a major vein) than women on placebo (35 cases vs. 22 cases). Blood clots occur more often in people with high blood pressure (hypertension) or diabetes, smokers, and in those who are obese.

Is there a relationship between tamoxifen use and the development of eye problems?

Women in the tamoxifen group, in general, had no more eye problems than women taking the placebo. However, women taking tamoxifen were at a slightly increased risk for developing cataracts (a clouding of the lens inside the eye) according to other research. Over the course of the study, 574 women in the tamoxifen group and 507 women in the placebo group developed cataracts; 114 and 73 women, respectively, had cataract surgery. As women age, they are more likely to develop cataracts whether or not they take tamoxifen.

Was tamoxifen associated with any other cancers?

Tamoxifen was not associated with an increased risk of any other cancer other than endometrial cancer.

What were the other adverse effects of tamoxifen?

Like most medications, whether over-the-counter medications, prescription drugs, or drugs in research studies, tamoxifen causes adverse effects in some women. The effects experienced most often by women in the tamoxifen group were hot flashes and vaginal discharge. Women in both groups reported sometimes having side effects—even though the placebo itself would not cause any symptoms. The side effects that some women in both groups reported included: vaginal dryness, itching, or bleeding; menstrual irregularities; depression; loss of appetite; nausea and/or vomiting; dizziness; headaches;

and fatigue. Treatments that could minimize or eliminate most side effects were available to the participants.

What is happening to the participants now?

All participants are being asked to continue with their follow-up examinations. Women who have been randomized to the tamoxifen group who have not completed five years of tamoxifen therapy will have the opportunity to continue on therapy. Postmenopausal women who had been taking the placebo are being invited to participate in the upcoming Study of Tamoxifen and Raloxifene that will compare tamoxifen to the osteoporosis drug raloxifene, which could have similar breast cancer prevention properties, but might be associated with fewer adverse effects. Women in the placebo group also have the option of seeking tamoxifen from their private health care providers.

How can a woman learn more about the Study of Tamoxifen and Raloxifene?

The NSABP is planning a new breast cancer prevention trial, scheduled to begin recruiting participants in 1999. The trial, known as STAR (Study of Tamoxifen and Raloxifene) would involve about 22,000 postmenopausal women who are at least 35 years old and are at increased risk for developing breast cancer. The study would compare tamoxifen to raloxifene, an osteoporosis drug that appears to have breast cancer prevention effects. Raloxifene (Evista®) is manufactured by Eli Lilly and Company, Indianapolis, Ind.

There are several ways to be placed on a mailing list for more information on this upcoming trial—by Internet, by mail, or by fax. On the Internet, the NSABP homepage (http://www.nsabp.pitt.edu/) has a form available. By regular mail, send a letter or post card with name, mailing address, and a note specifying interest in future breast cancer prevention trials to: NSABP, Box 21, Pittsburgh, PA 15261. Or fax the same information to NSABP at (412) 330-4660. When information about the next prevention trial is available, it will be mailed to the people on this list.

Would it be beneficial for women to take tamoxifen for more than five years?

Not necessarily: Results of another NSABP study in which women with early stage breast cancer took tamoxifen for five years vs. 10 years (called the B-14 trial) showed no greater benefit from the longer duration of tamoxifen and showed a trend toward more adverse effects.

Based on the BCPT results, should women who are at increased risk of breast cancer take tamoxifen?

Women who are at increased risk of breast cancer now have the option to consider taking tamoxifen to reduce their chances of developing breast cancer. As with any medical procedure or intervention, the decision to take tamoxifen is an individual one in which the benefits and risks of the therapy must be considered. The balance of these benefits and risks will vary depending on a woman's personal health history and how she weighs the benefits and risks. Therefore even if a woman is at increased risk of breast cancer, tamoxifen therapy may not be appropriate for her. Women who are considering tamoxifen therapy should talk with their health care provider.

How does a woman determine whether she is at increased risk of breast cancer?

A computer-based tool that allows health professionals to project a woman's individualized estimate of breast cancer risk is being released in a pilot program by the NCI this month. The Breast Cancer Risk Assessment Tool is a computer disk that women and their health care providers can use to estimate a woman's chances of developing breast cancer based on several established risk factors. Researchers from NCI and NSABP developed the tool. The disk is available at no charge and in personal computer (PC) and Macintosh computer formats. To order, call the NCI's Cancer Information Service at 1-800-4-CANCER or use the online sign-up form.

Will women with breast cancer gene alterations (BRCA1 and BRCA2) benefit from tamoxifen?

These two breast cancer gene alterations, which increase a woman's risk of the disease, were identified after the BCPT began. Using blood samples taken from participants, analyses are under way to determine whether tamoxifen has the same relative effects on women whether or not they carry alterations in these genes. To maintain strict confidentiality, samples in this study have no identifying labels that could link them to individual women. Therefore, researchers will not be able to give individual results to a participant or her health care provider.

Is tamoxifen a good substitute for hormone replacement therapy?

No. Every woman has individual health risks that affect her need for interventions such as hormone replacement therapy or tamoxifen therapy. Hormone replacement therapy is intended to help women maintain bone density. Many women benefit from a reduction in hot flashes and other problems that can affect quality of life. Some studies have suggested that hormone replacement therapy increases a woman's chances of developing breast cancer. The BCPT results show that tamoxifen reduces breast cancer risk and may help slow or reduce bone loss, as evidenced by the reduced number of bone fractures.

Should women who are not known to be at increased risk of breast cancer consider taking tamoxifen?

This question has not been studied. At this time, there is no evidence that tamoxifen is beneficial for women who do not have an increased risk of breast cancer.

Are there any women who should not take tamoxifen?

Animal studies have suggested that the use of tamoxifen during pregnancy might harm the fetus. Women who were pregnant or who planned to become pregnant were not eligible to participate in the BCPT. Premenopausal women participating in the BCPT were required to use some method of birth control other than oral contraceptives ("the pill") while taking tamoxifen. Oral contraceptives may change the effects of tamoxifen and may also affect the risk of breast cancer. Women with a history of blood clots, hypertension, diabetes, and cigarette smoking must also consider that tamoxifen increases the risk for serious blood clots.

Where were the study results published?

The study is published in the *Journal of the National Cancer Institute*, Vol. 90, No. 18, Sept. 16, 1998. The study is titled, "Tamoxifen for Prevention of Breast Cancer: Report of the National Surgical Adjuvant Breast and Bowel Project P-1 Study. The authors are B. Fisher, J.P. Costantino, D.L. Wickerham, C.K. Redmond, M. Kavanah, W.M. Cronin, V. Vogel, A. Robidoux, N. Dimitrov, J. Atkins, M. Daly, S. Wieand, E. Tan-Chiu, L. Ford, N. Wolmark, and other NSABP investigators.

413

What is the National Surgical Adjuvant Breast and Bowel Project?

The NSABP is a cooperative group with a 40-year-history of designing and conducting clinical trials, the results of which have changed the way breast cancer is treated, and now, potentially prevented. Results of research studies conducted by NSABP researchers have been the dominant force in altering the standard surgical treatment of breast cancer from radical mastectomy to lumpectomy plus radiation. This group was also the first to demonstrate that adjuvant therapy could alter the natural history of breast cancer, thus increasing survival rates. When a breast cancer prevention study was initially conceived, more than 30,000 women with breast cancer had participated in treatment studies conducted by NSABP investigators. Additional research studies to prevent cancer are a logical next step for this research group.

For More Information

For more information about cancer visit NCI's Web site for patients, public, and the mass media at http://rex.nci.nih.gov/ or NCI's main web site at http://www.nci.nih.gov/.

414

Chapter 48

Questions about Treating Small Tumors of the Breast

Small Breast Tumors: Does More Treatment Help?

Awareness of the most common type of cancer in American women, breast cancer, has grown significantly at the same time that screening has considerably improved. More patients than ever are diagnosed at an early stage, when tumors are still small and confined to a limited area. What is the best way to treat these very small tumors?

Patients with stage I breast tumors (less then two centimeters) in whom the underarm, or axillary, lymph nodes are free of cancer, have an excellent prognosis with surgery alone. Approximately 90 percent of women in this group will live five or more years without a recurrence of their cancer. Women with even smaller tumors (less than one centimeter) probably have an even better prognosis.

A subset of this latter group, however, may benefit from post-surgical, or adjuvant, therapy, despite the additional risk associated with potential side effects (including serious infections and heart failure). Determining which patients may gain from adjuvant treatments, including chemotherapy and hormone therapy, is a problem facing researchers and clinicians.

"Small Breast Tumors: Does More Treatment Help?" Cancer Trials, National Cancer Institute, February 2001.

Pooling Data

In early 2001, a new look at five clinical trials conducted between 1976 and 1993 strongly suggested that adjuvant therapy be considered as an option for some women with very small breast tumors. The report by Bernard Fisher, M.D., of the National Surgical Breast and Bowel Project (NSABP) in Pittsburgh, Penn., appeared in the Jan. 17, 2001, issue of the *Journal of the National Cancer Institute*.

The report's main finding: post-surgical treatment with chemotherapy, hormonal therapy (tamoxifen), or both, reduced the risk of recurrence in women with tumors measuring one centimeter or less that had no associated sign of cancer in axillary lymph nodes.

In an editorial in the same issue, however, Marc E. Lippman, M.D., professor and chair of the Department of Internal Medicine at the University of Michigan, urged caution before shifting the current treatment paradigm to more liberal recommendations for adjuvant systemic therapy, especially for chemotherapy. So what should patients who fall into the report's profile make of these results?

An important point to keep in mind is that the data in Fisher's report came not from a new clinical trial, but from a "meta-analysis" of five small trials. A meta-analysis re-examines existing data in order to improve the strength of scientific findings by comparing information from similar patients whose numbers in each individual study may be small. The method is a way to combine the results of separate studies, and to synthesize summaries and conclusions.

Meta-analyses can be helpful in evaluating the effectiveness of therapies or in generating ideas about where researchers should go next for answers, but they do not often change medical paradigms or practice. That's because the separate studies in a meta-analysis have often been conducted over a period of 10 to 15 years, in which diagnostic and treatment methods may have changed. Also, different studies are not set up the same way, so data comparisons may be made between similar but not identical variables, or between different variables altogether.

In supporting his report's conclusion that at least some women with very small breast tumors may benefit from adjuvant therapy, Fisher said the meta-analysis for the first time showed with reasonable data that not all women with small tumors will be free from recurrence after surgery without adjuvant therapy.

"There are indeed benefits with this group of patients," Fisher said. "The big question is which patient should get the benefits of this,"—that is, be given the opportunity to get the drugs—"and which ones shouldn't. This is a dilemma of all clinical trials. The question has to be considered very carefully and be based on the degree of benefit."

Better Prognostic Factors Needed

Part of the difficulty in deciding whether an early breast cancer patient would benefit from adjuvant therapy is that "in small tumors, prognosis changes millimeter by millimeter," Lippman wrote in the accompanying editorial. Where should the line be drawn?

In addition, if the women have no cancer in axillary lymph nodes, physicians can't use one of the strongest predictors of recurrence: the number of cancerous lymph nodes. Instead, physicians must rely on other indicators, such as hormone receptor status, age or menopausal status, all of which may be less reliable.

Another concern of Lippman's was that while the meta-analysis aimed to describe patients with tumors of one centimeter or less, many women in the pooled studies actually had larger tumors. That is, there might not be enough women of the right cancer profile in the pooled studies to support the call for a change in recommended treatment.

"This is a data- and evidence-based question," Lippman said. "The numbers in the study don't apply to most women with small tumors because most women in the study do not have tumors less than one centimeter, and it's not a randomized study."

In the end, wrote Lippman, "the small but real risks [associated with adjuvant therapy] of infection, hemorrhage, cardiomyopathy, deep-vein thrombosis, pulmonary emboli, uterine cancer, etc., may approach, if not exceed, therapy gains."

Jeff Abrams, M.D., coordinator of breast cancer treatment trials in the National Cancer Institute's Cancer Therapy Evaluation Program, said the meta-analysis' conclusion that adjuvant therapy may be beneficial to some early breast cancer patients appears consistent with recommendations from the National Institutes of Health's Consensus Development Conference in November 2000. But he agreed that questions remain.

There are potential pitfalls, he said, involved in combining data over many years. What's needed are additional studies to measure the interplay of factors such as patient's age, tumor size, grade and histological type, and the role of estrogen receptors, all of which must be factored into an assessment of the patient's overall health. Also, new research into genetic and molecular markers of breast cancer may help doctors better quantify the risk of recurrence on a person-by-person basis.

For the future, more studies will be needed to look at just this sub-group of patients. Doctors do not want to subject women who have such a low risk of recurrence to unnecessary therapy, nor do they want to neglect treating women for whom the risk of treatment may be worthy of the benefit.

"The only answer for these women with small tumors will actually come from clinical trials that directly test the question," Abrams said. A better understanding of molecular pathways might someday provide better answers, but those too, will need clinical testing to be sure they accurately predict the outcome for a given individual. "There is no shortcut around clinical trials," he added.

Chapter 49

The Study of Tamoxifen and Raloxifene (STAR)

Questions and Answers about the Study of Tamoxifen and Raloxifene (STAR)

What is the Study of Tamoxifen and Raloxifene (STAR)?

The Study of Tamoxifen and Raloxifene (STAR) is a clinical trial (a research study conducted with people) designed to see how the drug raloxifene (Evista®) compares with the drug tamoxifen (Nolvadex®) in reducing the incidence of breast cancer in women who are at an increased risk of developing the disease. Researchers with the National Surgical Adjuvant Breast and Bowel Project (NSABP) are conducting the study at more than 400 centers across the United States, Puerto Rico, and Canada. The study is primarily funded by the National Cancer Institute (NCI), the U.S. Government's main agency for cancer research.

What is tamoxifen?

Tamoxifen is a drug, taken by mouth as a pill. It has been used for more than 20 years to treat patients with breast cancer. Tamoxifen works against breast cancer, in part, by interfering with the activity

This chapter includes text from "Questions and Answers About the Study of Tamoxifen and Raloxifene (STAR)," Cancer Facts, National Cancer Institute, June 1999; and "STAR Enrolls 6,139 Women in First Year," Press Release, National Cancer Institute, July 27, 2000.

of estrogen, a female hormone that promotes the growth of breast cancer cells. In October 1998, the U.S. Food and Drug Administration (FDA) approved tamoxifen to reduce the incidence of breast cancer in women at high risk of the disease based on the results of the Breast Cancer Prevention Trial (BCPT). The BCPT is a study of more than 13,000 pre- and postmenopausal high-risk women ages 35 and older who took either tamoxifen or a placebo (an inactive pill that looked like tamoxifen) for up to 5 years. NSABP conducted the BCPT, which also showed that tamoxifen works like estrogen to preserve bone strength, decreasing fractures of the hip, wrist, and spine in the women who took the drug.

What is raloxifene?

Raloxifene is a drug, taken by mouth as a pill. In December 1997, it was approved by the FDA for the prevention of osteoporosis in postmenopausal women. Raloxifene is being studied because large studies testing its effectiveness against osteoporosis have shown that women taking the drug developed fewer breast cancers than women taking a placebo.

Who is eligible to participate in STAR?

Women at increased risk for developing breast cancer, who have gone through menopause and are at least 35 years old, can participate in STAR. All women must have an increased risk of breast cancer equivalent to or greater than that of an average 60- to 64-year-old woman. At that age, about 17 of every 1,000 women are expected to develop breast cancer within 5 years.

Why can't premenopausal women participate in STAR?

STAR is limited to postmenopausal women because the drug raloxifene has yet to be adequately tested for long-term safety in premenopausal women. NCI recently launched a separate study to evaluate the safety of raloxifene in premenopausal woman.

What factors are used to determine increased risk of breast cancer for the participants?

Increased risk of breast cancer is determined in one of two ways. The risk for most women is determined by a computer calculation based on the following factors:

- Current age;

- Number of first-degree relatives (mother, daughters, or sisters) diagnosed with breast cancer;

- Whether a woman had any children and her age at her first delivery;

- The number of breast biopsies a woman has had, especially if the tissue showed a condition known as atypical hyperplasia; and

- The woman's age at her first menstrual period.

Women diagnosed as having lobular carcinoma in situ (LCIS), a condition that is not cancer but indicates an increased chance of developing invasive breast cancer, are eligible based on that diagnosis alone, as long as any treatment for the condition was limited to local excision. Mastectomy, radiation, or systemic therapy would disqualify a woman with LCIS from the study.

How will a potential participant's risk of breast cancer be determined?

Each potential participant will complete a one-page questionnaire (risk assessment form), which will be forwarded to NSABP by the local STAR clinical staff. The NSABP will use computer software to generate an individualized risk profile based on the information provided and will return the profile to the local STAR site so that it can be given to the potential participant. The profile will estimate the woman's chance of developing breast cancer over the next 5 years and will also present the potential risks and benefits of the study drugs. The woman can then use this information to help her decide whether or not she is interested in participating in STAR.

What other factors affect eligibility for the study?

Certain existing health conditions affect eligibility for the study. Health professionals at the STAR site will discuss these with each potential participant. For example, women with a history of cancer (except basal or squamous cell skin cancer), blood clots, stroke, or certain types of heartbeat irregularities cannot participate. Women whose high blood pressure or diabetes is not controlled also cannot participate.

421

Also, women taking hormone replacement therapy (estrogen or an estrogen/progesterone combination) cannot take part in the trial unless they stop taking this medication. Those who stop taking these hormones are eligible for the study 3 months after they discontinue the drugs. Women who have taken tamoxifen or raloxifene for no more than 3 months are eligible for the study, but they must also stop the medication for 3 months before joining STAR.

What are the common side effects of tamoxifen and raloxifene?

Like most medications, including over-the-counter medications, prescription drugs, or drugs in clinical trials, tamoxifen and raloxifene cause adverse effects in some women. The effects experienced most often by women taking either drug are hot flashes and vaginal symptoms, including discharge, dryness, or itching. It is possible that some women may experience leg cramps, constipation, pain with intercourse, sinus irritation or infection, or problems controlling the bladder upon exertion. Treatments that may minimize or eliminate most of these side effects will be available to the participants.

Does tamoxifen have any serious side effects?

The best information available about the serious side effects of tamoxifen comes from 30 years of clinical trials, including the BCPT. In the BCPT, women taking tamoxifen had more than twice the chance of developing endometrial cancer (cancer of the lining of the uterus or womb) compared with women who took the placebo (36 of the 6,600 women taking tamoxifen versus 15 of the 6,600 women taking placebo). The risk was higher in women over the age of 50. The increased risk is in the same range as the risk for postmenopausal women taking single-agent estrogen replacement therapy. Like all cancers, endometrial cancer is potentially life-threatening. Women who have had a hysterectomy (surgery to remove the uterus) are not at risk for endometrial cancer.

Women taking tamoxifen in the BCPT had three times the chance of developing a pulmonary embolism (blood clot in the lung) as women who took the placebo (18 women taking tamoxifen versus 6 on placebo). Three women taking tamoxifen died from these embolisms. Women in the tamoxifen group were also more likely to have a deep vein thrombosis (a blood clot in a major vein) than women on placebo (35 women on tamoxifen versus 22 on placebo). Women taking tamoxifen also appeared to have an increased chance of stroke (38 women on tamoxifen versus 24 on placebo).

Does raloxifene have any serious side effects?

Information about raloxifene is limited compared with the data available on tamoxifen because of the shorter time it has been studied (about 5 years) and the smaller number of women who have been studied. Studies of raloxifene have generally involved women who received the drug to determine its effect on osteoporosis, and the duration of both therapy and followup have been short. Women taking raloxifene in clinical trials have about three times the chance of developing a deep vein thrombosis or pulmonary embolism as women on a placebo. In osteoporosis studies of raloxifene, the drug did not increase the risk of endometrial cancer. An important part of STAR will be to assess the long-term safety of raloxifene versus tamoxifen in women at increased risk of breast cancer.

Who will get which drug?

Participants in STAR will be randomized (assigned by chance) to receive either tamoxifen or raloxifene. In a process known as "double blinding", neither the participant nor her physician will know which pill she is receiving. Setting up a study in this way allows the researchers to directly compare the true benefits and side effects of each drug without the influence of other factors. All women in the study will take two pills a day for 5 years: half will take active tamoxifen and a raloxifene placebo (an inactive pill that looks like raloxifene); the other half will take active raloxifene and a tamoxifen placebo (an inactive pill that looks like tamoxifen). All women will receive one of the active drugs; no one in STAR will receive only the placebo. The dosages are 20 mg of tamoxifen and 60 mg raloxifene.

Why does everyone have to take two pills?

Tamoxifen and raloxifene have different shapes. The trial would not be double blinded if participants or physicians could tell which drug they were receiving because of its shape. The maker of tamoxifen, AstraZeneca Pharmaceuticals in Wilmington, Delaware, and the maker of raloxifene, Eli Lilly and Company in Indianapolis, Indiana, are providing the active pills and the look-alike placebos without charge.

Are participants required to have any medical exams? Who will pay for these exams?

Participants are required to have blood tests, a mammogram, a breast exam, and a gynecologic exam before they are accepted into the study. These tests will be repeated at intervals during the trial. Physicians' fees and the costs of medical tests will be charged to the participant in the same fashion as if she were not part of the trial; however, the costs for these tests generally are covered by insurance. Every effort is made to contain the costs specifically associated with participation in this trial, and financial assistance is available for some women.

How is the safety of participants ensured? Is the trial monitored?

The safety of participants is of primary importance to STAR investigators. There are strict requirements about who can join the trial as well as frequent monitoring of participants' health status. An independent Data Safety and Monitoring Committee (DSMC) will provide oversight of the trial. The DSMC includes medical and cancer specialists, biostatisticians, and bioethicists who have no other connection to NSABP. The DSMC will meet semiannually and review unblinded data from all participants. Two other committees will also provide oversight. The Participant Advisory Board (PAB) is made up of 16 women from the BCPT. As women join STAR, board membership will change to include STAR participants. The PAB meets semiannually with professionals from NSABP and NCI and provides feedback on many study-related functions such as informed consent, participant recruitment, and communications issues. The STAR Steering Committee is made up of NSABP investigators, breast cancer advocates, experts from other medical disciplines, as well as NCI and NSABP personnel. The committee, which also meets semiannually, is charged with providing overall administrative oversight of the trial.

In addition, NSABP provides the FDA, NCI, AstraZeneca Pharmaceuticals, and Eli Lilly and Company with annual reports on STAR that summarize the overall data collected to date (only the DSMC receives unblinded data).

What is the National Surgical Adjuvant Breast and Bowel Project?

The NSABP is a cooperative group with a 40-year history of designing and conducting clinical trials, the results of which have changed the way breast cancer is treated and, now, prevented. Results of clinical trials conducted by NSABP researchers have been the dominant force in altering the standard surgical treatment of breast cancer from radical mastectomy to lumpectomy plus radiation. This group was also the first to demonstrate that adjuvant therapy could alter the natural history of breast cancer, thus increasing survival rates.

STAR Enrolls 6,139 Women in First Year

The first year of the Study of Tamoxifen and Raloxifene (STAR) saw 6,139 postmenopausal women at increased risk of breast cancer enroll in this landmark prevention study—and more than 47,000 women went through an individualized, no-obligation risk assessment to determine their risk of breast cancer and weigh the pros and cons of joining the trial. Enrollment began July 1, 1999.

More than 500 centers across the United States, Puerto Rico, and Canada are enrolling participants in STAR. STAR is a study of the National Surgical Adjuvant Breast and Bowel Project (NSABP) and is supported by the U.S. National Cancer Institute (NCI).

NSABP Chairman Norman Wolmark, M.D., said, "We are pleased that so many women have joined this trial to help us answer this important medical question. We encourage women to go through the risk assessment process to learn more about their breast cancer risk and about STAR. In the end, each woman who joins does so for her own reasons, but every single woman plays a vital role."

As in the BCPT, women can join STAR if they have an increased risk of developing breast cancer equivalent to the risk of an average 60-year-old woman. These women have a 1.7 percent risk of breast cancer in five years, meaning that about 17 of them in 1,000 would be expected to develop breast cancer within five years. The women who are actually choosing to join the trial, as a group, exceed that minimum requirement.

Postmenopausal women of all ethnicities and races are encouraged to participate in STAR, and about 5 percent of the first 6,000 women in STAR are minorities. In this first year of STAR, a total of 6,636 minority women went through the risk assessment process, 1,812 had an increased risk of breast cancer that would qualify them for the study, and 281 have already decided to join.

In contrast, in the entire five years of enrollment for the BCPT, a total of 8,525 minority women went through the risk assessment process, 2,979 were risk-eligible, and 486 joined the trial.

The NSABP has undertaken several novel strategies to encourage minority women to participate in STAR, which include the STAR Community Outreach Program for Education (SCOPE) under way in ten cities in the United States. The goal of SCOPE is to educate minority women about breast cancer, which may ultimately lead to their more widespread participation in clinical trials.

Moreover, STAR is supported by the National Medical Association (NMA), a network of more than 20,000 African-American physicians. As a first effort, the NSABP is working closely with Region II of the NMA, which includes members in Pennsylvania, Delaware, Maryland, Virginia, West Virginia, and the District of Columbia, to pilot a unique outreach project. The initial participation is in Philadelphia with plans to extend outreach into the rest of Region II and eventually throughout the NMA organization.

Recent analyses of the use of tamoxifen in women with breast cancer show that tamoxifen works equally well in white and African-American women. Worta McCaskill-Stevens, M.D., of the NCI's Division of Cancer Prevention, who presented this research at the May 2000 meeting of the American Society of Clinical Oncology, notes that "The benefits and risks of tamoxifen are the same in African-American and white women. Women of all races can feel comfortable about considering STAR if they are at increased risk of breast cancer."

Women who participate in STAR must be postmenopausal, at least age 35, and have an increased risk of breast cancer as determined by their age, family history of breast cancer, personal medical history, age at first menstrual period, and age at first live birth. They will also go through a process known as informed consent, during which they will learn about the potential benefits and risks of tamoxifen and raloxifene before deciding whether to participate in STAR.

Tamoxifen and raloxifene may also increase a woman's chances of developing several rare, but potentially life-threatening health problems: deep vein thrombosis (blood clot in a large vein) and pulmonary embolism (blood clot in the lung). Tamoxifen use may also increase a woman's risk of stroke and endometrial cancer (cancer of the lining of the uterus) at a rate similar to estrogen replacement therapy. In ongoing studies, raloxifene has not been associated with an increased risk of endometrial cancer. STAR will help further define the risks and benefits of tamoxifen and raloxifene therapy.

Once a woman decides to participate, she is randomly assigned to receive either 20 mg tamoxifen or 60 mg raloxifene daily for five years and has regular follow-up examinations, including mammograms and gynecologic exams.

The maker of tamoxifen, AstraZeneca Pharmaceuticals, Wilmington, Delaware, and the maker of raloxifene, Eli Lilly and Company, Indianapolis, Indiana, are providing their drugs for the trial without charge. Eli Lilly and Company has also given NSABP a $36 million five-year grant to defray recruitment costs at the participating centers.

First Year Recruitment Data

- During the first year of the trial, which started enrolling women on July 1, 1999, 47,114 women went through the risk assessment process. Of these women, 29,303 were eligible for the trial based on breast cancer risk alone. Of those risk-eligible women, 6,139 chose to participate.

- In the first year, 3,786 African-American women went through the risk assessment process, 739 were risk-eligible, and 103 joined STAR. About 1.7 percent of the women on STAR are African-American.

- In the first year, 1,688 Hispanic/Latina women went through the risk assessment process, 464 were risk-eligible, and 81 joined STAR. About 1.3 percent of the women on STAR are Hispanic/Latina.

- In the first year, 1,162 women who defined themselves as representing another minority population, such as Native American or Asian American, went through the risk assessment process, 609 were risk-eligible, and 97 joined STAR. About 1.6 percent of the women on STAR are ethnic minorities other than African-American or Hispanic/Latina.

- Of the 6,139 women joining STAR, 1,126 were from the placebo group of the Breast Cancer Prevention Trial.

- More than half of the women joining STAR had had a hysterectomy prior to enrolling (52.3 percent). Women who have had a hysterectomy are not at risk for endometrial cancer.

- The breast cancer risk of women joining STAR in the first year has been above the minimum 1.7 percent risk of developing the disease within the next five years. (see Table 49.1.)

- Women joining STAR must be postmenopausal and at least 35 years of age. The ages of women joining STAR in the first year is shown in Table 49.2.

- In the first year, 7.9 percent of the women joining STAR had had a diagnosis of lobular carcinoma in situ (LCIS), a condition that is not cancer, but which indicates an increased chance of developing invasive breast cancer.

- Number of women who joined STAR by U.S. state and Canadian province is shown in Table 49.3.

- Tamoxifen (trade name Nolvadex®) was proven in the BCPT to reduce breast cancer incidence by 49 percent in women at increased risk of the disease. The FDA approved the use of tamoxifen to reduce the incidence of breast cancer in women at increased risk of the disease in October 1998. Tamoxifen has been approved by the FDA to treat women with breast cancer for more than 20 years and has been in clinical trials for about 30 years.

- Raloxifene (trade name Evista®) was shown to reduce the incidence of breast cancer in a large study of its use to prevent and treat osteoporosis. This drug was approved by the FDA to prevent osteoporosis in postmenopausal women in December 1997

Table 49.1. Cancer Risk among STAR participants

Five-Year Breast Cancer Risk	Percent of women in STAR
1.7- 2.0 percent	10.3 percent
2.0-2.9 percent	30.3 percent
3.0-4.9 percent	32.2 percent
Greater than 5.0 percent	27.2 percent

Table 49.2. Age of STAR participants

Age	Percent of women in STAR
35-49	9.4 percent
50-59	50.2 percent
60+	40.4 percent

Table 49.3. Residence of STAR participants.

U.S. States (and Puerto Rico)

Alabama	20	Indiana	119
Arizona	77	Iowa	136
Arkansas	8	Kansas	132
California	359	Kentucky	83
Colorado	110	Louisiana	76
Connecticut	96	Maine	27
Delaware	31	Maryland	72
District of Columbia	23	Massachusetts	155
Florida	159	Michigan	259
Georgia	55	Minnesota	151
Hawaii	41	Mississippi	27
Idaho	26	Missouri	255
Illinois	333	Montana	41
Nebraska	63	South Carolina	131
Nevada	38	South Dakota	47
New Hampshire	24	Tennessee	114
New Jersey	98	Texas	520
New Mexico	44	Utah	5
New York	231	Vermont	33
North Carolina	168	Virginia	54
North Dakota	49	Washington	154
Ohio	250	West Virginia	18
Oklahoma	94	Wisconsin	136
Oregon	63		
Pennsylvania	415		
Rhode Island	10	Puerto Rico	15

Canadian Provinces

Alberta	41	Ontario	93
British Columbia	37	Quebec	254
Manitoba	68	Saskatchewan	1

and to treat osteoporosis in postmenopausal women in September 1999. It has been under study for about seven years.

Contact Information

- Postmenopausal women in the United States and Puerto Rico who are interested in participating in STAR can call the NCI's Cancer Information Service at 1-800-4-CANCER (1-800-422-6237) for information in English or Spanish. The number for callers with TTY equipment is 1-800-332-8615.

- Postmenopausal women in Canada who are interested in participating in STAR can call the Canadian Cancer Society's Cancer Information Service at 1-888-939-3333 for information in English or French.

- For more information via the Internet, visit NSABP's Web site at http://www.nsabp.pitt.edu or NCI's clinical trials Web site at http://cancertrials.nci.nih.gov.

Chapter 50

Buserelin and Tamoxifen for Advanced Breast Cancer

A drug commonly used for prostate cancer, buserelin, helped pre-menopausal women with advanced breast cancer live longer, according to a report in the June 7, 2000 issue of the *Journal of the National Cancer Institute*.

When combined with tamoxifen, buserelin increased the average survival time of patients by almost a year. This combined therapy yielded an average survival time of 3.7 years, versus 2.9 years with tamoxifen alone or 2.5 years with buserelin alone.

Many premenopausal breast cancer patients have their ovaries removed to eliminate estrogen from their system. Estrogen is thought to cause some types of breast cancer to grow more quickly. But treating these same patients who have tumors classified as estrogen-receptor positive with tamoxifen is an accepted alternative to ovarian removal.

However, women treated with tamoxifen often develop high levels of estradiol, a sex hormone. Estradiol is thought by some researchers to inhibit the action of tamoxifen or even cause breast cancer to regrow. Buserelin suppresses ovarian production of estradiol, just as it blocks testosterone in prostate cancer patients.

The European Organization for the Research and Treatment of Cancer (EORTC) tested the drug combination in a phase III clinical trial that enrolled 161 patients in nine countries. All of the patients had locally advanced (spread to many lymph nodes) or metastatic

---

"Hormone Therapy Increases Survival for Some Breast Cancer Patients," CancerTrials, National Cancer Institute, June 2000.

(spread to other organs) breast cancer, and all had estrogen receptor positive tumors. Women taking buserelin alone had 6.6 milligrams implanted under their skin at 6-week intervals for the first 12 weeks, and then at 8-week intervals. Women on tamoxifen took 40 milligrams of the drug daily. Women in the combined-treatment group took both drugs at these same dosages.

After following the women for an average of 7.3 years, the researchers found the combined treatment superior in overall survival and progression-free survival. In another measure, the combined therapy group had an overall 5-year survival rate of 34 percent, compared with 15 to 18 percent for the single-agent groups. Blood levels of estradiol were suppressed equally in the combined treatment group and the buserelin-only group; in the tamoxifen-only group, levels of the hormone jumped threefold or higher.

These results open the door to more widespread use of hormone treatment for breast cancer, writes Nancy Davidson, M.D., of the Johns Hopkins Oncology Center in Baltimore, in an editorial. However, she cautions that the study was fairly small (due to problems accruing enough participants), and that newer hormone treatments under study may be more effective than buserelin.

Chapter 51

Two New Trials to Test Herceptin in Non-Metastatic Breast Cancer

Herceptin research took a giant step forward this spring with the opening of the first large randomized trials to test the novel biological drug in non-metastatic breast cancer.

Herceptin (trastuzumab) won Food and Drug Administration approval in Sept. 1998 for treatment of metastatic breast tumors that produce unusually large amounts of—or overexpress—the HER2 protein. The drug's success in advanced HER2-positive cancers raised hopes that it would prove at least as effective if used immediately after surgery in earlier-stage disease. Smaller phase II trials and pilot studies are already doing that, but the new trials, with thousands of patients, are the first major (phase III) studies of Herceptin in patients who do not have metastatic disease.

Both trials are taking place at multiple sites in the United States and Canada, and both are sponsored by the National Cancer Institute. One of the trials, being conducted by the National Surgical Adjuvant Breast and Bowel Project (NSABP), opened in March 2000. The other, led by the North Central Cancer Treatment Group, enrolled its first patient in June.

How best to design this next generation of trials has been a topic of much debate, according to Elizabeth Tan-Chiu, M.D., protocol officer of the NSABP trial. The paramount issue, she said, was Herceptin's effect on the heart. Earlier studies have shown that it can cause heart problems in some women, especially in combination with

---

Cancer Trials, National Cancer Institute, July 2000.

Adriamycin® (doxorubicin), a state-of-the-art chemotherapy treatment for breast cancer.

The NSABP trial will compare Adriamycin and Cytoxan® (cyclophosphamide) followed by Taxol® (paclitaxel) to the same regimen plus Herceptin. Tan-Chiu said that concerns about cardiac dysfunction led to NSABP's decision to break the protocol into two stages. In the first stage—the first 1,000 patients—investigators will evaluate the cardiac toxicity of the treatments. If the incidence of heart problems falls within established boundaries, the study will proceed to the second stage, in which the remaining 1,700 patients will be enrolled.

Potential heart problems were also a major concern in developing the NCCTG study, which is led by Edith Perez, M.D., of the Mayo Clinic in Jacksonville, Fla. It is addressing the cardiac issue by assessing different schedules for administering Herceptin—either with the chemotherapy drugs or following them.

In one arm of this 3000-patient trial, patients will receive Adriamycin and Cytoxan followed by weekly Taxol and Herceptin given at the same time. In a second arm, Herceptin will follow the Taxol. (Women on a third arm will receive Adriamycin and Cytoxan followed by weekly Taxol without Herceptin.)

Both trials require frequent tests to monitor heart function, and both prohibit radiation of the internal mammary lymph nodes because of the additional cardiac risk it may entail. Tan-Chiu and Perez said they have worked together on designing the two trials and plan to communicate regularly about toxicity data.

How to predict response to Herceptin is another intriguing problem that has influenced design of the trials. Because only a subset of HER2-positive women respond to the drug, the new studies include a raft of biological studies to search for markers that will predict who those patients are.

Investigators will look, for instance, at the presence of activated or phosphorylated HER2, other closely related molecules that may interact with HER2, chromosomal or gene copy abnormalities, and, in the words of the NSABP protocol, "any additional potentially predictive markers of response to Herceptin which may be discovered in the future."

Another major question woven into the study designs is that of tamoxifen: Do HER2-positive women have a poor response to the hormonal drug as some studies have suggested?

Both studies will include tamoxifen, which is now standard in early breast cancer for women who have hormone receptors. Patients will be stratified, or divided up, according to their hormone receptor status before they are randomized. This means that all trial arms will include patients who have hormone receptors and are taking tamoxifen. The strategy is expected to yield data on how women respond to tamoxifen with and without Herceptin.

How long will it take to get the answer to this question and others posed by the trials? It depends as always on how long it takes to enroll participants in the studies, and as Tan-Chiu noted, only a minority of newly diagnosed breast cancer patients are both node-positive and HER2-positive. Currently, the investigators estimate that it will take between three and five years to complete the trials.

Chapter 52

Sentinel Node Biopsy Trials

Questions and Answers about NCI's Sentinel Node Biopsy Trials

The National Cancer Institute (NCI) is sponsoring two large randomized clinical trials (research studies) comparing sentinel lymph node biopsy with conventional axillary lymph node dissection for breast cancer. The trials are being carried out by the National Surgical Adjuvant Breast and Bowel Project (NSABP) and the American College of Surgeons-Oncology Group (ACOS-OG). NSABP and ACOS-OG are both NCI-sponsored Clinical Trials Cooperative Groups, which are networks of institutions and physicians across the country who jointly conduct trials.

Below is general information about sentinel node biopsy followed by details of the two trials.

What is a sentinel node?

A sentinel node is the first lymph node to which a tumor drains, and therefore is the first place to which cancer is likely to spread. In some cases, there can be more than one sentinel node. In breast cancer, the sentinel node is usually located in the axillary nodes, the group of lymph nodes under the arm; however, in a small percentage of cases, the sentinel node is found elsewhere in the lymphatic system of the

---

Cancer Facts, National Cancer Institute, February 2000.

breast. If a doctor can feel lymph nodes during a physical exam of the breast and underarm area that he or she suspects may be cancerous, the patient is diagnosed as "clinically node-positive." If a patient is clinically node-negative, surgery and a laboratory analysis must be performed to determine whether there is microscopic evidence of cancer in the lymph nodes.

What is the conventional surgical treatment for breast cancer?

Standard treatment usually involves removing a breast tumor by either lumpectomy or mastectomy and removing most of the axillary nodes (axillary node dissection). Several complications can arise from removing the axillary nodes; some reports indicate that more than 80 percent of women who undergo a complete axillary dissection have at least one complication after surgery. These complications are of varying severity, but can include lymphedema (swelling in the arm caused by excess fluid buildup), numbness, a persistent burning sensation, infection, and limited movement of the shoulder.

What information is provided by the sentinel node biopsy procedure?

Previous research has suggested that the sentinel node can be used to determine if cancer cells have spread to the lymph nodes. In sentinel node biopsy, only one or a few lymph nodes are removed for laboratory analysis when a patient has a lumpectomy or mastectomy. Preliminary studies suggest that if an analysis finds no cancer cells in the sentinel node, the patient is unlikely to have tumor cells in the remaining axillary nodes.

How is the sentinel node found?

There are two methods for finding the sentinel node. One is to inject a blue dye near the breast tumor and track its path through the lymph nodes. The dye accumulates in the sentinel node. In a similar technique, doctors inject a safe, small amount of a radioactive solution near the tumor and then use a gamma detector to find the "hotspot," or the node in which the solution has accumulated. These two techniques can also be used together. Surgeons participating in the NSABP trial will use both methods together, and surgeons participating in the ACOS-OG trial may use either of the techniques or the combination.

Why is sentinel node biopsy being studied?

The sentinel node may provide valuable information about the status of a woman's cancer without the complications associated with axillary dissection. While several studies have examined the correlation between the sentinel node and the remaining axillary nodes, these are the first two randomized trials that will compare the long-term results of sentinel node dissection with full axillary node dissection. The two trials, while different in design, have similar goals. Both trials will examine the effect of sentinel node biopsy and full axillary dissection on long-term survival and disease-free survival. Both trials will also compare the side effects of the different surgeries.

Is sentinel node biopsy a new procedure?

Some surgeons already perform sentinel node biopsies in patients with breast cancer, although it is still considered an investigational procedure. The concept of mapping the sentinel node was first reported in 1977 by a researcher studying cancer of the penis. The technique was later used to study drainage patterns of melanoma, and was first reported for breast cancer in 1993. Since then, researchers have improved methods for finding the sentinel node, and several studies have shown that when the sentinel node is negative, the remaining nodes are also negative in a majority of cases. These studies were done in a small number of centers and overall survival was not examined in these trials. Surgeons participating in both the NSABP and ACOS-OG trials must be specially trained in identifying sentinel nodes and performing sentinel node biopsies. Side effects of sentinel node biopsy can include minor pain or bruising at the biopsy site and the rare possibility of an allergic reaction to the blue dye used in finding the sentinel node.

Why is the NCI supporting two different trials?

The two trials are asking different but important questions, and can be viewed as complementary. The NSABP study is examining whether sentinel lymph node biopsy can replace axillary lymph node dissection in the approximately 70 percent of breast cancer patients with negative sentinel nodes while the ACOS-OG study is examining the same issue in women with positive sentinel nodes.

NSABP Study of Sentinel Node Biopsy in Node-Negative Women

What will the NSABP study do?

This trial is designed to determine whether sentinel node biopsy provides the same information, control of the disease in the area around the breast, and survival as conventional axillary dissection while significantly reducing complications.

The study will randomize about 4,000 breast cancer patients who have clinically negative nodes into two groups. Group 1 will undergo sentinel node biopsy followed by axillary dissection. Group 2 will undergo sentinel node biopsy followed by axillary dissection only if the sentinel node is positive for cancer. If the sentinel node is negative, women in this group will have no further axillary dissection.

What surgical procedures are involved?

All patients will undergo breast-conserving surgery (lumpectomy), or mastectomy and removal of the sentinel nodes. Some will also have additional underarm lymph nodes removed, as described above.

What other treatments will patients receive?

In accordance with standard guidelines for cancer treatment, patients may receive chemotherapy and/or hormonal therapy following mastectomy or lumpectomy. Patients undergoing lumpectomy will also receive breast radiation treatments. Patients undergoing mastectomy who have positive sentinel nodes may receive radiation treatments to the chest wall or to the nodes under the arm at the discretion of their physician.

What issues will be examined?

The primary goals of this study are to determine if: 1) control of the regional spread of breast cancer is equivalent between the two procedures, 2) the overall survival and number of years without recurrence are comparable, and 3) the side effects associated with sentinel node removal are less severe than those from conventional axillary dissection.

The trial will also examine whether the sentinel node is as effective as the axillary nodes at determining if cancer has spread and whether sentinel nodes can properly identify patients with an increased risk of having their cancer recur. Investigators will use a special technique (immunohistochemistry or IHC) to detect very small amounts of cancer cells (micrometastases) in biopsy specimens from negative nodes. These micrometastases are not found during routine examination of biopsy specimens. With the IHC results, researchers hope to learn whether micrometastases are associated with breast cancer recurrence.

Who is eligible for the NSABP study?

Breast cancer patients may be eligible if:

- They have been diagnosed with breast cancer removable by lumpectomy or mastectomy.
- Their axillary lymph nodes cannot be felt during a physical exam.
- They have not had any treatment for their current breast cancer.
- They have a life expectancy of at least 10 years.

What is the National Surgical Adjuvant Breast and Bowel Project (NSABP)?

The NSABP is a cooperative group with a 40-year history of designing and conducting clinical trials, the results of which have changed the way breast cancer is treated. Results of research studies conducted by NSABP researchers have been the dominant force in altering the standard surgical treatment of breast cancer from radical mastectomy to lumpectomy plus radiation. This group was also the first to demonstrate that adjuvant therapy could alter the natural history of breast cancer, thus increasing survival rates.

ACOS-OG Study of Sentinel Node Biopsy in Women with Positive Biopsies

What will the ACOS-OG study do?

This trial will examine whether long-term survival for patients with positive sentinel nodes who do not receive an axillary node dissection or axillary radiation is any different from survival of those who do undergo a complete dissection.

For this trial, ACOS-OG is seeking to enroll about 7,600 women with early breast cancer. The researchers anticipate that about 1,900 of these patients will have positive sentinel node biopsies. These women with positive sentinel nodes will be randomized into two groups. One group will have a complete axillary node dissection, and the other group will have no further lymph nodes removed and no radiation to the axilla. For the women with negative sentinel nodes, no further axillary surgery will be performed.

What surgical procedures are involved?

All women in this trial will undergo breast-conserving surgery (lumpectomy) and sentinel lymph node biopsy. About half of the patients with positive sentinel nodes, as explained above, will have a complete axillary node dissection, while half will have no further axillary surgery.

What other treatments will patients receive?

Following standard guidelines for cancer treatment, women in both groups of the study will have breast radiation therapy, and may have chemotherapy and/or hormonal therapy as well.

What issues will be examined?

This trial is designed to determine if overall survival for patients with positive sentinel nodes who do not undergo axillary node dissection is different from survival for sentinel node-positive patients who do receive a complete axillary node dissection. The study will also compare the side effects of the two procedures. For women with negative sentinel nodes, recurrence of cancer in the breast and surrounding area will be monitored.

In addition, participants' sentinel nodes will be analyzed with special studies that are not routinely performed (immunohistochemistry) to search for any cancer cells that were not detected with routine methods. In this way, researchers hope to learn if minute amounts of tumor in the lymph nodes micrometastases have any significance in terms of the patient's outcome.

Is it dangerous to leave axillary lymph nodes in place if the sentinel node is positive?

This is a major unanswered question in breast cancer treatment. There is no firm evidence that removing involved lymph nodes improves survival, even though it is standard practice. Randomized studies suggest that lymph node removal may not improve survival, although it is valuable in determining the stage of the cancer. Sentinel node biopsy can be used to determine stage, so it may be all that is necessary, even in node-positive women. One of the aims of this study is to resolve the issue of whether axillary lymph node removal is necessary in node-positive women and justifies its long-term side effects. (Also, it is important to note that patients in the ACOS-OG study will receive post-surgical radiation therapy to the breast and may have chemotherapy and/or hormonal therapy as well.)

Who is eligible for the ACOS-OG study?

Breast cancer patients may be eligible if:

- They have stage I or II breast cancer with a tumor that can be removed by lumpectomy.
- Their axillary lymph nodes cannot be felt during a physical exam.
- They have not been previously treated with chemotherapy for their current breast cancer.
- They have a life expectancy of at least 10 years.

What is the American College of Surgeons (ACOS)?

ACOS is the largest professional organization of surgeons in the world. Established in 1913, it has for many years provided its members with standards of practice, credentialing for specialists, and educational materials. In a new venture in 1998, it formed the Oncology Group (ACOS-OG) which will perform clinical trials sponsored by the National Cancer Institute. The Group will be able to draw upon the organization's nationwide membership and its long experience with medical education. The sentinel node trial is one of the first clinical trials the group is conducting.

National Cancer Institute Information Resources

You may want more information for yourself, your family, and your doctor. The following National Cancer Institute (NCI) services are available to help you.

Telephone: Cancer Information Service (CIS) provides accurate, up-to-date information on cancer to patients and their families, health professionals, and the general public. Information specialists translate the latest scientific information into understandable language and respond in English, Spanish, or on TTY equipment.

Telephone 1-800-4-CANCER (1-800-422-6237)

TTY: 1-800-332-8615 (for deaf and hard of hearing callers)

Internet: These web sites may be useful:

NCI's primary web site; contains information about the Institute and its programs. http://www.nci.nih.gov/

CancerNet; contains material for health professionals, patients, and the public, including information from PDQ about cancer treatment, screening, prevention, genetics, supportive care, and clinical trials, and CANCERLIT, a bibliographic database. http://cancernet.nci.nih.gov/

cancerTrials; NCI's comprehensive clinical trials information center for patients, health professionals, and the public. Includes information on understanding trials, deciding whether to participate in trials, finding specific trials, plus research news and other resources. http://cancertrials.nci.nih.gov/

This site includes news, upcoming events, educational materials, and publications for patients, the public, and the mass media. http://rex. nci.nih.gov

Cancer Patient Education Database; provides information on cancer patient education resources for patients, their families, and health professionals. http://chid.nih.gov/ncichid/

E-mail: CancerMail includes NCI information about cancer treatment, screening, prevention, genetics, and supportive care. To obtain a contents list, send e-mail to cancermail@icicc.nci.nih.gov with the word "help" in the body of the message.

Fax: CancerFax includes NCI information about cancer treatment, screening, prevention, genetics, and supportive care. To obtain a contents list, dial 301-402-5874 or 1-800-624-2511 from a touch-tone telephone or fax machine hand set and follow the recorded instructions.

Chapter 53

Radiation and Chemotherapy Research Updates

Radiation Plus Tamoxifen Confirmed to Reduce Breast Cancer Recurrence

Since the late 1980s, radiation and the drug tamoxifen have been given to women who had surgery that removed early breast tumors. These therapies dramatically reduce the risk of cancer recurring.

To spare women a double-dose of side effects, though, researchers hoped that they could eliminate one of the treatments. But after a study of 1,000 women, presented at the annual meeting of the American Society of Clinical Oncology, the combination therapy remains the standard of care.

"The specific aims of the study were straight forward—can tamoxifen replace radiation?" said Norman Wolmark, M.D., of the National Surgical Breast and Bowel Project in Pittsburgh. "The data are clear in demonstrating that tamoxifen can not replace radio-therapy."

The study women were split into three groups: one received tamoxifen alone, the second radiation alone, and the third tamoxifen and radiation. At five years after treatment, the recurrence rate—or

---

Text in this chapter is from "Radiation Plus Tamoxifen Confirmed to Reduce Breast Cancer," Cancer Trials, National Cancer Institute (NCI), May 22, 2000; "Shorter Radiation Schedule Available for Breast Cancer," Cancer Trials, NCI, May 23, 2000; "High-Dose Chemotherapy for Breast Cancer at a Crossroads," Cancer Trials, NCI, April 12, 2000; and "Early Breast Cancer Patients Benefit from Shortened Chemotherapy," Cancer Trials, May 21, 2000.

the proportion of women who had their cancer return in the same breast—was 10.7% in the tamoxifen group; 4.8% in the radiotherapy group; and 2% in the combined therapy group.

"This means that the standard care remains unchanged even for these very small, favorable tumors," said Wolmark. All of the women in the study had tumors one centimeter or smaller in size.

The study also confirmed that tamoxifen reduces the occurrence of contralateral breast cancer, or disease in the second breast. The incidence of contralateral breast cancer in the group that did not receive tamoxifen was 3% compared to 0.6% in the groups that took tamoxifen.

Shorter Radiation Schedule Available for Breast Cancer Patients

Women who choose lumpectomy instead of the more disfiguring mastecomy surgery for breast cancer typically receive daily radiation therapy for five weeks, to help prevent cancer recurrence. A new study says that cutting that schedule to three weeks works just as well.

If the new schedule becomes widely adopted it will mean 10 fewer trips to the hospital for patients and substantial savings for health care providers.

"A shorter schedule will lessen the burden for women fighting breast cancer, in terms of convenience and personal costs and in terms of travel and time off work. It will also have important consequences for health care system, allowing more women to be treated with the same resources," said Timothy Whelan, M.D., of the Hamilton Regional Cancer Center in Canada, who conducted the study.

After following 1,200 Canadian women for five years, Whelan found that those who received the shortened schedule had the same low rate of recurrence as those on the five week schedule. About 3% of women in both groups had their cancer return. The total amount of radiation given was roughly equal in both groups, but those on the shortened schedule received higher doses each day.

Whelan and his colleagues also compared cosmetic outcomes in both groups, looking at signs like the appearance of small blood vessels and thickening of breast tissue. These side effects were again comparable in both groups, occurring in less than 25% of patients.

"The shorter treatment schedule is just as good as the longer schedule, and it may make the option of breast conserving therapy more attractive," said Whelan.

High-Dose Chemotherapy for Breast Cancer at a Crossroads

Over the past 20 years, more than 15,000 women with breast cancer have been treated with an arduous yet largely unproven procedure—high doses of chemotherapy followed by blood cell transplants (cells are removed from the patient before chemotherapy) to replace bone marrow damaged by the chemotherapy.

In the early 1990s, after a few encouraging preliminary reports, breast cancer patients and advocates began demanding the treatment. Some state legislatures responded by mandating that insurance companies pay for the lengthy procedure, which can cost up to $100,000 per case, much more than conventional treatments. By mid-decade, more people were receiving high-dose chemotherapy with transplants for breast cancer than for any other cancer.

But two recently published studies show that high doses of chemotherapy are no more effective than standard chemotherapy for women with advanced or high-risk breast cancer. And results from a third study—which was originally positive for the high-dose treatment—have been discounted after the lead South African researcher admitted serious fraud.

These developments leave the practice of high-dose chemotherapy for breast cancer in limbo. The American Society of Clinical Oncology recommends that women receive the treatment only if part of a "high-quality" clinical trial. Editorials in the March 18, 2000 *The Lancet* and the April 13, 2000 *New England Journal of Medicine* (*NEJM*) make the same argument. Researchers at the National Cancer Institute (NCI) have long supported this approach and NCI has sponsored four large national trials; three of these have completed enrollment and one is still ongoing.

These scientific sentiments have been echoed by one of the nation's largest insurers, Aetna/U.S. Healthcare, which in February announced that it will pay for high-dose chemotherapy plus transplants only for patients enrolled in federally-sponsored clinical trials. The company previously reimbursed expenses for women who were not in clinical trials.

The vast majority of women who received the high-dose regimens have not participated in clinical trials, which are required to rigorously test new cancer treatments. Results from well-conducted, carefully monitored randomized trials are urgently needed to figure out which breast cancer patients, if any, may benefit from high-dose therapy plus transplants, says Jeff Abrams, M.D., a breast cancer researcher at NCI.

Newly Published Studies

The early studies of high-dose chemotherapy plus transplant for breast cancer that caused so much attention were not randomized. That is, they did not compare patients who received the new treatment to patients who received standard treatment. The two new studies, one published in the *NEJM*, led by Edward Stadtmauer, M.D., University of Pennsylvania Cancer Center; the other in the *Journal of the National Cancer Institute* (*JNCI*) from Gabriel Hortobagyi, M.D. at the University of Texas M.D. Anderson Cancer Center, were randomized, meaning that they provide a truer measure of the treatment's effectiveness.

The Stadtmauer study enrolled 553 patients who had metastatic (spreading to other organs) breast cancer. All of the patients received four to six cycles of standard chemotherapy. The patients whose disease responded were then randomized; 89 received the standard chemotherapy (cyclophosphamide, methotrexate, and fluorouracil) and 110 the high-dose chemotherapy (cyclophosphamide, carboplatin, and thiotepa) plus transplant.

After following both groups for an average of three years, the researchers report no significant difference in overall survival times—32 percent of the high-dose group and 38 percent of the conventional chemotherapy group were alive at three years post-treatment. There also was no difference in the time it took for the disease to worsen—about 9 months post-treatment for each group. In addition, infection, vomiting, diarrhea, and other side effects were much more common in the high-dose group.

While the final study was smaller than originally planned, the authors state that there were still enough patients to detect even a small (6 month) survival time advantage. They conclude that they do not recommend high-dose chemotherapy for women with metastatic breast cancer.

The second study, from Hortobagyi, reached a similar conclusion for 78 patients with less severe breast cancer—cancer that had spread to the lymph nodes near the breast, but not to other organs. (This type of breast cancer is often called "high risk" because patients often relapse after surgery or chemotherapy.)

The three-year survival rate for the group receiving high-dose chemotherapy was 58 percent, compared to 77 percent for the standard chemotherapy group. Relapse-free survival rates were 48 percent and 62 percent respectively. Again, there were more severe side effects in the high-dose group. These results lead the authors to succinctly report that "high-dose chemotherapy is not indicated outside a clinical trial."

However, the Hortobagyi study was "much too small to detect even moderate differences" in survival times. That means that the study should not be considered definitive and that additional, larger studies are needed.

Ongoing Trials

While results from recent studies are discouraging for those who had hopes for high-dose chemotherapy for breast cancer, several larger studies need to be completed or analyzed before the treatment is completely discounted, says Abrams.

Preliminary findings of one of these trials (a study of 800 women with high-risk breast cancer), were presented at the 1999 meeting of the American Society of Clinical Oncology. Headed by William Peters, M.D., Ph.D., director of the Barbara Ann Karmanos Cancer Institute in Detroit, the study is comparing women who receive high doses of cyclophosphamide, cisplatin and BCNU [carmustine], followed by transplants, with women who receive "intermediate" doses of the same drugs without transplants.

Although early results show no difference in survival, patients receiving the high-dose therapy have about a 68 percent chance of being alive without breast cancer at three years, compared with a 64 percent chance for those receiving the intermediate-dose therapy. While the patients need to be followed for a few more years before any conclusions can be drawn, the early results provide encouragement for completion of ongoing trials.

The largest of these studies is designed to enroll 1000 patients at 100 centers nationwide. Women may be eligible if they have had breast surgery and have four to nine lymph nodes with cancer. Another study, based in Seattle, is looking at a different chemotherapy regimen in women with both high-risk and metastatic breast cancer. Other studies are ongoing in Australia, France, and Scotland.

A full list of current trials, with links to more information on patient eligibility criteria, is available on cancerTrials (http://cancertrials. nci.nih.gov).

References

"Where next with stem-cell-supported high-dose therapy for breast cancer?" J. Bergh, *The Lancet*, March 18, 2000, p. 944. [Text of this editorial is available on *The Lancet*'s website at www.thelancet. com]

"High-dose chemotherapy plus autologous bone marrow transplantation for metastatic breast cancer," M. Lippman, *The New England*

Journal of Medicine, April 13, 2000, p. 1119. [Text of this editorial is available on *NEJM*'s website at www.nejm.org]

"Conventional-dose chemotherapy compared with high-dose chemotherapy plus autologous hematopoietic stem-cell transplantation for metastatic breast cancer," E. A. Stadtmauer, et al., *The New England Journal of Medicine*, April 13, 2000, p. 1069. [Text of this article is available on *NEJM*'s website at www.nejm.org]

"Randomized trial of high-dose chemotherapy and blood cell autografts for high-risk primary breast cancer," G.N. Hortobagyi, et al., *Journal of the National Cancer Institute*, February 2, 2000, pp. 225-233. [An abstract of this article is available from the National Library of Medicine's PubMed database at www.nlm.nih.gov]

Early Breast Cancer Patients Benefit from Shortened Chemotherapy

Women with one type of early breast cancer get the same benefit from three months of one chemotherapy as they do from six months of another drug combination, according to a large study presented at the American Society for Clinical Oncology annual meeting on Sunday.

The results mean that breast cancer patients who do not benefit from the drug tamoxifen—which includes about half of all early cases—can halve the duration of their drug therapy without diminishing the chances for long-term survival.

The study compared the chemotherapy combination AC (adriamycin and cyclophosphamide) to the more widely used CMF (cyclophosphamide, methotrexate, and flurouracil) in 2,000 women whose cancer had not spread to their lymph nodes and who had tumors classified as estrogen receptor negative. Half received four cycles of AC over three months; the other half received six cycles of CMF over six months. Cancer-free survival after five years was 82% in both groups and overall survival was 89% in both.

"There has been a swing toward using the AC regimen, and these findings should accelerate that trend," said Bernard Fisher, M.D., the lead researcher on the study conducted by the National Surgical Adjuvant Breast and Bowel Project in Pittsburgh.

Lori Goldstein, M.D., of Fox Chase Cancer Center in Philadelphia, went a step further by saying, "This is one of the studies that will have a direct and immediate impact on patients being treated today."

That impact includes three fewer months of side effects that can include fatigue, nausea, and generally diminished quality of life.

Chapter 54

Possible Third Gene Involved in Hereditary Breast Cancer

Researchers in Finland, Iceland, and Sweden, working with scientists at the National Human Genome Research Institute (NHGRI) of the National Institutes of Health (NIH), have found evidence of a new gene that appears to increase susceptibility to hereditary breast cancer. The study examined women who live in Nordic countries and who have three or more female family members with breast cancer.

The finding, published in the August 15 issue of the *Proceedings of the National Academy of Sciences* (*PNAS*), may help explain why some women with a family history of hereditary breast cancer are at particularly high risk of developing the potentially fatal disease, even when they lack mutations in two previously identified breast cancer susceptibility genes, BRCA1 and BRCA2.

Initially, spelling errors in the genetic code of BRCA1 and BRCA2 were theorized to account for perhaps 90 percent of all hereditary breast cancers. However, more recent research suggests that these two genes account for a significantly smaller proportion of all hereditary breast cancers.

However, since all cancers are based on genetic mutations in body cells, whether they are inherited or triggered by aging or environmental factors, studies on cancer genetics can lead to improved diagnosis and treatment.

"Scientists Pinpoint Location of Possible Third Gene Involved in Hereditary Breast Cancer to Chromosome 13," National Institutes of Health (NIH) and National Human Genome Research Institute (NHGRI), NIH News Release dated August 14, 2000.

While scientists reporting in the current *PNAS* have not yet identified a third BRCA gene, they have succeeded in pinpointing its probable
location to chromosome 13, in an interval of about five million base
pairs. This is the same chromosome that also contains the previously
identified BRCA2 gene, discovered in 1995. (BRCA1, discovered in
1994, lies on chromosome 17.)

The human genome—the DNA on all chromosomes—contains
about 3 billion base pairs, misspellings and deletions of which can
increase susceptibility to diseases. Mutations of BRCA1 and BRCA2
impair the body cells' production of tumor suppressor proteins.

"We've located what looks like a very good region in the human
genome in which to search for a third breast cancer susceptibility
gene," said Dr. Olli Kallioniemi, senior scientist at NHGRI and cor-
responding author for the *PNAS* paper. He is one of 35 scientists in
14 laboratories in the United States, Finland, Sweden, Iceland and
Germany who collaborated on the study.

"Our results are preliminary results at this point," Dr. Kallioniemi
stressed. "More work must be done to confirm these results in other
populations, and we have yet to identify the DNA sequence of the gene.
But if these results are confirmed, this new gene could account for
up to one third of the hereditary breast cancer cases that cannot be
explained by BRCA1 or BRCA2 in the Nordic population."

"I greet these research findings with a combination of excitement
and caution," said NHGRI Director Dr. Francis Collins. "We've suspected for some time that hereditary breast cancer is triggered by
many susceptibility genes. Once we have most of them identified and
understood, we'll be able to tailor diagnosis and treatments much
more effectively than we are able to do now."

"However, lots of research still remains to be done," he added.

The possible location of the suspected gene was first identified by
applying a technique called comparative genomic hybridization, or
CGH, to breast cancer tumor tissues. The tissues came from 61 women
with hereditary breast cancer, whose BRCA1 and BRCA2 genes had
no detectable misspellings. All 61 women lived in Finland, Sweden,
and Iceland, and came from 37 families with three or more hereditary breast cancer-affected female relatives.

Results from the CGH analysis revealed that genetic material had
been deleted in this region of chromosome 13 at an early stage in the
development of the tumors, suggesting the presence of a new cancer-
causing gene there.

Further genetic studies were then carried out on a larger group—334
in number—of affected women representing even more (77) Finnish,

Icelandic, and Swedish families. These families were specifically chosen because their strong family history of breast cancer could not be attributed to the BRCA1 and BRCA2 genes. These studies employed linkage analysis, a complex statistical method designed to determine the likelihood that a gene is inherited, or passed along from one generation to the next, and to find the location of this gene. The linkage analysis, in turn, supported the CGH evidence for a new breast cancer susceptibility gene in the same region on chromosome 13.

"While the probability of seeing linkage evidence this strong just by chance is less than two out of a thousand, we still need confirmation of this linkage in an independent set of families," said Dr. Joan Bailey-Wilson, another co-author of the study and a statistical geneticist at NHGRI.

Although this latest finding cannot be applied now to diagnosis and treatment, it will help researchers narrow their search for a new breast cancer gene, said Dr. Heli Nevanlinna, one of the study's co-authors and a geneticist in the Department of Obstetrics and Gynaecology at Helsinki University Central Hospital in Finland.

"If a new gene is found, it will provide another important means of diagnosis for families who are at risk of developing hereditary breast cancer," Dr. Nevanlinna added.

If the scientists are able to identify a third BRCA gene in the chromosome 13 region that they are studying, they and other researchers will have to conduct much more research to determine the new gene's possible role in more heterogeneous populations, such as in the United States. Mutations in BRCA1 and BRCA2 can occur in very different frequencies in different populations, and it is likely the same would be true for any other breast cancer gene.

"There are probably other genes besides this one," suggested Dr. Ake Borg, another of the study's co-authors and a molecular geneticist in the Department of Oncology at University Hospital in Lund, Sweden. "And the importance of each of these genes may vary greatly, depending on the population."

The success of this study had much to do with the Nordic populations being studied, noted Dr. Rosa Bjork Barkardottir, a molecular biologist in the Department of Pathology at University Hospital of Iceland in Reykjavik.

"It might have been difficult to spot this candidate breast cancer region in other, more heterogeneous populations, since especially the Finnish population and Icelandic population are rather homogeneous," Dr. Barkardottir said. "Also, compared to other populations, it is easier to identify which families carry a mutation in BRCA1 or

BRCA2 and which families would be good in looking for a new BRCA gene."

In addition, Finland, Sweden, and Iceland have extensive population records and cancer registries dating back several generations. This information helps researchers determine inheritance patterns for genetic-related diseases such as cancer.

For NHGRI researcher Dr. Tommi Kainu, another co-author, much of the credit for the study should go both to the researchers in the Nordic countries who recruited the breast cancer families, and to the families themselves.

"When these families came through cancer clinics and were diagnosed with breast cancer, they were asked to fill out a family questionnaire on the presence of breast cancer in their relatives," Dr. Kainu said. "And even in this difficult time in dealing with their own disease, they took an active part in the project. So, this study is also a tribute to them."

The next stage in the U.S.-Nordic team's research will be to identify the precise sequence of DNA in the region on chromosome 13 believed to contain the gene. In that region are some five million base pairs—the chemical units of DNA. But within this region, there may still be 100 to 150 genes that must be evaluated one by one, in order to identify the precise gene responsible for the breast cancer risk.

Because the Human Genome Project has sequenced almost all of the human genetic code and made that data freely available to all researchers, the scientists have the templates from which to search, said Dr. Kallioniemi. "But that's not to say this will be an easy job. There's still a lot of work to be done," he added.

Institutions participating in the study include NHGRI; the National Center for Biotechnology Information (also part of NIH); Deutsches Krebsforschungzentrum, Heidelberg, Germany; Tampere University and University Hospital, Finland; University Hospital of Iceland, Reykjavik, Iceland; University Hospital, Lund, Sweden; University Hospital, Umea, Sweden; Helsinki University Central Hospital, Finland; and Turku University Hospital, Finland. (A complete list of authors is attached.)

Support for the study was provided by the NIH, the Nordic Cancer Society, the Finnish Cancer Society, the Academy of Finland, the Sigrid Juselius Foundation, the Clinical Research Funds of the Tampere and Helsinki University Hospitals, the Icelandic Research Council, the Icelandic University Hospital Research Fund, the Swedish Cancer Society, Mrs. Berta Kamprads Foundation, the G.A.E. Nilsson Foundation, the F&M Bergqvist Foundation, the King Gustav

V's Jubilee Foundation, the Finnish Cultural Foundation, the Emil Aaltonen Foundation, and the Maud Kuistila Foundation.

Co-authors

Five groups totaling 35 scientists, representing 14 laboratories at eight institutions in five countries, contributed to the paper titled, "Somatic deletions in hereditary breast cancers implicate 13q21 as a putative novel breast cancer susceptibility locus," published in the Aug. 15, 2000 issue of the *Proceedings of the National Academy of Sciences*. Here is a list of all the co-authors and their institutions:

Group 1: Tommi Kainu[1], Suh-Hang Hank Juo[2], Richard Desper[3], Alejandro A. Schäffer[4], Elizabeth Gillanders[1], Ester Rozenblum[1], Diana Freas-Lutz[1], Don Weaver[1], Dietrich Stephan[1], Joan Bailey-Wilson[2], and Olli-P. Kallioniemi[1].

[1]Cancer Genetics Branch, NHGRI, NIH, Bethesda, MD, USA. [2]Inherited Disease Research Branch, NHGRI, NIH, Baltimore, MD, USA. [3]Abteilung Theoretische Bioinformatik, Deutsches Krebsforschungzentrum (DKFZ), Heidelberg, Germany. [4]Computational Biology Branch, National Center for Biotechnology Information, NIH, Bethesda, MD, USA.

Group 2: Mika Tirkkonen*[1], Kirsi Syrjäkoski[1], Tuula Kuukasjärvi[2], Pasi Koivisto[1], Ritva Karhu[1], and Kaija Holli[3].

[1]Laboratory of Cancer Genetics, [2]Department of Pathology, and [3]Department of Oncology, Tampere University and University Hospital, Finland.

Group 3: Adalgeir Arason*, Gudrun Johannesdottir, Jon Thor Bergthorsson, Hrefna Johannsdottir, Valgardur Egilsson, and Rosa Björk Bardardottir. Laboratory of Cell Biology, Department of Pathology, University Hospital of Iceland, Reykjavik, Iceland.

Group 4: Oskar Johannsson*[1], Karin Haraldsson[1], Therese Sandberg[1], Eva Holmberg[3], Henrik Grönberg[3], Håkan Olsson1, and Åke Borg[1].

[1]Department of Oncology, University Hospital, Lund, Sweden; [2]Department of Clinical Genetics and [3]Department of Oncology, University Hospital, Umeå, Sweden.

Group 5: Paula Vehmanen*[1], Hannaleena Eerola[2], Päivi Heikkilä[3], Seppo Pyrhönen[4], and Heli Nevanlinna.

[1]Department of Obstetrics and Gynaecology, [2]Department of Oncology, and [3]Department of Pathology, Helsinki University Central Hospital, Finland. [4]Department of Oncology and Radiotherapy, Turku University Hospital, Finland.

* contributed equally to this work

Chapter 55

Researchers Develop Gene Test that Differentiates Breast Cancer Types

Technique Can Distinguish Hereditary from Non-Hereditary Tumors; May Lead to New Diagnostic Tests, Future Treatments

According to their report in the current issue of *The New England Journal of Medicine*, scientists at the National Human Genome Research Institute (NHGRI) at the National Institutes of Health (NIH) have developed a new genetic test that, for the first time, can easily distinguish between hereditary and sporadic forms of breast cancer. This new approach should make it possible for physicians to quickly and accurately diagnose the cause of an individual woman's disease and may ultimately guide decisions about the most effective treatment.

The international team of researchers, led by Dr. Jeffrey Trent, NHGRI's scientific director and head of the NHGRI Cancer Genetics laboratory, used a new technique called gene-expression profiling to differentiate between breast tumors that were caused by inherited genetic changes and those that were not. Based on a laboratory method that uses a type of DNA chip called a microarray, the researchers simultaneously assessed how active some 6,000 genes within breast cancer cells were, altogether making nearly 250,000 measurements.

"NHGRI Researchers Develop Gene Test that Differentiates Breast Cancer Types," National Institutes of Health and National Human Genome Research Institute, NIH News Release dated February 21, 2001.

The study revealed clear differences in the patterns of gene activity in breast tumors, patterns that can be as unique as a fingerprint, pinpointing into which group a woman's cancer belongs.

"This powerful new technology gives us a snapshot of exactly which genes are active in a tumor cell," Trent says. "Over the last few decades, scientists have made important progress in understanding the molecular origins of cancer by studying one gene at a time. Now we can look at thousands, and even tens of thousands of genes as they interact to produce a tumor. This capability will have important implications for both diagnosis and treatment."

Genetics of Breast Cancer

Earlier insights tended to give a fairly static view of the genetic changes that produced a tumor. The current study demonstrates the power of a dynamic analysis that shows the interaction of many genes within a cell's metabolic pathways. In what may become a new research and diagnostic trend, the team has established that it can differentiate between hereditary and non-hereditary breast cancer by studying thousands of genes simultaneously.

Physicians have long known that breast cancer can run in families. Approximately 5 to 10 percent of breast tumors are hereditary; the remaining cases are caused by genetic changes that occur during a woman's life and are commonly called sporadic. In the mid 1990s, scientists identified mutations in genes now called BRCA1 and BRCA2 that are the major cause of the hereditary form of the disease. Women inheriting these mutations have a 40 to 85 percent lifetime risk of developing breast cancer, as well as an increased risk of ovarian cancer.

Telling the tumor types apart is not easy with traditional techniques. "When you look at these tumors under a microscope, based on their shapes and other features, it is very difficult to tell which tumors are caused by BRCA1, and virtually impossible to distinguish cancer caused by BRCA2 from those caused by non-inherited mutations," says another of the study's senior authors, Dr. Ake Borg of the University of Lund. Furthermore, the BRCA1 and BRCA2 genes are very large, and searching through them for mutations is both complicated and expensive.

To determine whether gene profiling could tell the difference between sporadic tumors and those with BRCA1 or BRCA2 mutations, the research team examined samples of tumors that had been surgically removed from 22 breast cancer patients at the University of Lund in Lund, Sweden. Fifteen of the women were known to have hereditary breast cancer based on family history and other analyses. Of the 15, seven had mutations in BRCA1; eight had mutations in BRCA2. The control group was comprised of eight women with sporadic cases that had no evidence of any family history of the disease.

When the team examined the gene-expression profiles for the 22 patients using the microarray analyses, they were able to quickly and accurately differentiate the BRCA1 from the BRCA2 inherited changes as well as the non-inherited genetic changes. "We were surprised that we could separate the groups as well as we could," says Ingrid Hedenfalk, one of the two lead authors of the study and a doctoral student visiting NHGRI from the University of Lund. Placing patients in the proper diagnostic category can be critical to a successful treatment. For example, women shown to be carrying BRCA1 or BRCA2 mutations are at high risk for second breast cancers, and for ovarian cancer, and thus need very close follow-up.

Microarray Analysis

The team's approach relied on a cutting edge technology called a DNA microarray, or sometimes, a gene chip. The microarray itself is merely a glass slide with tiny dots of DNA from different genes arranged in a grid-like array. Using microarrays, the activity of thousands of known genes can be quickly tested in a cell sample.

To perform the analysis, scientists isolate a special collection of molecules from the test cells called messenger RNA or mRNA. These molecules are produced by active genes and indicate which of the estimated 30,000 genes are "turned on" in a cell. The information in the messenger RNAs can be converted into a form of DNA called complementary DNA or cDNA—kind of like copying a music CD to digital audiotape; same information, just in a different form. A fluorescent label can be added to the cDNA made from the test cells. A robot then systematically deposits a sample of the cDNA onto the glass slide. If the sample contains cDNA that matches a particular gene on the microarray, the cDNA sticks to that spot on the array, like two pieces of Velcro coming together. Unmatched cDNA is washed away.

Automated computerized detectors then measure the amount of fluorescence for each spot. The brighter the fluorescence, the more cDNA has attached to the known gene, and the more active the gene must be in that tissue sample. The result appears as a pattern of spots that are either bright or dark, showing whether the known gene is active or inactive in the tumor cell.

"Our gene expression profiling technology reveals a pattern, a kind of fingerprint for each tumor type," Dr. Trent says. "The fingerprint shows us key genes involved in tumor development and progression."

Because of the number of gene samples, and the number of patients tested, the study produced almost a quarter million data points. To handle the huge amounts of information generated by this process, the researchers turned to computer-based statistical analyses. With the help of statisticians from the NIH's National Cancer Institute, Agilent Laboratories, and Texas A & M University, the researchers were able to show that the differences between the groups of genes from the cancer cells were, indeed, statistically significant.

Diagnostic Impact

In a surprising twist, the scientists found their gene-profiling technique to be so good that it found a previously unrecognized rare event among the classically diagnosed tumors. Among the control tumors that had been originally diagnosed as non-hereditary, one tumor showed a gene-profile that made it look like a hereditary form of the disease caused by mutations in the BRCA1 gene.

After careful ethical advice was obtained, the researchers decided to re-contact the patient to ask for permission to do additional testing. The researchers then sequenced her BRCA1 gene and found no mutations. This puzzling result lead the team to test for a newly discovered mechanism that appears to contribute to the cause of some forms of cancer, even when a critical gene is not mutated. Instead, the gene is somehow abnormally turned off. Scientists call this recently discovered phenomenon gene silencing.

"We discovered that even though the spelling of her BRCA1 gene was normal, it was silenced due to a non-inherited mechanism called methylation," Dr. Trent says. Methylation previously has been identified as a way that a cell may temporarily or reversibly silence the activity of a gene. It remains unclear just what caused the methylation to silence this patient's BRCA1 gene and essentially turn it off. Nevertheless, Dr. Trent says, several recent studies by researchers elsewhere have shown that gene methylation may be involved in a number of different cancers, including breast and colon cancer, and may be a more common mechanism for tumor formation than previously thought.

Future Directions

Although the research team initially tested thousands of genes to find the pattern associated with the hereditary and nonhereditary forms of breast cancer, computational techniques helped them reduce the number of genes needed to a much more manageable number. "In fact," says co-lead author Hedenfalk, "we were able to narrow the number of genes needed to separate the three groups to just 50 or so."

"Not unexpectedly, these critical genes turn out to be involved in various aspects of cancer progression," says Dr. David Duggan, the study's other co-lead author. These aspects include mechanisms controlling the repair of damaged DNA, cell division, cell death, and other important cellular housekeeping functions.

These 50 or 60 genes are obvious candidates for further research to understand the molecular basis of cancer and are potential targets for the development of new drug treatments. "If you were trying to develop a therapeutic that selected hereditary breast cancer," Dr. Trent says, "these genes would be a good place to start."

The study also sheds new light on how breast cancer develops. "Even though BRCA1 and BRCA2 look nothing like each other in terms of their DNA sequence, they can cause the same net effect—increased susceptibility to both breast and ovarian cancer," Dr. Borg says. By looking at the kinds of cellular genes that are active in these cancer cells, "our results indicate that these two types of inherited genetic changes use quite different pathways, or series of biochemical steps, to cause the same devastation."

Results from the study may also help researchers find additional genes involved in breast cancer. In August 2000, an NHGRI-led team reported finding evidence for a third hereditary breast cancer gene in certain Nordic families. By using gene expression profiling to study these families, the researchers hope to narrow their search for this, and possibly, other genes involved in breast cancer.

Already, the research is being hailed by leading cancer specialists as a breakthrough in basic science with potentially broad clinical applications.

"This very important research by a superb group begins to better clarify the different functions of these hereditary breast cancer genes BRCA1 and BRCA2," said Dr. Dan Von Hoff, director of the Arizona Cancer Center in Tucson, Arizona. "This pioneering piece of microarray work will enable us to better design prevention and therapy strategies for patients with hereditary breast cancer and, I suspect, for many other cancers as their genetic basis becomes elucidated."

For NHGRI Director Dr. Francis Collins, the discovery provides a glimpse of the future of genome research. "This work is an excellent example of the kind of research that will characterize the next phase of the Human Genome Project, as scientists move from sequencing the entire human genetic code to understanding the functions of genes in health and disease," he says.

Authors

Members of the research team include (in order of the study's list of authors) NHGRI's Ingrid Hedenfalk, David Duggan, and Yidong Chen; Michael Radmacher of the National Cancer Institute (NCI); Michael Bittner of NHGRI; Richard Simon of NCI; Paul Meltzer of NHGRI; Barry Gusterson of the University of Glasgow, United Kingdom; Manel Esteller of the Johns Hopkins Oncology Center; Olli-P. Kallioniemi and Benjamin Wilfond of NHGRI; Ake Borg of the University of Lund, Sweden; and Jeffrey Trent, of NHGRI.

Other authors include Mark Raffeld of NCI; Zohar Yakhini and Amir Ben-Dor, both of Agilent Laboratories; Edward Dougherty of Texas A & M University; Juha Kononen of NHGRI; Lukas Bubendorf of NHGRI and the University of Basel, Switzerland; Wilfrid Fehrle and Stefania Pittaluga, both of NCI; Sofia Gruvberger, Niklas Loman, Oskar Johannsson, and Hakan Olsson, all of the University of Lund; and Guido Sauter of the University of Basel.

Their report, "Gene-Expression Profiles in Hereditary Breast Cancer," Hedenfalk, et. al., appears in the Feb. 22, 2001, issue of the *New England Journal of Medicine*, 244:539-548.

Chapter 56

Cancer Family Registry for Breast Cancer Studies

What is the Cancer Family Registry for Breast Cancer Studies?

The Cancer Family Registry for Breast Cancer Studies (CFRBCS) contains information and biospecimens on more than 5,000 families who have an inherited risk for breast and/or ovarian cancers. The Registry was established in 1995 with funding from the U.S. National Cancer Institute, and provides a comprehensive and collaborative infrastructure to facilitate interdisciplinary studies in the genetic epidemiology of breast and ovarian cancers. The Registry was formerly called the Cooperative Family Registry for Breast Cancer Studies.

Enrollment of families in the Registry is on-going, and researchers are welcome to apply to use its resources.

The Registry is an international consortium of six research institutions and an Informatics Support Center. The participating sites are located at the:

- University of Melbourne, Melbourne, Australia;
- Columbia University, New York, New York;
- Northern California Cancer Center, San Francisco, California;
- Cancer Care Ontario, Toronto, Canada;

Excerpted from "Cancer Family Registry for Breast Cancer Studies" and "Questions and Answers," Cancer Family Registries, Division of Cancer Control and Population Sciences, National Cancer Institute, 2000. The full text of these documents is available at http://www-dccps.ims.nci.nih.gov/CFRBCS.

- Fox Chase Cancer Center, Philadelphia, Pennsylvania; and
- Huntsman Cancer Institute, Salt Lake City, Utah.

The Informatics Support Center, which is located at the University of California, Irvine, is developing a comprehensive central database to include anonymized data from all participating sites. Summary statistics will be made available through the Center's Website.

The six Registry sites collect family history information, epidemiologic and clinical data, and related biological specimens from individuals with breast and/or ovarian cancers and Li-Fraumeni syndrome, and their families. The Registry is a resource for population-based, translational research in the genetic epidemiology of cancer. It is particularly suited to the identification and characterization of cancer-associated genes, because of the detailed data collected, parallel collection of biological specimens, the dual nature of the large collection of families ascertained (both high-risk and population-based), and the identification of a prospective cohort of probands and their families.

What kinds of research does the Registry support?

Registry supports research in the areas of:

1. Genetic epidemiology to: (a) search for undiscovered cancer susceptibility loci using linkage studies; (b) test for association and/or linkage with known "candidate" genes or metabolism genes; (c) ascertain the penetrance and modifiers of penetrance for each gene (gene-gene and gene-environment interactions); and to (d) develop and disseminate innovative analytical approaches and related software for cancer susceptibility gene identification and gene-gene and gene-environment interactions, through the Registry-associated Biostatistics, Genetics, and Epidemiology Consortium.

2. Clinical epidemiology to address issues related to prognosis and optimal treatment for genetically defined subgroups.

3. Social and behavioral epidemiology to address choices by, and behaviors of, genetically defined individuals and high-risk populations.

4. Health policy and public health research that focuses on inter-relationships among different legislative, health care, and social

structures with health policies related to genetic testing and research.

What is the scope of the Registry?

The scope of the Registry covers:

1. Collecting pedigree information, epidemiological and clinical data, and biological specimens from individuals and participants with a family history of breast and breast-ovarian cancers and breast cancer-related syndromes, who are ascertained from a variety of populations in the United States, Canada, and Australia.

2. Providing a resource and infrastructure for interdisciplinary and translational studies on the etiology of breast and ovarian cancers.

3. Identifying populations at risk for breast and/or ovarian cancers that could benefit from development of new preventive and therapeutic strategies, and from appropriate counseling.

What types of information and biospecimens are available?

The Registry can provide family history (pedigrees), and clinical, demographic, and epidemiologic data on risk factors. Families are also periodically recontacted in order to obtain follow-up epidemiologic data, and data on cancer recurrence, new morbidity, and mortality. The types of biological specimens obtainable are: tissue sections from paraffin embedded breast and ovarian cancers; peripheral blood lymphocytes, serum, fresh frozen tissue (when available); and from some Registry sites, other biological fluids may be available.

The Registry includes families who have a family history of breast and/or ovarian cancers, and who have Li-Fraumeni syndrome. The families are ascertained through high-risk clinic settings, as well as through population-based recruitment. Three Registry sites focus on enrolling high-risk families: Columbia University, Fox Chase Cancer Center, and the Huntsman Cancer Institute. The other three sites are population-based registries: University of Melbourne, Northern California Cancer Center, and Cancer Care Ontario.

Families representing the whole continuum of risk for breast and ovarian cancers are enrolled. Population groups include Non-Hispanic whites, Hispanics, African Americans, and Asians. Some sites are also ascertaining population-based control families.

The confidentiality of participants is protected. Participation in approved studies that involve additional contact is optional, and these contacts are handled by the Registry sites.

Who can obtain specimens?

Registry specimens and data are available to the entire scientific community for meritorious studies. Researchers apply to the Advisory Committee for use of resources.

Why is the Registry important?

The Registry, which continues to grow, provides researchers a valuable resource for conducting important investigations on genetic and environmental susceptibility for these cancers. Researchers are invited to apply to the Registry for use of its resources, and eligible families are welcome to enroll.

Without such registries and the help of many at-risk individuals and families who participate, it would take years for a researcher to be able to identify enough families and collect the key information needed to even begin a study.

This Registry will quicken the pace of research and support investigations in genetic epidemiology. It also is designed to support clinical investigations, such as on methods to improve prognosis and provide optimal treatment for patients; social and behavior epidemiology, such as on the choices and behaviors of at-risk groups; and health policy and public health research.

For More Information

For more information about the Cancer Family Registry for Breast Cancer Studies, visit the CFRBCS Website at http://www-dccps.ims. nci.nih.gov/CFRBCS.

Part Seven

Coping with Breast Cancer

Chapter 57

Dealing with a Cancer Diagnosis

If you have recently been diagnosed with breast cancer or with any other cancer you may be experiencing a wide variety of emotions: fear, anger, sadness, guilt, helplessness, and anxiety. You may wonder, 'Why me?'. Often patients are unsure about what to do next and at times have to sort out contradictory medical information and treatment advice.

In the very near future you will need to acquire some new skills including how to best communicate with doctors and other medical personal; how to choose your best treatment options and how to manage your own responses and those of your family and friends. Today there is strong research data that your emotional well-being and having good support from others can be important to physical recovery.

Your Health Team

Cancer is a serious and complex disease, to beat it you will need a team of health professionals all bringing their own specific specialties to your recovery. Oncologists specialize in cancer treatment, your primary care physician will also be a part of your team. You are also likely to see a surgeon and perhaps other specialists as well. A mental health professional is an important team player as well. Psychologists and other mental health professionals work directly with the patient and his/her family as well as with the entire medical team to help personalize the patient's

"Getting Beyond 'Why Me?': Dealing with a Cancer Diagnosis," from the American Psychological Association's HelpCenter at http://www.apa.org. © 1997 by the American Psychological Association. Reprinted with permission.

medical decisions, manage treatment side effects, improve communication, provide support, and enhance emotional recovery and well-being.

Cancer Treatment Can Be as Difficult as the Disease Itself

Conventional cancer treatments from surgery to chemotherapy are themselves traumatic to the patient. However, in many cases they are known to save lives. Some patients may decide to pursue dietary and lifestyle changes as part of their primary treatment regimen. Psychologists have techniques to make adherence to these new behaviors easier and more successful.

Psychological interventions have also proven to be extremely effective in helping patients handle the pain and symptoms of the disease and the side effects of treatment. For example, techniques used by psychologists can significantly reduce anxiety before surgery and decrease the nausea that often precedes and accompanies chemotherapy. Psychological interventions can also help the majority of cancer patients who report debilitating pain. Psychological techniques can be used to create positive imagery, to increase the motivation to adhere to new behaviors and to facilitate reentry into the real world once treatment has been completed.

The post-treatment period is usually ignored. Emotional recovery from the trauma of cancer treatment takes longer than physical recovery. Psychological services can help mitigate the long term effects of cancer treatment.

Cancer Affects Whole Families

When one member of a family has cancer, the whole family is effected and, in fact, psychologists consider these family members to be 'secondary patients.' Cancer affects an entire family, not only because there are genetic links to cancer and cancer risk but because when one member of a family has cancer the whole family must deal with the illness. If you or a loved one has been diagnosed with cancer, help for the entire family may be in order. When a woman is diagnosed with breast cancer for example roles suddenly change: spouses will need to take on new responsibilities at home; relatives and friends may be needed to participate in the day-to-day running of the household; and the children involved will need special attention. Communication amongst all the players and protecting against caregiver burnout is imperative. Psychologists help construct a game plan that works for all family members during every phase of the illness.

Chapter 58

How Your Mind Can Help Your Body

Each year 185,000 women in this country learn that they have breast cancer. Because less than a quarter of them have genetic or other known risk factors, the diagnosis often comes as a devastating surprise. The emotional turmoil that results can affect women's physical health as well as their psychological well-being. This question-and-answer text explains how psychological treatment can help these women harness the healing powers of their own minds.

What impact does a breast cancer diagnosis have on psychological well-being?

Receiving a diagnosis of breast cancer can be one of the most distressing events women ever experience. And women may not know where to turn for help.

Distress typically continues even after the initial shock of diagnosis has passed. As women begin what is often a lengthy treatment process, they may find themselves faced with new problems. They may find their personal relationships in turmoil, for instance. They may feel tired all the time. They may be very worried about their symptoms, treatment, and mortality. They may face discrimination from

"Breast Cancer: How Your Mind Can Help Your Body," from the American Psychological Association's HelpCenter at http://www.apa.org. © 1997 by the American Psychological Association. Reprinted with permission. The American Psychological Association Practice Directorate gratefully acknowledges the assistance of Alice F. Chang, PhD, and Sandra B. Haber, PhD, in developing this material.

employers or insurance companies. Factors like these can contribute to chronic stress, anxiety and depression.

Why is it important to seek psychological help?

Feeling overwhelmed is a perfectly normal response to a breast cancer diagnosis. But negative emotions can cause women to stop doing things that are good for them and start doing things that are bad for anyone but especially worrisome for those with a serious disease. Women with breast cancer may start eating poorly, for instance, eating fewer meals and choosing foods of lower nutritional value. They may cut back on their exercise. They may have trouble getting a good night's sleep. And they may withdraw from family and friends. At the same time, these women may use alcohol, cigarettes, caffeine or other drugs in an attempt to soothe themselves.

A breast cancer diagnosis can also lead to more severe problems. Researchers estimate that anywhere from 20 to 60 percent of cancer patients experience depressive symptoms, which can make it more difficult for women to adjust, participate optimally in treatment activities, and take advantage of whatever sources of social support are available. Some women become so disheartened by the ordeal of having cancer that they refuse to undergo surgery or simply stop going to radiation or chemotherapy appointments. As a result, they may get even sicker. In fact, studies show that missing as few as 15 percent of chemotherapy appointments results in significantly poorer outcomes.

How can psychological treatment help women adjust?

Licensed psychologists and other mental health professionals with experience in breast cancer treatment can help a great deal. Their primary goal is to help women learn how to cope with the physical, emotional, and lifestyle changes associated with cancer as well as with medical treatments that can be painful and traumatic. For some women, the focus may be on how to explain their illness to their children or how to deal with a partner's response. For others, it may be on how to choose the right hospital or medical treatment. For still others, it may be on how to control stress, anxiety, or depression. By teaching patients problem-solving strategies in a supportive environment, psychologists help women work through their grief, fear, and other emotions. For many women, this life-threatening crisis eventually proves to be an opportunity for life-enhancing personal growth.

Breast cancer patients themselves aren't the only ones who can benefit from psychological treatment. Psychologists often help spouses who must offer both emotional and practical support while dealing with their own feelings, for instance. Children, parents, and friends involved in caretaking can also benefit from psychological interventions.

The need for psychological treatment may not end when medical treatment does. In fact, emotional recovery may take longer than physical recovery and is sometimes less predictable. Although societal pressure to get everything back to normal is intense, breast cancer survivors need time to create a new self-image that incorporates both the experience and their changed bodies. Psychologists can help women achieve that goal and learn to cope with such issues as fears about recurrence and impatience with life's more mundane problems.

Can psychological treatment help the body, too?

Absolutely. Take the nausea and vomiting that often accompany chemotherapy, for example. For some women, these side effects can be severe enough to make them reject further treatment efforts. Psychologists can teach women relaxation exercises, meditation, self-hypnosis, imagery, or other skills that can effectively relieve nausea without the side effects of pharmaceutical approaches.

Psychological treatment has indirect effects on physical health as well. Researchers already know that stress suppresses the body's ability to protect itself. What they now suspect is that the coping skills that psychologists teach may actually boost the immune system's strength. In one well-known study, for example, patients with advanced breast cancer who underwent group therapy lived longer than those who did not.

Research also suggests that patients who ask questions and are assertive with their physicians have better health outcomes than patients who passively accept proposed treatment regimens. Psychologists can empower women to make more informed choices in the face of often-conflicting advice and can help them communicate more effectively with their health care providers. In short, psychologists can help women become more fully engaged in their own treatment. The result is an enhanced understanding of the disease and its treatment and a greater willingness to do what needs to be done to get well again.

What type of psychological treatment is helpful?

A combination of individual and group treatment sometimes works best. Individual sessions with a licensed psychologist typically emphasize the understanding and modification of patterns of thinking and behavior. Group psychological treatment with others who have breast cancer gives women a chance to give and receive emotional support and learn from the experiences of others. To be most effective, groups should be made up of women at similar stages of the disease and led by psychologists or other mental health professionals with experience in breast cancer treatment.

Whether aimed at individuals or groups, psychological interventions strive to help women adjust to their diagnoses, cope with treatment, and come to terms with the disease's impact on their lives. These interventions offer psychologists an opportunity to help women better understand breast cancer and its treatment. Psychologists typically ask women open-ended questions about their assumptions, ideas for living life more fully, and other matters. Although negative thoughts and feelings are addressed, most psychological interventions focus on problem-solving as women meet each new challenge.

A breast cancer diagnosis can severely impair women's psychological functioning, which in turn can jeopardize their physical health. It doesn't have to be that way. Women who seek help from licensed psychologists with experience in breast cancer treatment can actually use the mind-body connection to their advantage to enhance both mental and physical health.

Chapter 59

Common Reactions of Children to Their Mother's Breast Cancer

Some of the most common reactions of children to their mother's cancer are fear and insecurity, anger, sadness, isolation, and curiosity.

Fear

Fears can take many forms: fear of death of their parent, fear because their parents have fear, fear of separation, fear cancer is contagious and that they will catch it, fear that they caused the cancer, fear that the life they know will change.

Fear of death. Because our society frequently hides the diagnosis of cancer, often a child's or teen's only exposure to cancer is people who have died. Therefore cancer means death. This may be the first time that the possibility of death of someone close has ever become a consideration. They may sense your fear of death. A younger child may think death is near at hand, an older child may interpret therapies as only postponing death.

Fear because their parents have fear: Children of all age groups can sense a parent's anxiety and fear. In turn they can then become more afraid and insecure. Smaller children may cling to you and want more than usual attention.

"Breast Cancer: Common Reactions of Children and How to Help," by Jane Brazy, MD and Mary Ircink, RN, Breast Problem Clinic, University of Wisconsin Medical School, January 2000; reprinted with permission. This document is available online at http://www2.medsch.wisc.edu/childrenshosp/childrens.html. The University of Wisconsin-Madison, Department of Surgery's Website is available online at http://www.surgery.wisc.edu.

Fear of separation. When small children realize that their mother may be hospitalized, they have fear that they will be separated from you. They have little sense of time and they live in the "now". A few days may be interpreted as permanent. They may also experience separation frequently when you have radiation treatments or chemotherapy as these take up a significant fraction of their day.

Fear cancer is contagious. Many children think cancer is contagious, that they can catch it from you. After all, most of the colds and illnesses that they have had they did get from someone else. It is very important to assure children of all ages that cancer of all kinds is *not* contagious, that they can't catch it. Assure them that breast cancer doesn't happen to children. Their friends may also think cancer is contagious and may stop playing with your child because of the fear of catching it or spreading it to their mother.

Fear that they caused cancer. Magical thinking is normal in children, and is extremely common in preschool and grade school children. Magical thinking is the idea that they can make their thoughts and wishes come true. Last week they may have been mad at you and thought, "I'm mad at Mommy; I want to hurt her." Now you have cancer and you hurt, more than they ever thought possible. They fear they caused the cancer and the impact of their wishes is now beyond their control. They feel very guilty and afraid.

Fear that their life will change. Children derive a great deal of security in knowing what to expect day by day and in the future. Suddenly their life is upset and they don't know what to expect today or from now on. Their family security is at risk of disappearing.

Anger

Anger can also take on many forms: anger at you for getting cancer, anger at the cancer for attacking you, anger at what this event is doing to their life now and what it might do to them in the future. Since anger is a normal response for you too, they may sense or see your anger and frustration.

Often the anger is misplaced. They are angry at what this event is doing to their life and take it out on you or other family members. Sometimes children act out and become more demanding and unruly. They may do less well in school or do things they would not do otherwise. There may be more conflict between siblings. We always teach children to be fair...they therefore expect life to be fair. This may be their first exposure to the unfairness in life and they respond with anger.

Sadness

Because you may cry often when you are holding your young children, they may think they are causing you to be sad. Acknowledge that you are sad because of your illness, but be sure they understand that they did not make you sad.

Occasionally older children will share in your sadness or grief and openly cry with you, but often they do not. Some will try to be cheerful when around you, but express their sadness/grief when they are alone or with friends. Others will not appear to express any sadness or emotion; for them the whole ordeal is too overwhelming and they will appear to ignore it.

Isolation/Separation

You and you spouse or other support person need to and will spend time together to work out your feelings and provide mutual support. Your children may feel left out. Your children may also feel isolated because other kids avoid them, either because they are afraid of the concept of cancer or because they think they might catch it. Small children may experience separation from you. These feelings of isolation become realities when you go to the hospital, and again each day that you have radiation treatments or chemotherapy.

Curiosity

Most children will be very curious about your surgery and what your breast or chest looks like afterward. If, when and how you choose to show your children your breast is highly individual and may depend on the age and sex of your child and how comfortable you feel about showing them. Usually, however, what they imagine is far worse than the reality. The time to address questions with small children is when they ask them. Try to make comparisons with their past experiences. For example, the incision can be compared to cuts that they have had on their fingers or knees. This may not seem as a valid comparison to you but to them little cuts on their bodies are very important. Assure them that cut edges will grow back together again. When they ask about drains and drainage, show how the fluid goes down the tube and then to the bulb. After it gets to the bulb, you measure it and throw it out. It is a way to get rid of the extra fluid that you don't need. It is good to get rid of it. "Where did your breast or lump go?" You may want to say they kept it at the hospital to learn more about your lump. Assure them that you are fine without it, you don't need it anymore.

If your children are older, you can pick a time that is more suitable to you and when you perceive they are ready to handle it. Very early after surgery (especially mastectomy) may not always be the best time, first because you may not be ready and are unadjusted to its appearance, second, because it looks worse with drains in, and third, the early drainage is bloody and the sight of blood is often scary and/ or repulsive to school age children. If you show it to them early, then be sure to show it again when the drains are out and it is healing. If you feel uncomfortable showing your own breast to your son or daughter, you may want to show him/her a picture or diagram from a book. Don't be surprised, however, if someday your son or daughter sneaks a peek by coming into your bedroom when you are dressing to ask a question which could have easily waited. Just act natural, don't get angry and don't be too quick to cover up (let them get their peek); their timing was probably not an accident.

Approaches

Preschool, Early Grade School

This is a time of family stress when your children need extra love and attention. It is difficult to meet all the additional needs of children when you have many unmet needs yourself. Try to find someone else who can help give your children special attention. This should be someone who is very familiar to them. If possible have their dad spend more time with them. Studies have shown that increased time with the non-ill parent helps in the child's adjustment to cancer. You may want to have their favorite baby-sitter come over for the sole purpose of entertaining them and giving them extra attention. If grandparents or close relatives live nearby, they can be of great help in this respect. If your child has a special friend, try to arrange for his mother to have your child over to play during this period. Interrupt your children's normal routine as little as possible. Do activities together as a family. Let your children do things for you if they wish, but don't force tasks on them. If your child is in day care or school, be sure to let the teacher know about your cancer. Suggest that she/he alert you to changes in your child's behavior that are of concern. If you are having radiation therapy or chemotherapy, let the teacher know that you will not be available for classroom projects or field trips. Ask her to alert you if contagious diseases (such as chicken pox) begin circulating in your child's classroom.

If your children are too young to understand the concept of cancer refer to it as "my sickness". Be sure that your children understand that they had nothing to do with your sickness (or you getting cancer), and that wishes and thoughts cannot make people sick (or get cancer). Assure them that they are not going to get your sickness (or cancer), "children and daddies can't get my kind of sickness (breast cancer); no one can get it from me". If your child seems angry, anxious or frustrated, encourage him/her to play with a toy that will allow expression of anger e.g. a pound-the-peg-board, a drum, or a fierce animal puppet or toy (tiger, shark etc.). Encourage them to draw pictures. Ask them to tell you about their pictures. Observe when your children draw or play with stuffed animals or dolls. Things that they say or do may give you clues to their thinking and emotions. Don't criticize if they have aggressive play toward their toys, but if they are doing unacceptable things, help them redirect their energies to more acceptable activities. Assure them that its okay to be sad or mad (if they are); you are sad and feel angry too. But, continue to be consistent in your parenting approach. You may find that your children regress to more immature behavior. This is normal. When they feel secure again, they will return to more age appropriate behavior.

Answer questions that they have simply. Don't offer explanations that are more complicated than the questions they ask. Keep it at their level. Let them know that Mommy will be gone to the hospital for a few days. Be sure they know who will care for them when you're not there. If possible have them visit when you are in the hospital. Make their visit as entertaining and positive as possible. Show them how to adjust the bed by pushing the buttons and make you more comfortable. A TV suspended from the wall may be novel. Answer their curiosity questions about equipment simply. Have them bring in special pictures for you, including things that they have drawn or made for you. Be sure that they bring a photo of them and a photo of the whole family for you to have in your room. See if they can think of other things to bring you to make you feel better, like a small bouquet of flowers from your garden or even dandelions from the lawn. These tokens of love will make both of you feel better and important. *But, be sure they keep their own security object at home, not with you; they will need it.*

If you are having radiation or chemotherapy, you may want to take them to visit the facility so they know where you go and what it is like. You might want to select a day that you do not have treatments so it is just a short trip and you are with them the whole time. You might want to give them a picture of you or something from your purse to keep with them and care for while you are away. Tell them you will be back for them and provide a time frame that is meaningful to them, for example, after a specific activity or TV show.

Junior High, Teens, Early 20's

The responses of older children to their mothers diagnosis of breast cancer are highly variable. Almost all children feel some anger, fear, a sense of unfairness, loss and insecurity. For some the whole thing is too overwhelming and they will choose to deal with it by trying to ignore it. They may show little or no emotion and will appear to go about their activities as if nothing happened. This may be hard for you because they seem very unfeeling to you. Some will share your sadness openly, but others will keep their sadness to themselves or share it only with their friends or other relatives and not with you. Regardless of the response, acknowledge that cancer is difficult to deal with, offer to answer questions, and be supportive. Suggest that they might want to share their feelings with some other person(s); make suggestions such as an adult relative, teacher, coach, school nurse, pediatrician or one of their peers, but let them choose who and let them regulate their closeness or distance from you and from cancer. Encourage activities that might help them vent anger and frustration safely such as shoot-the-object computer games, shooting baskets or playing other sports. Provide for family time together, every day if possible. As soon as you are able, do your favorite family activities together.

Try to be honest with your children but don't force more information on them than they are ready to handle. Sometimes leaving age-appropriate information out on the counter for them will let them get information at a time and in amounts that they can handle. Let them know it is there for them to read if they want to and that you want to be sure they get answers to any questions that they might have. It is often a good idea to have a family discussion of your cancer. During this time you could go over some of the basic information regarding breast cancer. It is a good time to share mutual feelings. You may want to discuss the data on your own case with your children. Be optimistic. Be sure your children know what is being planned for you in the near future (therapy) and how that will effect your life (i.e. side effects such as tiredness, possible loss of hair) and most important, how it might effect their lives. However, one should strive to interrupt their life style and activities as little as possible.

A few studies have investigated children's reactions to their mother's breast cancer. Most mother-child relationships stayed strong or became stronger, but some mother-child relationships deteriorated. Problems were more common if the mother had a poor prognosis, if there was extensive surgery, or if there was a prior history of poor relations between the mother and child. Mother's relationships with daughters were more stressed than relationships with their sons. Pre-adolescent daughters were more likely to show signs of fearfulness. Daughters in their later teens and early 20's sometimes showed the most dramatic responses characterized by being distant, aversive to discussions of breast cancer, and demonstrating signs of rejection of their mother. The authors speculated that perhaps the greater reactions in daughters arose from greater fears of developing the disease themselves and the greater responsibilities placed on them. Another study identified the following factors as increasing anxiety in children when a parent had cancer: inability to discuss the diagnosis with the parents, decreased time with their friends, decreased time available for sports and leisure activity, and deterioration of their schoolwork. Stress makes it difficult to concentrate. If your child's school work is deteriorating, make the teacher aware of the situation at home so that the teacher can provide extra help and support for your child.

Teenagers, especially daughters, are very image conscious. Aspects of your therapy may embarrass them, especially in the presence of their friends. These include baldness, going without a prosthesis, or even such a minor thing as not having your "breasts" perfectly even when going out in public. Try discussing these things openly with your children and come to some agreement about what is acceptable to both of you in the presence of their friends or when out in public with them. Also, although you and other close adults may use a little humor as a way to deal with your situation, teenagers may find this very disturbing. They are likely to view it as "gross" or disgusting and not see it as a way of coping and adjusting.

Daughters and the Future Risk of Breast Cancer

As a group, daughters of women with breast cancer are at increased risk of sometime developing breast cancer. Actually, only a few daughters are at very high risk and the rest are at nearly the same risk as the general public. Risk increases if the mother developed breast cancer before menopause, had breast cancer in both breasts, and/or had the combination of ovarian cancer and breast cancer. There are several genes related to breast cancer risk. Unfortunately all the tests are not yet available that can tell you into which group your daughter falls. This is an area of very active research and within the next several years such tests will be more available. Pay attention to news regarding breast cancer genes, and the risks and benefits of screening. There are potential hidden risks in screening such as ability to get health or life insurance, guilt, etc. Discuss all aspects of screening with a professional before you decide about it.

It is *very important* that all daughters with breast development learn to correctly perform a self-breast examination. Be sure that your daughter learns it by the time she gets out of high school. There are pamphlets and tapes that can provide her with the basics. Then it is important that a health professional *show* her how to perform the examination correctly on herself. This can be your regular physician, her pediatrician, or one of your cancer specialists. Help your daughter get into the habit of performing it once a month, just after her period.

Summary for Helping Your Children

1. Be sure your children have adequate opportunities to discuss your cancer and express their feelings. You may or may not be the person they feel most comfortable talking to. They may prefer expressing their thoughts and feelings to a close friend, your spouse, a teacher, or a relative. Don't isolate them by not letting them talk to the person they feel most comfortable with, even if it is a peer. If you don't feel comfortable with too many people knowing about your cancer, help them select which friend(s) they may want to tell.

2. Be honest with them; provide them with the amount of information that they seek. Keep it at their level of education and understanding. Be sure someone answers their questions, even if you have to write them down and ask your doctor.

3. Don't be afraid to show your emotions in their presence. This will demonstrate to them that it is okay for everyone to have and show emotions.

4. Provide more family time. Do things together. Talk about activities and ideas. Discuss your cancer and your feelings as a family.

5. Be sure that they understand that cancer is not contagious; cancer can be cured; and it is normal for them to be frightened, angry, and sad.

6. Try to change their daily routine as little as possible. Encourage them to play with their friends, participate in their usual activities. If possible don't put extra work demands on them at home. But, if they volunteer to do things to help you or make you more comfortable, accept them gratefully.

7. Have your spouse or another significant person spend more time with them.

8. Once your daughter is past puberty, be sure she learns self breast examination.

Internet Resources

Kidscope—a site to help children cope with a parent's cancer
http://www.kidscope.org

Breast Cancer: Help Me Understand It!
http://www.surgery.wisc.edu/breast_info/laybreastca.html

Dr. Wolberg's Breast Tutorial—information about breast cancer and other breast problems
http://www.surgery.wisc.edu/wolberg

References

Armsden GC and Lewis FM. Behavioral adjustment and self-esteem of school-age children of women with breast cancer. *Oncol Nurs Forum* 21:39-45, 1994.

Christ GH, Siegel K, Greund B, Lanosch D, Hendersen S, Sperber D and Weinstein L. Impact of parental terminal cancer on latency-age children. *Amer J Orthopsychiatr* 63:417-425, 1993.

Issel LM, Ersek M Lewis FM. How children cope with mother's breast cancer. *Oncology Nursing Forum* 17:15-13, 1990.

Lichtman RR, Taylor SE, Wood JV, Bluming AZ, Dosik GM and Leibowitz RL. Relations with children after breast cancer: The mother-daughter relationship at risk. *Journal of Psychosocial Oncology* 2:1-19, 1985.

Nelson E, Sloper P, Charlton A and While D. Children who have a parent with cancer: A pilot study. *J Cancer Edu* 9:30-36, 1994.

Wellisch DK, Gritz ER, Schain W, Wang HJ, and Siau J. Psychological functioning of daughters of breast cancer patients. Part II: Characterizing the distressed daughter of the breast cancer patient. *Psychosomatics* 32:324-336, 1991.

Additional Resources

McCue K. and Bonn R. (1994). *How to Help Children through a Parent's Serious Illness*, St. Martin's Press, New York, NY.

Stearns Parkinson V. (1991) *My Mommy Has Cancer*, (booklet for children) Solace Publishing, Inc., Box 567 Folson, CA, 95763-0567 1-800-984-9015.

Torrey L. (1999). *Michael's Mommy has Breast Cancer* (book for children 5-10 years) Hibiscus Press, PO Box 770666, Corel Springs, FL 33077-0666 1-800-468-4004.

Resources for Children whose Parent has a Terminal Illness

Fernside: A Center for Grieving Children. http//fernside.org

Brisson, Pat. (1999) *Sky Memories,* Random House Children's Books, New York, NY. Story of 10-year-old Emily, whose mother is diagnosed with cancer and how the two find a way to ready themselves for the coming loss while celebrating life and cherishing their time left together. Comes with parent-child discussion guide. Ages 8 and up.

Goldman L. (1994). *Life and Loss, A Guide to Help Grieving Children*. Accelerated Development, A member of the Taylor and Francis Groups, Accelerated Development, Inc. Bristol, PA.

Jewell Jarratt C, (1982). *Helping Children Cope with Separation and Loss*, The Harvard Common Press, Boston, Massachusetts.

Papenbrock P and Voss R. (1988). *Children's Grief, How to Help the Child Whose Parent Has Died*, (booklet) Medic Publishing Company, Box 89 Redmond, WA. 98073. 206-881-2883.

Other books for children about Parents Dying: from the bibliography of Life and Loss, A Guide to Help Grieving Children (See above)

Blume J. (1981). *Tiger Eyes*. New York, NY: Macmillan Children's Group. Fifteen-year-old Davey works through the feelings of his father's murder in a store hold-up. Ages 11 and up.

Douglas, E. (1990). *Rachel and the Upside Down Heart*. Los Angeles, CA: Price Stern Sloan. The true story of four-year-old Rachel, and how her father's death affects her life. Ages 5-9.

Frost, D. (1991). *DAD! Why'd You Leave Me?* Scottdale, PA; Herald Press. This is a story about ten-year-old Ronnie who can't understand why his dad died. Ages 8-12.

Greenfield E. (1993). *Nathanial Talking*. New York, NY: Black Butterfly Children's Group. Nathanial, an energetic nine-year-old, helps us understand a black child's world after his mom dies. He uses rap and rhyme to express his feelings. Ages 7-11.

Krementz J. (1981). *How It Feels When a Parent Dies*. New York, NY: Knoph Publishing Co. Eighteen children (ages 7-16) speak openly words about their feelings and experiences after the death of a parent.

Lanton, S. (1991). *Daddy's Chair*. Rockville, MD: Kar-Ben Copies, Inc., Michael's dad died. This follows the Shiva, the Jewish week of mourning. He doesn't want anyone to sit in Daddy's chair. Ages 5-10.

LeShan, E. (1975). *Learning to Say Goodbye When a Parent Dies*. New York, NY: Macmillan Publishing Co. Written directly to children about problems to be recognized and overcome when a parent dies. Ages 8 and up.

Levine J. (1992). *Forever in My Heart*. Burnsville, NC: Mt. Rainbow Publications. A story and workbook that helps children participate in life when their parent is dying. Ages 5-9.

Powell S. (1990). *Geranium Morning*. Minneapolis, MN: Carol Rhoda Books, Inc. A boy's dad is killed in a car accident and a girl's mom is dying. These children share their feelings within a special friendship. Ages 6 and up.

Tiffault, B. (1992). *A Quilt for Elizabeth*. Omaha, NE: Centering Co-operation, Inc. Elizabeth's grandmother helps her understand her feelings after her father dies. This is a good story to initiate an open dialogue with children. Ages 7 and up.

Thaut P. (1991). *Spike and Ben*. Deerfield Beach, FCL; Health Communication, Inc. The story of a boy whose friend's mom dies. Ages 5-9.

Vigna J. (1991). *Saying Goodbye to Daddy*. Niles, IL: Albert Whitman and Co. A sensitive story about a dad's death and the healing that takes place in the weeks that follow. Ages 5-8.

—Jane Brazy, MD and Mary Ircink, RN

Dr. Brazy is Professor of Pediatrics, University of Wisconsin. Her speciality is Newborn Intensive Care. Ms. Ircink is a pediatric nurse who works with Dr. Brazy in patient care and in research. Both are mothers and developed breast cancer before age 50. They are authors of another web site, *For Parents of Preemies: Answers to Commonly Asked Questions* at http://www2.medsch.wisc/edu/childrenshosp/parents_of_premies/index.html

Chapter 60

The Women's Health and Cancer Rights Act of 1998

Annual Notice Requirements Update

The Women's Health and Cancer Rights Act (WHCRA) was signed into law on October 21, 1998. The law includes important new protections for mastectomy patients who elect breast reconstruction in connection with a mastectomy. WHCRA amended the Employee Retirement Income Security Act of 1974 (ERISA) and the Public Health Service Act (PHS Act) and is administered by the Departments of Labor and Health and Human Services.

Among other things, WHCRA requires that group health plans and health insurance issuers, including insurance companies and HMOs, notify individuals at three separate instances (after the enactment of the Act, upon enrollment, and annually) regarding the coverage required by WHCRA. The one-time notification provision required plans and issuers to inform participants and beneficiaries no later than January 1, 1999 ·of the coverage required by WHCRA. The permanent notification provision requires plans and issuers to notify participants upon enrollment and annually thereafter of the benefits required under WHCRA.

The Department of Labor and the Department of Health and Human Services have received numerous inquiries from the public focusing on the enrollment and annual notice requirements under WHCRA. In November 1998, to assist consumers and the regulated community,

The Department of Labor and the Department of Health and Human Services, *The Women's Health and Cancer Rights Act of 1998; Questions and Answers Annual Notice Requirements* Update, October 1999.

the Departments issued *questions and answers concerning WHCRA*. Additionally, in May 1999, the Departments issued a Request for Information (RFI) seeking public comment on the coverage and notice requirements of WHCRA. In response to the RFI, the Departments have received many questions from the public focusing on the annual notice requirement under WHCRA.

The Departments believe that the WHCRA notices distributed by plans, insurance companies and HMOs should educate participants and beneficiaries who had a mastectomy or will have a mastectomy about the benefits available under their plan (or health coverage) for reconstructive surgery and for complications related to a mastectomy. The Departments are also targeting their own outreach efforts and utilizing their health benefits campaigns, in partnership with a diverse group of companies and other interested parties, to most effectively educate the population protected by WHCRA.

The Departments also believe that employers, unions, and health insurance issuers play a key role in educating participants, beneficiaries, and covered individuals and should have some flexibility in determining how best to educate consumers about their rights under WHCRA.

To this end, the following information is intended to provide general guidance on frequently asked questions about the enrollment and annual notice requirements under the provisions of WHCRA that amend ERISA.

Are all group health plans, and their insurance companies or HMOs, required to satisfy the notice requirements under WHCRA?

All group health plans, and their health insurance issuers, that offer coverage for medical and surgical benefits with respect to a mastectomy are subject to the notice requirements under WHCRA.

What are the notice requirements under WHCRA?

There are three separate notices required under WHCRA. The first notice is a one-time requirement under which group health plans, and their insurance companies or HMOs, must have furnished a written description of the benefits that WHCRA requires to participants and beneficiaries no later than January 1, 1999. The second notice must also describe the benefits required under WHCRA but it must be provided to participants upon enrollment in the plan. The third notice is required to be furnished annually to participants under the plan.

When must the annual notice be delivered?

As mentioned above, WHCRA requires a written notice of the availability of such coverage to be delivered to the participant upon enrollment and annually thereafter. A plan or health insurance issuer satisfies the annual requirement if the plan delivers the annual notice anytime during a plan year.

During a plan year, must both an annual notice and an enrollment notice be provided to participants enrolling in the plan?

No. If a plan or health insurance issuer provides appropriate enrollment notice to a participant upon enrollment in the plan, then the plan or issuer does not have to provide that participant with an annual notice for the plan year during which that participant enrolled.

How must the annual notice be delivered?

The plan or health insurance issuer must use measures reasonably calculated to ensure actual receipt of the annual notice by plan participants and the notice must be sent by a method or methods of delivery likely to result in full distribution consistent with 29 CFR 2520.104b-1. For example, the notice may be provided by first class mail, via e-mail, or any other means of delivery prescribed in the regulation. For additional information and requirements relating to disclosure through electronic media see 64 Federal Register 4506 (January 28, 1999).

Does WHCRA require plans to send the annual notice separately?

No. The annual notice may be sent by itself or may, for example, be included in any of the following (provided that the conditions in 29 CFR 2520.104b-1 are met):

- a summary plan description (SPD), a summary of material modifications (SMM), or a summary annual report (SAR);
- a union newsletter (or a benefits newsletter);
- open enrollment materials; or
- any other written communication by the plan.

Can a plan satisfy the annual notice requirement by using the same notice as the one used to satisfy the enrollment notice?

Yes. Although WHCRA does not require plans to use the same notice to fulfill the enrollment and annual notice requirements, plans may satisfy the annual notice requirement by using the enrollment notice and delivering it to participants on an annual basis.

The enrollment notice must describe the benefits that WHCRA requires the group health plan, and its insurance companies or HMOs, to cover. The enrollment notice must indicate that, in the case of a participant or beneficiary who is receiving benefits in connection with a mastectomy, coverage will be provided in a manner determined in consultation with the attending physician and the patient, for:

- all stages of reconstruction of the breast on which the mastectomy was performed;

- surgery and reconstruction of the other breast to produce a symmetrical appearance; and

- prostheses and treatment of physical complications of the mastectomy, including lymphedema.

- The enrollment notice must also describe any deductibles and co-insurance limitations applicable to such coverage. Under WHCRA, coverage of breast reconstruction benefits may be subject only to deductibles and coinsurance limitations consistent with those established for other benefits under the plan or coverage.

If a plan does not use the enrollment notice to satisfy the annual notice requirement, is there another way to fulfill the annual notice requirement?

Yes. Instead of distributing the enrollment notice annually, a plan may choose to distribute annually a notice informing participants of the following:

- the availability of benefits for the treatment of mastectomy-related services, including reconstructive surgery, prosthesis, and lymphedema under the plan; and

- information (telephone number, web address, etc.) on how to obtain a detailed description of the mastectomy-related benefits available under the plan.

See model annual notice that may be used to satisfy WHCRA's annual notice requirement at the end of this chapter.

> **Example.** A group health plan provides benefits for mastectomies and is subject to the requirements of WHCRA. In October of every year, the plan delivers to each participant (including those on COBRA) an issue of a periodical benefits newsletter with the following statement in a prominent place on the front page: "IMPORTANT NOTICE ABOUT YOUR RIGHTS UNDER YOUR GROUP HEALTH PLAN: October is National Breast Cancer Awareness Month. Your plan, [or identify plan by name], provides benefits for mastectomy-related services including reconstruction and surgery to achieve symmetry between the breasts, prostheses, and complications resulting from a mastectomy (including lymphedema). Keep this notice for your records and call your Plan Administrator for more information."

In this example, the plan fulfills the annual notification requirement. Additionally, the plan could satisfy the annual notice requirement if the plan instead furnished its SPD, which includes the WHCRA information, on an annual basis to plan participants along with a notice that the SPD distribution is intended to satisfy the WHCRA annual notice requirement regarding mastectomy-related services available under the plan.

Must a group health plan, and their insurance companies or HMOs, furnish separate notices under WHCRA?

No. To avoid duplication of notices, a group health plan or health insurance issuers, including insurance companies or HMOs, can satisfy the notice requirements of WHCRA by contracting with another party that provides the required notice. For example, in the case of a group health plan funded through an insurance policy, the group health plan will satisfy the notice requirements with respect to a participant or beneficiary if the insurance company or HMO actually provides the notice that includes the information required by WHCRA.

For additional information see *Questions and Answers: Notice Requirements under WHCRA* (November 1998). Individuals interested in obtaining a copy of this publication may call a toll free number, 800-998-7542, or access the publication on-line at www.dol.gov/dol/pwba, the Department of Labor's website. Questions and answers pertaining to WHCRA are also available on-line at www.hcfa.gov/hipaa, the Health Care Financing Administration's website.

Women's Health and Cancer Rights Act of 1998 Model Annual Notice

"Did you know that your plan, as required by the Women's Health and Cancer Rights Act of 1998, provides benefits for mastectomy-related services including reconstruction and surgery to achieve symmetry between the breasts, prostheses, and complications resulting from a mastectomy (including lymphedema)? Call your Plan Administrator [insert phone number] for more information."

Part Eight

Additional Help
and Information

Chapter 61

Glossary of Breast and Cancer Terms

A

Abnormal: Not normal. May be cancerous or premalignant.

Adjuvant therapy: Treatment given after the primary treatment to make it work better. Adjuvant therapy may include chemotherapy, radiation therapy, or hormone therapy.

Alteration, altered: Change; different from original.

Anesthesia: Drugs or gases given before and during surgery so the patient won't feel pain. The patient may be awake or asleep.

Anesthesiologist: A doctor who gives drugs or gases that keep you comfortable during surgery.

Areola: The area of dark-colored skin on the breast that surrounds the nipple.

Aspirate: Fluid withdrawn from a lump, often a cyst.

Aspiration: Removal of fluid from a lump, often a cyst, with a needle and a syringe.

Atypical hyperplasia: A benign (noncancerous) condition in which cells have abnormal features and are increased in number.

Definitions provided in this glossary were compiled from National Institutes of Health (NIH) Pub. Nos. 98-1556, 98-4251, 00-1556, and 00-1566.

Autologous bone marrow transplantation: A procedure in which bone marrow is removed from a person, stored, and then given back to the person following intensive treatment.

Axilla: The underarm or armpit.

Axillary: Having to do with the armpit.

Axillary lymph node dissection: Surgery to remove lymph nodes found in the armpit region.

B

Benign: Not malignant; does not invade nearby tissue or spread to other parts of the body.

Biological therapy: Treatment that uses the body's immune system to fight cancer or to lessen the side effects that may be caused by some cancer treatments. Also known as immunotherapy.

Biopsy: A procedure used to remove cells or tissues in order to look at them under a microscope to check for signs of disease. When an entire tumor or lesion is removed, the procedure is called an excisional biopsy. When only a sample of tissue is removed, the procedure is called an incisional biopsy or core biopsy. When a sample of tissue or fluid is removed with a needle, the procedure is called a needle biopsy or fine-needle aspiration.

Bone marrow: The soft material inside bones. Blood cells are produced in the bone marrow.

Brachytherapy: A procedure in which radioactive material sealed in needles, seeds, wires, or catheters is placed directly into or near a tumor. Also called internal radiation, implant radiation, or interstitial radiation therapy.

Breast cancer in situ: Very early or noninvasive abnormal cells that are confined to the ducts or lobules in the breast. Also known as DCIS or LCIS.

Breast reconstruction: Surgery to rebuild a breast's shape after a mastectomy.

Breast-conserving surgery: An operation to remove the breast cancer but not the breast itself. Types of breast-conserving surgery include lumpectomy (removal of the lump), quadrantectomy (removal of one quarter of the breast), and segmental mastectomy (removal of the cancer as well as some of the breast tissue around the tumor and the lining over the chest muscles below the tumor).

C

Cancer: A term for diseases in which abnormal cells divide without control or order. Cancer cells can invade nearby tissues and can spread through the bloodstream and lymphatic systems to other parts of the body.

Carcinogen: Any substance that causes cancer.

Carcinoma: Cancer that begins in the lining or covering of an organ.

Cell: The smallest unit of tissues that make up any living thing. Cells have very specialized structure and function and are able to reproduce when needed.

Chemotherapy: Treatment with drugs to kill or slow the growth of cancer cells; also used to shrink tumors before surgery.

Clavicle: Collarbone.

Clear margins: An area of normal tissue that surrounds cancerous tissue, as seen during examination under a microscope.

Clinical trials: Research studies, where patients help scientist find the best way to prevent, detect, diagnose or treat diseases.

Colony-stimulating factors: Substances that stimulate the production of blood cells. Colony-stimulating factors include granulocyte colony-stimulating factors (also called G-CSF and filgrastim), granulocyte-macrophage colony-stimulating factors (also called GM-CSF and sargramostim), and promegapoietin.

Computed tomography: A series of detailed pictures of areas inside the body; the pictures are created by a computer linked to an x-ray machine. Also called computed tomography (CT) scan or computerized axial tomography (CAT) scan.

Cyst: A sac or capsule filled with fluid.

D

DCIS, ductal carcinoma in situ (intraductal carcinoma): Abnormal cells that involve only the lining of a milk duct.

Duct: A small channel in the breast through which milk passes from the lobes to the nipple.

Dysplasia: Cells that look abnormal under a microscope but are not cancer.

E

Erythrocytes: Red blood cells that carry oxygen from the lungs to cells in all parts of the body, and carry carbon dioxide from the cells back to the lungs.

Estrogen: A female hormone; one of the hormones that can help some breast cancer tumors grow.

Estrogen receptor test: Lab test to determine if breast cancer depends on estrogen for growth.

Excisional biopsy: A surgical procedure in which an entire lump or suspicious area is removed for diagnosis. The tissue is then examined under a microscope.

External radiation: Radiation therapy that uses a machine to aim high-energy rays at the cancer. Also called external-beam radiation.

F

Fertility: The ability to produce children.

Fine-needle aspiration: The removal of tissue or fluid with a needle for examination under a microscope. Also called needle biopsy.

G

Gene: The functional and physical unit of heredity passed from parent to offspring. Genes are pieces of DNA, and most genes contain the information for making a specific protein.

Gynecologist: A doctor who specializes in the care and treatment of women's reproductive systems.

H

Hormonal therapy: The use of hormones to treat cancer patients by removing, blocking, or adding to the effects of a hormone on an organ or part of the body.

Hormone receptor tests: Lab tests that determine if a breast cancer depends on female hormones (estrogen and progesterone) for growth.

Hormone replacement therapy (HRT): Hormones (estrogen, progesterone, or both) given to postmenopausal women or women who have had their ovaries surgically removed, to replace the estrogen no longer produced by the ovaries.

Hormones: Chemical substances in the body that affect the function of organs and tissues.

Hysterectomy: An operation in which the uterus is removed.

I

Immune system: The complex group of organs and cells that defends the body against infection or disease.

Immunotherapy: Treatment to stimulate or restore the ability of the immune system to fight infection and disease. Also used to lessen side effects that may be caused by some cancer treatments. Also called biological therapy or biological response modifier (BRM) therapy.

Implant: A silicone gel-filled or saline-filled sac inserted under the chest muscle to restore breast shape.

Incision: A cut made in the body during surgery.

Incisional biopsy: A surgical procedure in which a portion of a lump or suspicious area is removed for diagnosis. The tissue is then examined under a microscope.

Infertility: The inability to produce children.

Infiltrating breast cancer: Cancer that has spread to nearby tissue, lymph nodes under the arm, or other parts of the body. Also called invasive breast cancer.

Inflammatory breast cancer: A type of breast cancer in which the breast looks red and swollen, and feels warm. The skin of the breast may also show the pitted appearance called peau d'orange (like the skin of an orange). The redness and warmth occur because the cancer cells block the lymph vessels in the skin.

Internal radiation: A procedure in which radioactive material sealed in needles, seeds, wires, or catheters is placed directly into or near the tumor. Also called brachytherapy, implant radiation, or interstitial radiation therapy.

Intraductal carcinoma: Abnormal cells that are contained within the milk duct and have not spread outside the duct. Also known as DCIS (ductal carcinoma in situ).

Intravenous (IV): Injection into a vein.

Invasive cancer: Cancer that has spread beyond the layer of tissue in which it developed and is growing into surrounding, healthy tissues. Also called infiltrating cancer.

L

Leukocytes: White blood cells that defend the body against infections and other diseases.

Lobe, lobule: Located at the end of a breast duct, the part of the breast where milk is made. Each breast contains 15 to 20 sections, called lobes, each with many smaller lobules.

Lobular carcinoma in situ (LCIS): Abnormal cells found in the lobules of the breast. This condition seldom becomes invasive cancer; however, having lobular carcinoma in situ increases one's risk of developing breast cancer in either breast.

Local therapy: Treatment that affects cells in the tumor and the area close to it.

Lumpectomy: Surgery to remove the tumor and a small amount of normal tissue around it.

Lymph: The almost colorless fluid that travels through the lymphatic system and carries cells that help fight infection and disease.

Lymph nodes: Small bean-shaped organs (sometimes called lymph glands); part of the lymphatic system. Lymph nodes under the arm drain fluid from the chest and arm. During surgery, some underarm lymph nodes are removed to help determine the stage of breast cancer.

Lymphatic system: The system that removes wastes from body tissues and filters the fluids that help the body fight infection.

Lymphedema: Swelling in the arm caused by fluid that can build up when underarm lymph nodes are removed during breast cancer surgery or damaged by radiation.

M

Magnetic resonance imaging (MRI): A procedure in which a magnet linked to a computer is used to create detailed pictures of areas inside the body.

Malignant: Cancerous; capable of invading, spreading and destroying tissue.

Mammogram: An x-ray of the breast.

Mammography: The use of x-rays to create a picture of the breast.

Mastectomy: Surgery to remove the breast (or as much of the breast tissue as possible).

Medical oncologist: A doctor who specializes in diagnosing and treating cancer using chemotherapy, hormonal therapy, and biological therapy. A medical oncologist often serves as the main caretaker of someone who has cancer and coordinates treatment provided by other specialists.

Menopause: The time of life when a woman stops having monthly menstrual periods.

Metastasis or **metastatic:** Spread of cancer from the original part of the body to another. Cells that have metastasized are like those in the original (primary) tumor.

Microcalcifications: Tiny deposits of calcium that can be detected by mammography. A cluster of small specks of calcium may indicate that cancer is present.

Modified radical mastectomy: Surgical procedure in which the breast, some of the lymph nodes in the armpit, and the lining over the chest muscles are removed.

501

Monoclonal antibodies: Laboratory-produced substances that can locate and bind to cancer cells wherever they are in the body. Many monoclonal antibodies are used in cancer detection or therapy; each one recognizes a different protein on certain cancer cells. Monoclonal antibodies can be used alone, or they can be used to deliver drugs, toxins, or radioactive material directly to a tumor.

Mutation: Any change in the DNA of a cell. Mutations may be caused by mistakes during cell division, or they may be caused by exposure to DNA-damaging agents in the environment. Mutations can be harmful, beneficial, or have no effect. If they occur in cells that make eggs or sperm, they can be inherited; if mutations occur in other types of cells, they are not inherited. Certain mutations may lead to cancer or other diseases.

N

Negative: A lab test result that is normal; failing to show a positive result for the specific disease or condition for which the test is being done.

Neoadjuvant therapy: Treatment given before the primary treatment. Neoadjuvant therapy can be chemotherapy, radiation therapy, or hormone therapy.

Nipple discharge: Fluid coming from the nipple.

Nutritionist: A health professional with specialized training in nutrition, who can offer help and choices about the foods you eat.

O

Oncologist: Cancer specialist; a doctor who uses chemotherapy or hormonal therapy to treat cancer.

Oncology nurse: A nurse with special training in caring for cancer patients.

Oncology pharmacy specialist: A person who prepares anticancer drugs in consultation with an oncologist.

Ovaries: The pair of female reproductive organs that produce eggs and hormones.

P

Palpation: Examination by pressing on the surface of the body to feel the organs or tissues underneath.

Pathologist: A doctor who examines tissues and cells under a microscope to determine if they are normal or abnormal.

Pathology report: Diagnosis made by a pathologist based on microscopic evidence.

PDQ: National Cancer Institute's computer database that contains up-to-date cancer information for scientists, health professionals, patients, and the public.

Peripheral stem cell transplantation: A method of replacing blood-forming cells destroyed by cancer treatment. Immature blood cells (stem cells) in the circulating blood that are similar to those in the bone marrow are given to the person after treatment to help the bone marrow recover and continue producing healthy blood cells. Transplantation may be autologous (the person's blood cells saved earlier), allogeneic (blood cells donated by someone else), or syngeneic (blood cells donated by an identical twin). Also called peripheral stem cell support.

Physical therapist: A health professional who teaches exercises that help restore arm and shoulder movement and build back strength after breast cancer surgery.

Plastic surgeon: A surgeon who specializes in reducing scarring or disfigurement that may occur as a result of accidents, birth defects, or treatment for diseases.

Platelets: The part of a blood cell that helps prevent bleeding by causing blood clots to form at the site of an injury.

Positive: A lab test result that reveals the presence of a specific disease or condition for which the test is being done.

Positron emission tomography (PET) scan: A computerized image of the metabolic activity of body tissues used to determine the presence of disease.

Primary care doctor: A doctor who usually manages your health care and can discuss cancer treatment choices with you.

Progesterone: A female hormone; one of the hormones that can help some breast cancers grow.

Progesterone receptor test: Lab test to determine if a breast cancer depends on progesterone for growth.

Prognosis: The likely outcome or course of a disease; the chance of recovery.

Prosthesis: An artificial replacement of a part of the body. A breast prosthesis is a breast form that may be worn under clothing. Also, a technical name for an implant that is placed under the chest muscle in breast reconstruction.

Psychologist: A specialist who can talk with you and your family about emotional and personal matters, and can help you make decisions.

R

Radiation oncologist: A doctor who uses radiation therapy to treat cancer.

Radiation therapist: A health professional who gives radiation treatment.

Radiation therapy: The use of high-energy radiation from x-rays, neutrons, and other sources to kill cancer cells and shrink tumors. Radiation may come from a machine outside the body (external-beam radiation therapy) or from material called radioisotopes. Radioisotopes produce radiation and can be placed in or near a tumor or near cancer cells. This type of radiation treatment is called internal radiation therapy, implant radiation, or brachytherapy. Systemic radiation therapy uses a radioactive substance such as a radiolabeled monoclonal antibody that circulates throughout the body. Also called radiotherapy.

Radical mastectomy: Surgery for breast cancer in which the breast, chest muscles, and all of the lymph nodes under the arm are removed. For many years, this was the operation most used, but it is used now only when the tumor has spread to the chest muscles. Also called the Halsted radical mastectomy.

Radiologist: A doctor with special training in reading x-rays and performing specialized x-ray procedures.

Recur: To occur again. Recurrence is the return of cancer, at the same site as the original (primary) tumor or in another location, after the tumor had disappeared.

Remission: Disappearance of the signs and symptoms of cancer. When this happens, the disease is said to be "in remission." A remission may be temporary or permanent.

Risk factor: A habit, trait, condition, or genetic alteration that increases a person's chance of developing a disease.

S

Screening: Checking for disease when there are no symptoms.

Segmental mastectomy: The removal of the cancer as well as some of the breast tissue around the tumor and the lining over the chest muscles below the tumor. Usually some of the lymph nodes under the arm are also taken out. Sometimes called partial mastectomy.

Sentinel lymph node: The first lymph node(s) to which cancer cells spread after leaving the area of the primary tumor. Presence of cancer cells in this node alerts the doctor that the tumor has spread to the lymphatic system.

Side effects: Problems that occur when treatment affects healthy cells. Common side effects of cancer treatment are fatigue, nausea, vomiting, decreased blood cell counts, hair loss, and mouth sores.

Silicone: A synthetic gel that is used as an outer coating on breast implants and to make up the inside filling of some implants.

Social worker: A professional who can talk with you and your family about your emotional or physical needs and can help you find support services.

Stage or **staging:** Classification of breast cancer according to its size and extent of spread.

Standard: Usual, common, customary.

Stem cell: The immature cells in blood and bone marrow from which all mature blood cells develop.

Surgeon or **surgical oncologist:** A doctor who performs biopsies and other surgical procedures such as removing a lump or a breast.

Surgery: An operation; a procedure to remove or repair a part of the body or to find out whether disease is present.

Systemic: Affecting the entire body.

T

Therapy: Treatment.

Tissue: A group or layer of cells that together perform a specific function.

Tissue flap reconstruction: A flap of tissues is surgically relocated from another area of the body to the chest, and formed into a new breast mound.

Total mastectomy: Removal of the breast. Also called simple mastectomy.

Tumor: An abnormal growth of tissue. Tumors may be either benign (not cancer) or malignant (cancer).

U

Ultrasonography: A study in which sound waves (called ultrasound) are bounced off tissues and the echoes are converted into a picture (sonogram).

X

X-ray: A high-energy form of radiation; used in low doses for diagnosing diseases and in high doses to treat cancer.

Chapter 62

Directory of Organizations for Breast Cancer Patients

Breast Cancer Organizations and Internet Resources

American Society of Breast Disease
P.O. Box 140186
Dallas, TX 75214
Phone: 214-368-6836
Fax: 214-368-5719
Website: http://www.asbd.org
E-Mail: asbd1@aol.com

Breast Cancer Action
55 New Montgomery Street
Suite 323
San Francisco, CA 94105
Toll Free: 877-278-6722
Phone: 415-243-9301
Fax: 415-243-3996
Website: http://www.bcaction.org/home.html
E-Mail: info@bcaction.org

Information in this chapter was compiled from many sources deemed reliable; inclusion does not constitute endorsement. All contact information was verified in April 2001.

Breast Cancer Answers
University of Wisconsin Comprehensive Cancer Center
K4/658
600 Highland Avenue
Madison, WI 53792-0001
Phone: 608-263-8600
Fax: 608-263-8613
Website: http://www.medsch.wisc.edu/bca

Breast Cancer Awareness
U.S. Department of Defense TRICAR
Website: http://www.tricaresw.af.mil/breastcd/index.html

Breast Cancer and Environmental Risk Factors Program
Cornell University
112 Rice Hall
Ithaca, NY 14853-5601
Phone: 607-254-2893
Fax: 607-255-8207
E-mail: breastcancer@cornell.edu
Website: http://www.cfe.cornell.edu/bcerf

Breast Cancer Online
Website: http://www.bco.org

ENCOREPlus
YWCA of the USA
Office of Women's Health Advocacy
1015 18th Street, NW
Suite 700
Washington, DC 20036
Toll Free: 800-95E-PLUS (1-800-953-7587)
Phone: 202-467-0801
E-mail: cgould@ywca.org
Website: http://www.ywca.org

Inflammatory Breast Cancer Research Foundation
Toll Free: 877-Stop IBC (786-7422)
Website: http://www.ibcresearch.org/home

Komen Breast Cancer Foundation
5005 LBJ Freeway
Suite 370
Dallas, TX 75244
Toll Free: 1-800-IM-AWARE or 1-800-462-9273
Phone: 972-855-1600
Fax: 972-855-1605
Website: http://www.komen.org
E-Mail: helpline@komen.org

Kushner Breast Cancer Advisory Center
P.O. Box 224
Kensington, MD 20895
Phone: 301-897-3445
Fax: 301-897-3444

National Breast Cancer Coalition
1707 L Street NW, Suite 1060
Washington, DC 20036
Toll Free: 800-622-2838
Phone: 202-296-7477
Fax: 202-265-6854
Website: http://www.natlbcc.org
Website: http://www.stopbreastcancer.org

National Action Plan on Breast Cancer
U.S. Public Health Service's Office on Women's Health
U.S. Department of Health and Human Services
200 Independence Ave., S.W., Room 718F
Washington, D.C. 20201
Website: http://www.4woman.gov/napbc
E-Mail: napbcinfo@soza.com

National Alliance of Breast Cancer Organizations (NABCO)
9 E. 37th St., 10th Floor
New York, NY 10016
Toll Free: 1-888-806-2226
Phone: 212-889-0606
Website: http://www.nabco.org
E-Mail: nabcoinfo@aol.com

Sisters Network
8787 Woodway Drive
Suite 4206
Houston, TX 77063
Phone: 713-781-0255
Fax: 713-780-8998
Website: http://www.sistersnetworkinc.org

Y-ME National Breast Cancer Hotline
212 West Van Buren, 5th Floor
Chicago, IL 60607-3907
Toll Free: 1-800-221-2141 (English)
Toll Free: 800-986-9505 (Spanish)
Phone: 312-986-8338
E-mail: help@y-me.org
Website: http://www.y-me.org

National Cancer Organizations

American Association for Cancer Education
9500 Euclid Avenue
Cleveland, Ohio 44195
Phone: 216-444-9827
Fax: 216-444-8685
Website: http://www.aaceonline.com

American Association for Cancer Research
150 South Independence Mall W
Suite 826
Philadelphia, PA 19106
Phone: 215-440-9300
Fax: 215-440-9313
Website: http://www.aacr.org

American Cancer Society
1599 Clifton Road, N.E.
Atlanta, GA 30329-4251
Toll Free: 1-800-ACS-2345 (1-800-227-2345)
Website: http://www.cancer.org

American Institute for Cancer Research (AICR)
1759 R Street, NW.
Washington, DC 20009
Toll Free: 1-800-843-8114
Phone: 202-328-7744
E-mail: aicrweb@aicr.org
Website: http://www.aicr.org

Association of Community Cancer Centers
11600 Nebel Street, Suite 201
Rockville, MD 20852
Phone: 301-984-9496
Fax: 301-770-1949
Website: http://www.accc-cancer.org

R. A. Bloch Cancer Foundation, Inc.
4435 Main Street, Suite 500
Kansas City, MO 64111
Toll Free: 800-433-0464
Phone: 816-WE-BUILD (816-932-8453)
E-mail: hotline@hrbloch.com
Website: http://www.blochcancer.org

Cancer Care, Inc.
275 Seventh Avenue
New York, NY 10001
Toll Free: 1-800-813-HOPE (1-800-813-4673)
Phone: 212-302-2400
E-mail: info@cancercare.org
Website: http://www.cancercare.org

CancerFatigue
Website: http://www.cancerfatigue.org

Cancer Hope Network
Two North Road, Suite A
Chester, NJ 07930
Toll Free: 1-877-HOPENET (1-877-467-3638)
Phone: 908-879-4039
Fax: 908-879-6578
E-mail: info@cancerhopenetwork.org
Website: http://www.cancerhopenetwork.org

511

Cancer Research Foundation of America
1600 Duke Street, Suite 110
Alexandria, VA 22314
Toll Free: 1-800-227-2732
Phone: 703-836-4412
Fax: 703-836-4413
Website: http://www.preventcancer.org

Gilda's Club Worldwide
322 Eighth Avenue, 14th Floor
New York, NY 10001
Phone: 917-305-1200
Fax: 917-305-0549
Website: http://www.gildasclub.org

HOSPICELINK
Hospice Education Institute
190 Westbrook Road
Essex, CT 06426-1510
Toll Free: 800-331-1620
Phone: 860-767-1620
Fax: 860-767-2746
E-mail: HOSPICEALL@aol.com
Website: http://www.hospiceworld.org

Intercultural Cancer Council
PMB-C
1720 Dryden
Houston, TX 77030
Phone: 713-798-4617
Fax: 713-798-3990
http://icc.bcm.tmc.edu/home.htm
E-Mail: icc@bcm.tmc.edu

Karmanos Cancer Institute
4100 John R.
Detroit, MI 48201
Toll Free: 800-527-6266
Fax: 313-966-0722
Website: http://www.karmanos.org
E-Mail: info@karmanos.org

National Cancer Institute
31 Center Drive, MSC 2580
Bethesda, MD 20892-2580
Toll Free: 1-800-4-CANCER (1-800-422-6237)
Website: http://www.nci.nih.gov
CancerNet website: http://cancernet.nci.nih.gov
Cancer Trials website: http://cancertrials.nci.nih.gov

National Coalition for Cancer Survivorship (NCCS)
1010 Wayne Avenue, Suite 770
Silver Spring, MD 20910-5600
Toll Free: 877-NCCS-YES (877-622-7937)
Phone: 301-650-9127
Fax: 301-565-9670
E-mail: info@cansearch.org
Website: http://www.cansearch.org

National Foundation for Cancer Research
4600 East-West Highway, Suite 525
Bethesda, MD 20814
Toll Free: 800-321-2873
Phone: 301-654-1250
Fax: 301-654-5824
Website: http://www.nfcr.org

National Hospice and Palliative Care Organization (NHPCO)
1700 Diagonal Road, Suite 300
Alexandria, VA 22314
Toll Free: 800-658-8898 (Helpline)
Phone: 703-243-5900
Fax: 703-525-5762
E-mail: helpline@nhpco.org
Website: http://www.nhpco.org

National Marrow Donor Program
3001 Broadway Street, NE, Suite 500
Minneapolis, MN 55413
Toll Free: 800-MARROW-2 (1-800-627-7692)
Office of Patient Advocacy: 888-999-6743
Phone: 612-627-5800
Website: http://www.marrow.org

Patient Advocate Foundation (PAF)
753 Thimble Shoals Boulevard, Suite B
Newport News, VA 23606
Toll Free: 800-532-5274
Phone: 757-873-6668
Fax: 757-873-8999
E-mail: help@patientadvocate.org
Website: http://www.patientadvocate.org

The Wellness Community
35 East Seventh Street, Suite 412
Cincinnati, OH 45202
Toll Free: 888-793-WELL (888-793-9355)
Phone: 513-421-7111
Fax: 513-421-7119
E-mail: help@wellness-community.org
Website: http://www.wellness-community.org

Vital Options International and "The Group Room" Cancer Radio Talk Show
P.O. Box 19233
Encino, CA 91416-9233
Toll Free: 800-GRP-ROOM (800-477-7666)
Phone: 818-508-5657
Fax: 818-788-5260
E-mail: geninfo@vitaloptions.org
Website: http://www.vitaloptions.org

Chapter 63

Finding Cancer Support Groups

People with cancer and their families face many challenges that may leave them feeling overwhelmed, afraid, and alone. Sometimes it can be difficult to cope with these challenges or to talk to even the most supportive family and friends. However, members of the health care team and support groups can help the person feel less alone and can improve their ability to deal with the uncertainties and challenges cancer brings.

How can support groups help?

People with cancer sometimes find they need assistance coping with the emotional as well as the practical aspects of their disease. In fact, attention to the emotional burden of having cancer is sometimes part of a patient's treatment plan. Cancer support groups are designed to provide a confidential atmosphere where cancer patients or cancer survivors can discuss the challenges that accompany the illness with others who may be having similar experiences. For example, people gather to discuss the emotional needs created by cancer, to exchange information about their disease, including practical problems such as getting to and from treatment or managing side effects, and to share their feelings. Support groups have helped thousands of people cope with these and similar situations.

"Questions and Answers about Finding Cancer Support Groups," Cancer Facts, National Cancer Institute (NCI), March 1997. Contact information verified in March 2001.

Can family members and friends participate in support groups?

Family and friends are also affected when cancer touches someone they love. In addition to supporting the person with cancer, family members and friends may need help in dealing with stresses such as family disruptions, financial worries, and changing roles within the family. To help meet these needs, some support groups are designed just for family members of people with cancer; the groups encourage families and friends to participate with the patient.

How can people find support groups?

Many organizations offer support groups for individuals with cancer and family members or friends of those who are ill. The doctor, nurse, or hospital social worker will have information about support groups, such as their location, size, type, and how often they meet. Moreover, most hospitals have social services departments that provide information about cancer support programs. Many newspapers carry a special health supplement containing information about where to find support groups.

What types of support groups are available?

There are several kinds of support groups to meet individual needs. Support groups may be led by a professional, such as a psychiatrist, psychologist, or social worker, or by other patients. These groups may be for a particular disease, for teens or young adults, for family members, or for more general support. Many groups are free, but some require a fee (check to see if insurance will cover the cost). In addition, support groups can vary in approach, size, and how often they meet. It is important that individuals find an atmosphere that they are comfortable with and meets their individual needs.

Sources of Support

The following organizations help provide support for cancer patients through networking groups, support groups, and other resources.

American Cancer Society
1599 Clifton Road, NE
Atlanta, GA 30329-4251
Toll Free: 800-227-2345

Phone: 404-320-3333
Website: http://www.cancer.org

Cancer Care, Inc.
275 Seventh Avenue
New York, NY 10001
Toll Free: 800-813-4673
Phone: 212-302-2400
Fax: 212-719-0263
Website: http://www.cancercare.org
E-Mail: info@cancercare.org

Cancer Hope Network
2 North Road, Suite A
Chester, NJ 07930
Toll Free: 877-467-3638
Website: http://www.cancerhopenetwork.org
E-Mail: info@cancerhopenetwork.org

Gilda's Club Worldwide
322 Eighth Avenue, 14th Floor
New York, NY 10001
Phone: 917-305-1200
Fax: 917-305-0549
Website: http://www.gildasclub.org

National Coalition for Cancer Survivorship (NCCS)
1010 Wayne Avenue, Suite 707
Silver Spring, MD 20910-5600
Toll Free: 877-622-7937
Phone: 301-650-9127
Fax: 301-565-9670
Website: http://www.cansearch.org
E-Mail: info@cansearch.org

The Wellness Community
35 East Seventh Street, Suite 412
Cincinnato, OH 45202
Toll Free: 888-793-9355
Phone: 513-421-7111
Fax: 513-421-7119
Website: http://www.wellness-community.org
E-Mail: help@wellness-community.org

Chapter 64

Financial Assistance for Cancer Care

Cancer imposes heavy economic burdens on both patients and their families. For many people, a portion of medical expenses is paid by their health insurance plan. For individuals who do not have health insurance or who need financial assistance to cover health care costs, resources are available, including Government-sponsored programs and services supported by voluntary organizations.

Cancer patients and their families should discuss any concerns they may have about health care costs with their physician, medical social worker, or the business office of their hospital or clinic.

The organizations and resources listed below may offer financial assistance. Organizations that provide publications in Spanish or have Spanish-speaking staff have been identified.

The national **American Cancer Society (ACS)** office can provide the telephone number of the local ACS office serving your area. The local ACS office may offer reimbursement for expenses related to cancer treatment including transportation, medicine, and medical supplies. The ACS also offers programs that help cancer patients, family members, and friends cope with the emotional challenges they face. Some publications are available in Spanish. Spanish-speaking staff are available.

Telephone: 1-800-ACS-2345 (1-800-227-2345)

Web site: http://www.cancer.org

Cancer Facts, National Cancer Institute, September 2000.

519

The **AVONCares Program for Medically Underserved Women** provides financial assistance and relevant education and support to low income, under- and uninsured, underserved women throughout the country in need of diagnostic and/or related services (transportation, child care, and social support) for the treatment of breast, cervical, and ovarian cancers.

Telephone: 1-800-813-HOPE (1-800-813-4673)

Web site: http://www.cancercare.org

The **Candlelighters Childhood Cancer Foundation (CCCF)** is a nonprofit organization that provides information, peer support, and advocacy through publications, an information clearinghouse, and a network of local support groups. CCCF maintains a list of organizations to which eligible families may apply for financial assistance.

Telephone: 1-800-366-CCCF (1-800-366-2223)

Web site: http://www.candlelighters.org

Community voluntary agencies and service organizations such as the Salvation Army, Lutheran Social Services, Jewish Social Services, Catholic Charities, and the Lions Club may offer help. These organizations are listed in your local phone directory. Some churches and synagogues may provide financial help or services to their members.

Fundraising is another mechanism to consider. Some patients find that friends, family, and community members are willing to contribute financially if they are aware of a difficult situation. Contact your local library for information about how to organize fundraising efforts.

General Assistance programs provide food, housing, prescription drugs, and other medical expenses for those who are not eligible for other programs. Funds are often limited. Information can be obtained by contacting your state or local Department of Social Services; this number is found in the local telephone directory.

Hill-Burton is a program through which hospitals receive construction funds from the Federal Government. Hospitals that receive Hill-Burton funds are required by law to provide some services to people who cannot afford to pay for their hospitalization. A brochure about the program is available in Spanish.

Telephone: 1-800-638-0742

Web site: http://www.hrsa.dhhs.gov/osp/dfcr/obtain/consfaq.htm

Income Tax Deductions: Medical costs that are not covered by insurance policies sometimes can be deducted from annual income before taxes. Examples of tax deductible expenses might include mileage for trips to and from medical appointments, out-of-pocket costs for treatment, prescription drugs or equipment, and the cost of meals during lengthy medical visits. The local Internal Revenue Service office, tax consultants, or certified public accountants can determine medical costs that are tax deductible. These telephone numbers are available in the local telephone directory.
Web site: http://www.irs.ustreas.gov

The Leukemia and Lymphoma Society (LLS) offers information and financial aid to patients who have leukemia, non-Hodgkin's lymphoma, Hodgkin's disease, or multiple myeloma. Callers may request a booklet describing LLS's Patient Aid Program or the telephone number for their local LLS office. Some publications are available in Spanish.

Telephone: 1-800-955-4572

Web site: http://www.leukemia-lymphoma.org

Medicaid (Medical Assistance) a jointly funded, Federal-State health insurance program for people who need financial assistance for medical expenses, is coordinated by the **Health Care Financing Administration (HCFA)**. At a minimum, states must provide home care services to people who receive Federal income assistance such as Social Security Income and Aid to Families with Dependent Children. Medicaid coverage includes part-time nursing, home care aide services, and medical supplies and equipment. Information about coverage is available from local state welfare offices, state health departments, state social services agencies, or the state Medicaid office. Check the local telephone directory for the number to call. Information about specific state locations is also available on the HCFA Web site. Spanish-speaking staff are available in some offices.
Web site: http://www.hcfa.gov/medicaid/medicaid.htm

Medicare is a Federal health insurance program also administered by HCFA. Eligible individuals include those who are 65 or older, people of any age with permanent kidney failure, and disabled people under age 65. Medicare may offer reimbursement for some home care services. Cancer patients who qualify for Medicare may also be eligible for coverage of hospice services if they are accepted into a Medicare-certified hospice program. To receive information on eligibility, explanations of coverage, and related publications, call Medicare at the number listed below or visit their Web site. Some publications are available in Spanish.

Toll Free: 1-800-MEDICARE (1-800-633-4227)

TTY (for deaf and hard of hearing callers): 1-877-486-2048

Web site: http://www.medicare.gov

The Patient Advocate Foundation (PAF) is a national nonprofit organization that provides education, legal counseling, and referrals to cancer patients and survivors concerning managed care, insurance, financial issues, job discrimination, and debt crisis matters.

Telephone: 1-800-532-5274

Web site: http://www.patientadvocate.org

Patient Assistance Programs are offered by some pharmaceutical manufacturers to help pay for medications. To learn whether a specific drug might be available at reduced cost through such a program, talk with a physician or a medical social worker.

Social Security Administration (SSA) is the Government agency that oversees Social Security and Supplemental Security Income. A description of each of these programs follows. More information about these and other SSA programs is available by calling the toll-free number listed below. Spanish-speaking staff are available.

Telephone: 1-800-772-1213

TTY (for deaf and hard of hearing callers): 1-800-325-0778

> **Social Security** provides a monthly income for eligible elderly and disabled individuals. Information on eligibility, coverage, and how to apply for benefits is available from the Social Security Administration.
>
> Web site: http://www.ssa.gov/SSA_Home.html
>
> **Supplemental Security Income (SSI)** supplements Social Security payments for individuals who have certain income and resource levels. SSI is administered by the Social Security Administration. Information on eligibility, coverage, and how to file a claim is available from the Social Security Administration.
>
> Web site: http://www.ssa.gov/SSA_Home.html

The State Children's Health Insurance Program (SCHIP) is a Federal-State partnership that offers low-cost or free health insurance coverage to uninsured children of low-wage, working parents. Callers will be referred to the SCHIP program in their state for further information about what the program covers, who is eligible, and the minimum qualifications.

Telephone: 1-877-KIDS-NOW (1-877-543-7669)

Web site: http://www.insurekidsnow.gov

Transportation: There are nonprofit organizations that arrange free or reduced cost air transportation for cancer patients going to or from cancer treatment centers. Financial need is not always a requirement. To find out about these programs, talk with a medical social worker. Ground transportation services may be offered or mileage reimbursed through the local ACS or your state or local Department of Social Services.

Veterans Benefits: Eligible veterans and their dependents may receive cancer treatment at a Veterans Administration Medical Center. Treatment for service-connected conditions is provided, and treatment for other conditions may be available based on the veteran's financial need. Some publications are available in Spanish. Spanish-speaking staff are available in some offices.

Telephone: 1-800-827-1000

Web site: http://www.va.gov/vbs

Chapter 65

Additional Reading and Other Resources

Books

The following books, which are listed alphabetically by title, may be available at your local library or bookstore:

Title: *Be A Survivor: Your Guide to Breast Cancer Treatment*
Author: Vladimir Lange
Publisher: Lange Productions
Year: 1999
ISBN: 0966361008

Title: *Breast Cancer: The Complete Guide, 3rd edition*
Author: Yashar Hirshaut and Peter I. Pressman
Publisher: Bantam Books, Inc.
Year: 2000
ISBN: 0553380818

Title: *Breast Cancer Journey: Your Personal Guidebook*
Publisher: American Cancer Society, Inc.
Year: 2001
ISBN: 094423528X

Resources listed in this chapter were compiled from many sources deemed reliable; inclusion does not constitute endorsement.

Title: *The Breast Cancer Survival Manual, 2nd edition*
Author: John Link
Publisher: Owl Books
Year: 2000
ISBN: 0805064001

Title: *Dr. Susan Love's Breast Book, 3rd edition*
Author: Susan M. Love, Karen Lindsey, and Marcia Williams (Illustrator)
Publisher: Perseus Book Group
Year: 2000
ISBN: 0738202355

Title: *Helping Your Mate Face Breast Cancer, 3rd edition*
Author: Judy C. Kneece
Publisher: EduCare Publishing
Year: 1999
ISBN: 1886665117

Title: *The Informed Woman's Guide to Breast Health, 3rd edition*
Author: Kerry Anne McGinn
Publisher: Bull Publishing Co.
Year: 2001
ISBN: 0923521615

Title: *Just Get Me Through This!*
Author: Deborah A. Cohen and Robert M. Gelfand
Publisher: Kensington Publishing Corp.
Year: 2000
ISBN: 1575665514

Title: *Living Beyond Breast Cancer*
Author: Marisa C. Weiss and Ellen Weiss
Publisher: Times Books
Year: 1998
ISBN: 0812930665

Title: *Our Mom Has Cancer*
Author: Abigail and Adrienne Ackermann
Publisher: American Cancer Society
Year: 2001
ISBN: 094423531X

Title: *Your Breast Cancer Treatment Handbook, 3rd edition*
Author: Judy C. Kneece
Publisher: EduCare Publishing
Year: 1998
ISBN: 1886665109

Title: *Your Life in Your Hands*
Author: Jane A. Plant
Publisher: Thomas Dunne Books/St. Martin's Press
Year: 2001
ISBN: 0312275617

Brochures, Booklets, and Fact Sheets

The documents listed below represent a sampling of each organization's publications. Contact the producing organization for ordering or downloading information:

Agency on Healthcare Research and Quality (800-358-9295; www.ahrq.gov)

- Clinical Practice Guideline on Mammography

- Quick Reference Guide for Clinicians

- Quick Reference Guide for Women

American Psychological Association (800-374-2721; www.apa.org)

- Breast Cancer: How Your Mind Can Help Your Body

- Breast Cancer Patients Who Actively Express Their Emotions Do Better

- Coping with Serious Illness

- Getting Beyond "Why Me?"

Community Breast Health Project (650-326-6686; www.med. stanford.edu/cbhp)

- Depression and Breast Cancer

- Psychotherapy and Breast Cancer

- What Friends Can Do to Help and What Friends Should Avoid

Cornell University Program Breast Cancer and Environmental Risk Factors (607-254-2893; www.cfe.cornell.edu/bcerf)

- The Biology of Breast Cancer
- Meat, Poultry Fish and the Risk of Breast Cancer
- Phytoestrogens and the Risk of Breast Cancer

Susan G. Komen Breast Cancer Foundation (800-462-9273; www.breastcancerinfo.com)

- After Treatment: Living with Breast Cancer
- The Breast and Breast Cancer
- Risk Factors and Prevention

Mothers Supporting Daughters with Breast Cancer (410-778-1892; www.azstarnet.com/~pud/msdbc)

- Daughter's Brochure
- Mother's Handbook

National Action Plan on Breast Cancer (202-690-7650; www.4women.gov/napbc)

- Video: Genetic Testing for Breast Cancer Risk: It's Your Choice

National Breast Cancer Coalition (800-622-2838; www.natlbcc.org

- End the Breast Cancer Epidemic

National Coalition for Cancer Survivorship (301-650-8868; www.cansearch.org)

- Charting the Journey: An Almanac of Resources for Cancer Survivors
- Teamwork: The Cancer Patient's Guide to Talking with Your Doctor

National Institute of Environmental Health Sciences (919-541-3201; www.niehs.nih.gov)

Breast Cancer: Susceptibility and the Environment

National Institute for Occupational Safety and Health (NIOSH) (800-35-NIOSH; www.cdc.gov/niosh)

- Breast Cancer Research at NIOSH

U.S. Food and Drug Administration (888-463-6332; www.fda.gov/cdrh)

- Breast Implants: An Information Update
- Mammography Today

Y-Me National Breast Cancer Organization (800-221-2141; www.y-me.org)

- A Women's Guide to Breast Care
- For Single Women with Breast Cancer
- I Still Buy Green Bananas: Living with Hope
- Just for Teens
- When the Woman You Love Has Breast Cancer

National Cancer Institute

National Cancer Institute Information Resources

The following National Cancer Institute (NCI) services are available to help you.

- *Cancer Information Service (CIS):* Provides accurate, up-to-date information on cancer to patients and their families, health professionals, and the general public. Information specialists translate the latest scientific information into understandable language and respond in English, Spanish, or on TTY equipment.

  Toll-free: 1-800-4-CANCER (1-800-422-6237)

  TTY: 1-800-332-8615

- *Internet Resources:* These websites may be useful:

  http://www.nci.nih.gov —NCI's primary web site; contains information about the Institute and its programs.
  http://cancernet.nci.nih.gov —CancerNet; contains material for health professionals, patients, and the public, including information from PDQ about cancer treatment, screening,

prevention, genetics, supportive care, and clinical trials, and CANCERLIT, a bibliographic database.

http://cancertrials.nci.nih.gov —cancerTrials; NCI's comprehensive clinical trials information center for patients, health professionals, and the public. Includes information on understanding trials, deciding whether to participate in trials, finding specific trials, plus research news and other resources.

- *CancerMail:* Includes NCI information about cancer treatment, screening, prevention, genetics, and supportive care. To obtain a contents list, send e-mail to cancermail@icicc.nci.nih.gov with the word "help" in the body of the message.

- *CancerFax:* Includes NCI information about cancer treatment, screening, prevention, genetics, and supportive care. To obtain a contents list, dial 301-402-5874 or 1-800-624-2511 from a touch-tone telephone or fax machine hand set and follow the recorded instructions.

Reading Material Available from NCI

You may order printed copies of the following NCI booklets by calling 1-800-4-CANCER. Many are also available on the National Cancer Institute's Website (www.nci.nih.gov).

- Advanced Cancer

- Chemotherapy and You: A Guide to Self-Help During Treatment

- Eating Hints For Cancer Patients

- Facing Forward: A Guide for Cancer Survivors

- Genetic Testing for Breast Cancer Risk: It's Your Choice

- Get Relief From Cancer Pain

- Helping Yourself During Chemotherapy: 4 Steps for Patients

- Managing Cancer Pain

- Questions and Answers About Pain Control

- Radiation Therapy and You: A Guide to Self-Help During Treatment

- Taking Part in Clinical Trials: What Cancer Patients Need To Know

- Taking Time: Support for People With Cancer and the People Who Care for Them

- Understanding Breast Changes: A Health Guide for All Women

- Understanding Gene Testing

- What You Need To Know About Breast Cancer

- What You Need To Know About Cancer

- When Cancer Recurs: Meeting the Challenge Again

Spanish Publications Available from NCI

- El tratamiento de radioterapia: Guía para el paciente durante el tratamiento (Radiation Therapy: a Guide for Patients During Treatment)

- ¿En qué consisten los estudios clínicos? Un folleto para los pacientes de cáncer (What Are Clinical Trials All About? A Guide for Cancer Patients)

- Datos sobre el tratamiento de quimioterapia contra el cáncer (Facts About Chemotherapy)

PDQ

PDQ is a computer system that gives up-to-date information on cancer and its prevention, detection, treatment, and supportive care. It is a service of the National Cancer Institute (NCI) for people with cancer and their families and for doctors, nurses, and other health care professionals.

To ensure that it remains current, the information in PDQ is reviewed and updated each month by experts in the fields of cancer treatment, prevention, screening, and supportive care. PDQ also provides information about research on new treatments (clinical trials), doctors who treat cancer, and hospitals with cancer programs.

PDQ can be used to learn more about current treatment of different kinds of cancer. You may find it helpful to discuss this information with your doctor, who knows you and has the facts about your disease. PDQ can also provide the names of additional health care professionals who specialize in treating patients with cancer.

Before you start treatment, you also may want to think about taking part in a clinical trial. PDQ can be used to learn more about these trials. A clinical trial is a research study that attempts to improve current treatments or finds information on new treatments for patients with cancer. Clinical trials are based on past studies and information discovered in the laboratory. Each trial answers certain scientific questions in order to find new and better ways to help patients with cancer. Information is collected about new treatments, their risks, and how well they do or do not work. When clinical trials show that a new treatment is better than the treatment currently used as "standard" treatment, the new treatment may become the standard treatment. Listings of current clinical trials are available on PDQ. Many cancer doctors who take part in clinical trials are listed in PDQ.

To learn more about cancer and how it is treated, or to learn more about clinical trials for your kind of cancer, call the National Cancer Institute's Cancer Information Service. The number is 1-800-4-CANCER (1-800-422-6237); TTY at 1-800-332-8615. The call is free and a trained information specialist will be available to answer cancer-related questions.

Information from PDQ can also be accessed through the National Cancer Institute's CancerNet website at http://cancernet.nci.nih.gov.

PDQ is updated whenever there is new information. Check with the Cancer Information Service to be sure that you have the most up-to-date information.

American Cancer Society Supported Programs

Contact the American Cancer Society (800-227-2345; www.cancer. org) for more information about the following programs:

- *I Can Cope:* I Can Cope is a patient education program that is designed to help patients, families, and friends cope with the day-to-day issues of living with cancer.

- *Look Good. . .Feel Better:* This program was developed by the Cosmetic, Toiletry, and Fragrance Association Foundation in cooperation with ACS and the National Cosmetology Association. It focuses on techniques that can help people undergoing cancer treatment improve their appearance.

- *Reach to Recovery:* The Reach to Recovery Program is a rehabilitation program for women who have or have had breast cancer. The program helps breast cancer patients meet the physical, emotional, and cosmetic needs related to their disease and its treatment.

Information on the Internet

Breast Cancer Information on the Internet

Breast Cancer and Environmental Risk Factors Project
Website: http://www.cfe.cornell.edu/bcerf

This site provides fact sheets, critical evaluations, bibliographies, and a searchable database on breast cancer and environmental risk factors.

Breast Cancer Answers
Website: http://www.medsch.wisc.edu/bca

This is a service of the University of Wisconsin Comprehensive Cancer Center, providing accurate and up-to-date information from reliable sources on breast cancer prevention, detection, diagnosis, stage, and treatment.

Breast Cancer Awareness
Website: http://www.tricaresw.af.mil/breastcd/index.html

This interactive site from the U.S. Department of Defense TRICARE provides useful information on a broad range of issues concerning breast health.

Breast Cancer Online
Website: http://www.bco.org

Breast Cancer Online is an independent educational service and information source for professionals working in the field of breast cancer. It includes conference information and reports, news, links, case studies and questions for self-assessment.

Buddy Program for Breast Cancer Clinical Trials
Website: http://www.gis.net/~allisonm/buddies.html

This program links women who are eligible for a breast cancer clinical trial with a trained "buddy"—a woman who has been in a similar breast cancer clinical trial, and can tell about her experience.

Community Breast Health Project
Website: http://www-med.stanford.edu/CBHP

This site offers breast cancer information to patients and survivors of breast cancer. It includes practical advice and links to other Web sites that have breast cancer information.

ENCORE
Website: http://www.ywca.org

ENCORE is the YWCA's discussion and exercise program for women who have had breast cancer surgery. It is designed to help restore physical strength and emotional well-being. A local branch of the YWCA, listed in the telephone directory, can provide more information about ENCORE.

Inflammatory Breast Cancer Research Foundation
Website: http://www.ibcresearch.org

This Web site is dedicated to the advancement of research on inflammatory breast cancer.

The National Alliance of Breast Cancer Organizations (NABCO)
Website: http://www.nabco.org

NABCO is a coalition of more than 370 organizations that provide breast cancer detection, treatment, and care to thousands of women. This site provides information on clinical trials, a resource router to cancer information resources on the Internet, and links to local breast cancer support groups.

National Breast Cancer Coalition
Website: http://www.natlbcc.org

This organization focuses on three main goals in the fight against breast cancer: increasing cancer research, increasing access for all women to quality treatment and clinical trials, and increasing the influence of women living with breast cancer.

Susan G. Komen Breast Cancer Foundation
Website: http://www.breastcancerinfo.com

This Organization fights to eradicate breast cancer by funding national grants, education, and screening and treatment projects in communities throughout the U.S.

Y-ME National Breast Cancer Organization
Website: http://www.y-me.org

Y-ME National Breast Cancer Organization has a commitment to provide information and support to anyone who has been affected by breast cancer. This site includes general information about breast cancer and information on screening and detection; information for women and men who have breast cancer; and information for family members and loved ones. Some of this information is also presented in Spanish.

General Cancer Information on the Internet

American Association for Cancer Research (AACR)
Website: http://www.aacr.org

This site allows users to search for information in four AACR journals and in annual meeting abstracts.

American Cancer Society (ACS)
Website: http://www.cancer.org

This site provides information to patients on cancer treatment, early detection and prevention, as well as information on a variety of services available to cancer patients and their families.

American Society of Clinical Oncology (ASCO)
Website: http://www.asco.org

This site allows users to search the *Journal of Clinical Oncology* and the ASCO annual meeting abstracts.

Cancer 411
Website: http://www.cancer411.org

Cancer 411 is the website of the Rory Foundation whose mission is to help cancer patients and their families get information through chat shows, listings of clinical trials and cancer types, and other cancer information.

CancerEducation.com
Website: http://www.cancereducation.com

This website provides oncology professionals and their patients access to the latest advances in over 20 types of cancer, from prevention strategies and diagnostic procedures to new treatment options and advice on coping with cancer.

cancerfacts.com
Website: http://www.cancerfacts.com

The consumer portion of the site includes interactive tools that match an individual's medical history and test results with the medical literature and generate personalized reports of treatment options, side effects, and outcomes. In addition, the consumer portion includes e-mail discussion groups and a list of cancer support groups. The physician portion includes cancer literature, drug information, clinical trials, news, and online discussion forums.

CancerGuide: Steve Dunn's Cancer Information Page
Website: http://www.cancerguide.org

Maintained through the efforts of a cancer survivor, CancerGuide provides links to a variety of cancer information resources and offers helpful advice about using the information retrieved.

cancerpage.com
Website: http://www.cancerpage.com

This site has the latest news and general information, including stage specific treatment guidelines, support chat rooms, message boards and e-mail access to oncology nurses covering 46 cancer information areas.

Cancer News on the Net
Website: http://www.cancernews.com

This site features original articles about many types of cancer. Cancer News also links to sites that contain patient information on cancer.

CancerSource.com
Website: http://www.cancersource.com

CancerSource.com provides comprehensive, accurate and timely disease and treatment information in a personalized and tailored manner to consumers and health professionals with drug information, news, feature articles, community features, and relevant resources.

CancerTrack
Website: http://www.cancertrack.com

CancerTrack provides an excellent source of cancer news which is updated every 15 minutes. It provides information on books and links for all types of cancer.

Cansearch: A Guide to Cancer Resources on the Internet
Website: http://www.cansearch.org/canserch/canserch.htm

Cansearch is produced by the National Coalition for Cancer Survivorship (NCCS) to provide survivors and patients with a step-by-step guide to the many cancer resources found on the Web.

Centers for Disease Control and Prevention (CDC) National Program of Cancer Registries (NPCR)
Website: http://www.cdc.gov/nccdphp/dcpc/npcr/index.htm

Established by Congress in 1992, NPCR supports states and territories of the Untied States to initiate and improve cancer registries, and establish a computerized reporting and data-processing system.

Electronic Journal of Oncology
Website: http://ejo.univ-lyon1.fr

This exclusively on-line journal contains peer-reviewed original publications in the fields of oncology and hematology.

healthfinder
Website: http://www.healthfinder.gov

The U.S. Department of Health and Human Services' healthfinder® is a free gateway to reliable consumer health information. healthfinder links to online publications, clearinghouses, databases, websites, and support and self-help groups, as well as to government agencies and not-for-profit organizations that produce reliable information for the public.

MEDLINEplus
Website: http://www.nlm.nih.gov/medlineplus/cancers.html

This Web site provides information on many cancer topics by providing information and medical literature from the National Library of Medicine and multiple links to other Web sites.

National Cancer Institute (NCI) Publications Locator
Website: http://cancer.gov/publications

This site accesses National Cancer Institute publications. It allows Web users to order printed materials to be mailed to them, and also links NCI materials that may be viewed and downloaded from the Web.

National Foundation for Cancer Research (NFCR)
Website: http://www.nfcr.org

NFCR's website is devoted to providing information about prevention, detection, and treatment of cancers, as well as up-to-date content in the fields of research for a cancer cure.

Oncology.com
Website: http://www.oncology.com

Oncology.com offers information to cancer patients, families and health care professionals. It includes disease summaries, news stories, events and discussions on most major cancers.

OncoLink
Website: http://oncolink.upenn.edu

Sponsored by the University of Pennsylvania, OncoLink offers a comprehensive, well-organized source of cancer information for patients and health care professionals.

Surveillance, Epidemiology and End Results (SEER)
http://www-seer.ims.nci.nih.gov

The SEER program of the National Cancer Institute collects and publishes cancer incidence and survival data from population-based cancer registries that include approximately 14 percent of the U.S. population.

Sustaining Oncology Studies (SOS) Europe
Website: http://sos.unige.it/soseuro.html

This Web site contains information on support, training and research in cancer and includes links to international meetings, cancer-related publications, and international associations.

TeleSCAN Telematics Services in Cancer (European)
Website: http://telescan.nki.nl

This site contains European cancer research information for patients, health care professionals, and researchers.

Index

Index

Page numbers followed by 'n' indicate a footnote. Page numbers in *italics* indicate a table or illustration.

A

541

alkaloids 357

alteration, defined 495

alternative medicine, breast cancer treatment 339–40

American Academy of Pediatrics, breastfeeding recommendations 38

American Academy of Radiology 227

American Association for Cancer Education, contact information 510

American Association for Cancer Research (AACR)
contact information 510
web site 535

American Board of Medical Specialists (ABMS) 63

American Cancer Society (ACS)
cancer programs 532
contact information 229, 256, 510, 516–17
financial assistance 519
web site 535

American College of Surgeons (ACOS) 443

American College of Surgeons-Oncology Group (ACOS-OG) 437, 441–42, 535

American Institute for Cancer Research (AICR), contact information 511

American Psychological Association (APA), publications 469n, 471n, 527

American Registry of Radiological Technologists 12

American Society of Breast Disease, contact information 507

American Society of Clinical Oncology (ASCO), web site 535

aminoglutethimide, male breast cancer treatment 98

anesthesia, defined 495

anesthesiologist
defined 495
described 267

angiogenesis inhibitors 254

antineoplastons 362–63

antioxidants 353

antiperspirants, breast cancer risk 189–90

APA *see* American Psychological Association

areola, defined 16, 495

ASCO *see* American Society of Clinical Oncology

aspirate, defined 495

aspiration, defined 495
see also fine-needle aspiration

Association of Community Cancer Centers, contact information 511

AstraZeneca Pharmaceuticals 252, 337, 423, 424, 427

Atkinson, Holly 233

atypia 20, 85

atypical hyperplasia
breast cancer risk 20, 57
defined 495
see also hyperplasia

autologous bone marrow transplantation, defined 496

AVONCares Program for Medically Underserved Women, contact information 520

axilla
defined 496
lymph nodes 56

axillary, defined 496

axillary lymph node dissection
clinical trials 437, 442–43
defined 496
described 64

B

Bailey-Wilson, Joan 453

Baker grading, described 306–7

Barkardottir, Rosa Bjork 453

Bassett, Lawrence W. 375

BCPT *see* Breast Cancer Prevention Trial

Beam, Craig 373

Be a Survivor: Your Guide to Breast Cancer Treatment (Lange) 525

benign, defined 401, 496

benign breast disease 17

benign tumors 56, 85

bias, defined 387, 401

biological therapy
breast cancer treatment 68, 284
defined 269, 496

immuno-augmentative therapy 364–65

"Immuno-Augmentive Therapy" (NCI) 364

immunotherapy
    defined 269, 499
    described 284
    see also biological therapy

implant, defined 499

implant radiation 496
    see also internal radiation

"Improving Imaging Methods for Breast Cancer Detection and Diagnosis" (NCI) 237n

incidence, defined 205

incision, defined 499

incisional biopsy
    defined 499
    described 22, 496
    see also biopsy

infection
    breast implants 304, 310–11
    chemotherapy 279–80

infertility, defined 499

infiltrating breast cancer, defined 499

inflammatory breast cancer
    defined 71, 500
    described 93–94
    men 95

Inflammatory Breast Cancer Research Foundation, contact information 508

informed consent, defined 110, 387, 395–96, 402

The Informed Woman's Guide to Breast Health (McGinn) 526

in situ carcinoma 85

Institute for Comparative and Environmental Toxicology *see* Cornell University: Center for the Environment

institutional review board (IRB)
    clinical trials 380
    defined 387, 402–3

insulin-dependent growth factor-1 (IGF-1) 164–65

insurance coverage, cancer 487–92

integrative medicine, described 344

Intercultural Cancer Council, contact information 512

internal radiation
    defined 500
    see also brachytherapy

Internal Revenue Service, financial assistance 521

International Union Against Cancer (UICC) 190

Internet information *see* web sites

interstitial radiation therapy 496
    see also internal radiation

intervention group, defined 403

intraductal carcinoma
    defined 498, 500
    men 95

intraductal papilloma 19, 20

intravenous (IV), defined 500

invasive cancer
    defined 500
    diagnosis 62
    see also breast cancer; infiltrating breast cancer

investigator, defined 387, 403

IRB *see* institutional review board

Ircink, Mary 475n, 486

Iscador 357

isoflavones 146

Isorel 357

J

Jibaja, Mari 372

Jim's Juice *see* Cancell

Journal of Clinical Oncology 535

Journal of the National Cancer Institute 182

JS-101 *see* Cancell

JS-114 *see* Cancell

K

Kainu, Tommi 454

Kallioniemi, Olli 452, 454

Karmanos Cancer Institute, contact information 512

"Keep in Touch: Do BSE" 43n

Y

Yee-Tak Cheng, Elaine 158
Y-ME National Breast Cancer
  Hotline
    contact information 256, 510
    publications 529
    web site 534
Your Breast Cancer Treatment Handbook (Kneece) 527

Z

Zeneca Pharmaceuticals *see*
  AstraZeneca Pharmaceuticals
zeranol 161–63
Zujewski, JoAnne 336–37

Health Reference Series
COMPLETE CATALOG

AIDS Sourcebook, 1st Edition

Basic Information about AIDS and HIV Infection, Featuring Historical and Statistical Data, Current Research, Prevention, and Other Special Topics of Interest for Persons Living with AIDS

Along with Source Listings for Further Assistance

Edited by Karen Bellenir and Peter D. Dresser. 831 pages. 1995. 0-7808-0031-1. $78.

"One strength of this book is its practical emphasis. The intended audience is the lay reader . . . useful as an educational tool for health care providers who work with AIDS patients. Recommended for public libraries as well as hospital or academic libraries that collect consumer materials."
— *Bulletin of the Medical Library Association, Jan '96*

"This is the most comprehensive volume of its kind on an important medical topic. Highly recommended for all libraries."
— *Reference Book Review, '96*

"Very useful reference for all libraries."
— *Choice, Association of College and Research Libraries, Oct '95*

"There is a wealth of information here that can provide much educational assistance. It is a must book for all libraries and should be on the desk of each and every congressional leader. Highly recommended."
— *AIDS Book Review Journal, Aug '95*

"Recommended for most collections."
— *Library Journal, Jul '95*

■

AIDS Sourcebook, 2nd Edition

Basic Consumer Health Information about Acquired Immune Deficiency Syndrome (AIDS) and Human Immunodeficiency Virus (HIV) Infection, Featuring Updated Statistical Data, Reports on Recent Research and Prevention Initiatives, and Other Special Topics of Interest for Persons Living with AIDS, Including New Antiretroviral Treatment Options, Strategies for Combating Opportunistic Infections, Information about Clinical Trials, and More

Along with a Glossary of Important Terms and Resource Listings for Further Help and Information

Edited by Karen Bellenir. 751 pages. 1999. 0-7808-0225-X. $78.

"Highly recommended."
— *American Reference Books Annual, 2000*

"Excellent sourcebook. This continues to be a highly recommended book. There is no other book that provides as much information as this book provides."
— *AIDS Book Review Journal, Dec-Jan 2000*

"Recommended reference source."
— *Booklist, American Library Association, Dec '99*

"A solid text for college-level health libraries."
— *The Bookwatch, Aug '99*

Cited in *Reference Sources for Small and Medium-Sized Libraries, American Library Association, 1999*

■

Alcoholism Sourcebook

Basic Consumer Health Information about the Physical and Mental Consequences of Alcohol Abuse, Including Liver Disease, Pancreatitis, Wernicke-Korsakoff Syndrome (Alcoholic Dementia), Fetal Alcohol Syndrome, Heart Disease, Kidney Disorders, Gastrointestinal Problems, and Immune System Compromise and Featuring Facts about Addiction, Detoxification, Alcohol Withdrawal, Recovery, and the Maintenance of Sobriety

Along with a Glossary and Directories of Resources for Further Help and Information

Edited by Karen Bellenir. 613 pages. 2000. 0-7808-0325-6. $78.

"This title is one of the few reference works on alcoholism for general readers. For some readers this will be a welcome complement to the many self-help books on the market. Recommended for collections serving general readers and consumer health collections."
— *E-Streams, Mar '01*

"This book is an excellent choice for public and academic libraries."
— *American Reference Books Annual, 2001*

"Recommended reference source."
— *Booklist, American Library Association, Dec '00*

"Presents a wealth of information on alcohol use and abuse and its effects on the body and mind, treatment, and prevention."
— *SciTech Book News, Dec '00*

"Important new health guide which packs in the latest consumer information about the problems of alcoholism."
— *Reviewer's Bookwatch, Nov '00*

SEE ALSO *Drug Abuse Sourcebook, Substance Abuse Sourcebook*

■

Allergies Sourcebook, 1st Edition

Basic Information about Major Forms and Mechanisms of Common Allergic Reactions, Sensitivities, and Intolerances, Including Anaphylaxis, Asthma, Hives and Other Dermatologic Symptoms, Rhinitis, and Sinusitis

Along with Their Usual Triggers Like Animal Fur, Chemicals, Drugs, Dust, Foods, Insects, Latex, Pollen, and Poison Ivy, Oak, and Sumac; Plus Information on Prevention, Identification, and Treatment

Edited by Allan R. Cook. 611 pages. 1997. 0-7808-0036-2. $78.

Allergies Sourcebook, 2nd Edition

Basic Consumer Health Information about Allergic Disorders, Triggers, Reactions, and Related Symptoms, Including Anaphylaxis, Rhinitis, Sinusitis, Asthma, Dermatitis, Conjunctivitis, and Multiple Chemical Sensitivity

Along with Tips on Diagnosis, Prevention, and Treatment, Statistical Data, a Glossary, and a Directory of Sources for Further Help and Information

Edited by Annemarie S. Muth. 600 pages. 2001. 0-7808-0376-0. $78.

■

Alternative Medicine Sourcebook

Basic Consumer Health Information about Alternatives to Conventional Medicine, Including Acupressure, Acupuncture, Aromatherapy, Ayurveda, Bioelectromagnetics, Environmental Medicine, Essence Therapy, Food and Nutrition Therapy, Herbal Therapy, Homeopathy, Imaging, Massage, Naturopathy, Reflexology, Relaxation and Meditation, Sound Therapy, Vitamin and Mineral Therapy, and Yoga, and More

Edited by Allan R. Cook. 737 pages. 1999. 0-7808-0200-4. $78.

"Recommended reference source."
—Booklist, American Library Association, Feb '00

"A great addition to the reference collection of every type of library." *—American Reference Books Annual, 2000*

■

Alzheimer's, Stroke & 29 Other Neurological Disorders Sourcebook, 1st Edition

.Basic Information for the Layperson on 31 Diseases or Disorders Affecting the Brain and Nervous System, First Describing the Illness, Then Listing Symptoms, Diagnostic Methods, and Treatment Options, and Including Statistics on Incidences and Causes

Edited by Frank E. Bair. 579 pages. 1993. 1-55888-748-2. $78.

"Nontechnical reference book that provides reader-friendly information."
—Family Caregiver Alliance Update, Winter '96

"Should be included in any library's patient education section." *—American Reference Books Annual, 1994*

"Written in an approachable and accessible style. Recommended for patient education and consumer health collections in health science center and public libraries." *—Academic Library Book Review, Dec '93*

"It is very handy to have information on more than thirty neurological disorders under one cover, and there is no recent source like it." *—Reference Quarterly, American Library Association, Fall '93*

SEE ALSO *Brain Disorders Sourcebook*

Alzheimer's Disease Sourcebook, 2nd Edition

Basic Consumer Health Information about Alzheimer's Disease, Related Disorders, and Other Dementias, Including Multi-Infarct Dementia, AIDS-Related Dementia, Alcoholic Dementia, Huntington's Disease, Delirium, and Confusional States

Along with Reports Detailing Current Research Efforts in Prevention and Treatment, Long-Term Care Issues, and Listings of Sources for Additional Help and Information

Edited by Karen Bellenir. 524 pages. 1999. 0-7808-0223-3. $78.

"Provides a wealth of useful information not otherwise available in one place. This resource is recommended for all types of libraries."
—American Reference Books Annual, 2000

"Recommended reference source."
—Booklist, American Library Association, Oct '99

■

Arthritis Sourcebook

Basic Consumer Health Information about Specific Forms of Arthritis and Related Disorders, Including Rheumatoid Arthritis, Osteoarthritis, Gout, Polymyalgia Rheumatica, Psoriatic Arthritis, Spondyloarthropathies, Juvenile Rheumatoid Arthritis, and Juvenile Ankylosing Spondylitis

Along with Information about Medical, Surgical, and Alternative Treatment Options, and Including Strategies for Coping with Pain, Fatigue, and Stress

Edited by Allan R. Cook. 550 pages. 1998. 0-7808-0201-2. $78.

". . . accessible to the layperson."
—Reference and Research Book News, Feb '99

■

Asthma Sourcebook

Basic Consumer Health Information about Asthma, Including Symptoms, Traditional and Nontraditional Remedies, Treatment Advances, Quality-of-Life Aids, Medical Research Updates, and the Role of Allergies, Exercise, Age, the Environment, and Genetics in the Development of Asthma

Along with Statistical Data, a Glossary, and Directories of Support Groups, and Other Resources for Further Information

Edited by Annemarie S. Muth. 628 pages. 2000. 0-7808-0381-7. $78.

"A worthwhile reference acquisition for public libraries and academic medical libraries whose readers desire a quick introduction to the wide range of asthma information." *—Choice, Association of College and Research Libraries, Jun '01*

"Recommended reference source."
—Booklist, American Library Association, Feb '01

Back & Neck Disorders Sourcebook

Basic Information about Disorders and Injuries of the Spinal Cord and Vertebrae, Including Facts on Chiropractic Treatment, Surgical Interventions, Paralysis, and Rehabilitation

Along with Advice for Preventing Back Trouble

Edited by Karen Bellenir. 548 pages. 1997. 0-7808-0202-0. $78.

Blood & Circulatory Disorders Sourcebook

Basic Information about Blood and Its Components, Anemias, Leukemias, Bleeding Disorders, and Circulatory Disorders, Including Aplastic Anemia, Thalassemia, Sickle-Cell Disease, Hemochromatosis, Hemophilia, Von Willebrand Disease, and Vascular Diseases

Along with a Special Section on Blood Transfusions and Blood Supply Safety, a Glossary, and Source Listings for Further Help and Information

Edited by Karen Bellenir and Linda M. Shin. 554 pages. 1998. 0-7808-0203-9. $78.

Brain Disorders Sourcebook

Basic Consumer Health Information about Strokes, Epilepsy, Amyotrophic Lateral Sclerosis (ALS/Lou Gehrig's Disease), Parkinson's Disease, Brain Tumors, Cerebral Palsy, Headache, Tourette Syndrome, and More

Along with Statistical Data, Treatment and Rehabilitation Options, Coping Strategies, Reports on Current Research Initiatives, a Glossary, and Resource Listings for Additional Help and Information

Edited by Karen Bellenir. 481 pages. 1999. 0-7808-0229-2. $78.

SEE ALSO *Alzheimer's, Stroke & 29 Other Neurological Disorders Sourcebook, 1st Edition*

Breast Cancer Sourcebook

Basic Consumer Health Information about Breast Cancer, Including Diagnostic Methods, Treatment Options, Alternative Therapies, Self-Help Information, Related Health Concerns, Statistical and Demographic Data, and Facts for Men with Breast Cancer

Along with Reports on Current Research Initiatives, a Glossary of Related Medical Terms, and a Directory of Sources for Further Help and Information

Edited by Edward J. Prucha and Karen Bellenir. 580 pages. 2001. 0-7808-0244-6. $78.

SEE ALSO *Cancer Sourcebook for Women, 1st and 2nd Editions, Women's Health Concerns Sourcebook*

Breastfeeding Sourcebook

Basic Consumer Health Information about the Benefits of Breastmilk, Preparing to Breastfeed, Breastfeeding as a Baby Grows, Nutrition, and More, Including Information on Special Situations and Concerns, Such as Mastitis, Illness, Medications, Allergies, Multiple Births, Prematurity, Special Needs, and Adoption

Along with a Glossary and Resources for Additional Help and Information

Edited by Jenni Lynn Colson. 350 pages. 2001. 0-7808-0332-9. $48.

SEE ALSO *Pregnancy & Birth Sourcebook*

Burns Sourcebook

Basic Consumer Health Information about Various Types of Burns and Scalds, Including Flame, Heat, Cold, Electrical, Chemical, and Sun Burns

Along with Information on Short-Term and Long-Term Treatments, Tissue Reconstruction, Plastic Surgery, Prevention Suggestions, and First Aid

Edited by Allan R. Cook. 604 pages. 1999. 0-7808-0204-7. $78.

"This is an exceptional addition to the series and is highly recommended for all consumer health collections, hospital libraries, and academic medical centers." — *E-Streams, Mar '00*

"Recommended reference source."
— *Booklist, American Library Association, Dec '99*

SEE ALSO *Skin Disorders Sourcebook*

■

Cancer Sourcebook, 1st Edition

Basic Information on Cancer Types, Symptoms, Diagnostic Methods, and Treatments, Including Statistics on Cancer Occurrences Worldwide and the Risks Associated with Known Carcinogens and Activities

Edited by Frank E. Bair. 932 pages. 1990. 1-55888-888-8. $78.

Cited in *Reference Sources for Small and Medium-Sized Libraries, American Library Association, 1999*

"Written in nontechnical language. Useful for patients, their families, medical professionals, and librarians."
— *Guide to Reference Books, 1996*

"Designed with the non-medical professional in mind. Libraries and medical facilities interested in patient education should certainly consider adding the *Cancer Sourcebook* to their holdings. This compact collection of reliable information . . . is an invaluable tool for helping patients and patients' families and friends to take the first steps in coping with the many difficulties of cancer."
— *Medical Reference Services Quarterly, Winter '91*

"Specifically created for the nontechnical reader . . . an important resource for the general reader trying to understand the complexities of cancer."
— *American Reference Books Annual, 1991*

"This publication's nontechnical nature and very comprehensive format make it useful for both the general public and undergraduate students."
— *Choice, Association of College and Research Libraries, Oct '90*

■

New Cancer Sourcebook, 2nd Edition

Basic Information about Major Forms and Stages of Cancer, Featuring Facts about Primary and Secondary Tumors of the Respiratory, Nervous, Lymphatic, Circulatory, Skeletal, and Gastrointestinal Systems, and Specific Organs; Statistical and Demographic Data; Treatment Options; and Strategies for Coping

Edited by Allan R. Cook. 1,313 pages. 1996. 0-7808-0041-9. $78.

"An excellent resource for patients with newly diagnosed cancer and their families. The dialogue is simple, direct, and comprehensive. Highly recommended for patients and families to aid in their understanding of cancer and its treatment."
— *Booklist Health Sciences Supplement, American Library Association, Oct '97*

"The amount of factual and useful information is extensive. The writing is very clear, geared to general readers. Recommended for all levels."
— *Choice, Association of College and Research Libraries, Jan '97*

■

Cancer Sourcebook, 3rd Edition

Basic Consumer Health Information about Major Forms and Stages of Cancer, Featuring Facts about Primary and Secondary Tumors of the Respiratory, Nervous, Lymphatic, Circulatory, Skeletal, and Gastrointestinal Systems, and Specific Organs

Along with Statistical and Demographic Data, Treatment Options, Strategies for Coping, a Glossary, and a Directory of Sources for Additional Help and Information

Edited by Edward J. Prucha. 1,069 pages. 2000. 0-7808-0227-6. $78.

"This title is recommended for health sciences and public libraries with consumer health collections."
— *E-Streams, Feb '01*

". . . can be effectively used by cancer patients and their families who are looking for answers in a language they can understand. Public and hospital libraries should have it on their shelves."
— *American Reference Books Annual, 2001*

"Recommended reference source."
— *Booklist, American Library Association, Dec '00*

■

Cancer Sourcebook for Women, 1st Edition

Basic Information about Specific Forms of Cancer That Affect Women, Featuring Facts about Breast Cancer, Cervical Cancer, Ovarian Cancer, Cancer of the Uterus and Uterine Sarcoma, Cancer of the Vagina, and Cancer of the Vulva; Statistical and Demographic Data; Treatments, Self-Help Management Suggestions, and Current Research Initiatives

Edited by Allan R. Cook and Peter D. Dresser. 524 pages. 1996. 0-7808-0076-1. $78.

". . . written in easily understandable, non-technical language. Recommended for public libraries or hospital and academic libraries that collect patient education or consumer health materials."
— *Medical Reference Services Quarterly, Spring '97*

"Would be of value in a consumer health library. . . . written with the health care consumer in mind. Medical jargon is at a minimum, and medical terms are explained in clear, understandable sentences."
— *Bulletin of the Medical Library Association, Oct '96*

"The availability under one cover of all these pertinent publications, grouped under cohesive headings, makes this certainly a most useful sourcebook."
— *Choice, Association of College and Research Libraries, Jun '96*

"Presents a comprehensive knowledge base for general readers. Men and women both benefit from the gold mine of information nestled between the two covers of this book. Recommended."
—*Academic Library Book Review, Summer '96*

"This timely book is highly recommended for consumer health and patient education collections in all libraries." — *Library Journal, Apr '96*

SEE ALSO *Breast Cancer Sourcebook, Women's Health Concerns Sourcebook*

■

Cancer Sourcebook for Women, 2nd Edition

Basic Consumer Health Information about Specific Forms of Cancer That Affect Women, Including Cervical Cancer, Ovarian Cancer, Endometrial Cancer, Uterine Sarcoma, Vaginal Cancer, Vulvar Cancer, and Gestational Trophoblastic Tumor; and Featuring Statistical Information, Facts about Tests and Treatments, a Glossary of Cancer Terms, and an Extensive List of Additional Resources

Edited by Karen Bellenir. 600 pages. 2001. 0-7808-0226-8. $78.

SEE ALSO *Breast Cancer Sourcebook, Women's Health Concerns Sourcebook*

■

Cardiovascular Diseases & Disorders Sourcebook, 1st Edition

Basic Information about Cardiovascular Diseases and Disorders, Featuring Facts about the Cardiovascular System, Demographic and Statistical Data, Descriptions of Pharmacological and Surgical Interventions, Lifestyle Modifications, and a Special Section Focusing on Heart Disorders in Children

Edited by Karen Bellenir and Peter D. Dresser. 683 pages. 1995. 0-7808-0032-X. $78.

". . . comprehensive format provides an extensive overview on this subject."
—*Choice, Association of College and Research Libraries, Jun '96*

". . . an easily understood, complete, up-to-date resource. This well executed public health tool will make valuable information available to those that need it most, patients and their families. The typeface, sturdy non-reflective paper, and library binding add a feel of quality found wanting in other publications. Highly recommended for academic and general libraries. "
—*Academic Library Book Review, Summer '96*

SEE ALSO *Healthy Heart Sourcebook for Women, Heart Diseases & Disorders Sourcebook, 2nd Edition*

Caregiving Sourcebook

Basic Consumer Health Information for Caregivers, Including a Profile of Caregivers, Caregiving Responsibilities and Concerns, Tips for Specific Conditions, Care Environments, and the Effects of Caregiving

Along with Facts about Legal Issues, Financial Information, and Future Planning, a Glossary, and a Listing of Additional Resources

Edited by Joyce Brennfleck Shannon. 600 pages. 2001. 0-7808-0331-0. $78.

■

Colds, Flu & Other Common Ailments Sourcebook

Basic Consumer Health Information about Common Ailments and Injuries, Including Colds, Coughs, the Flu, Sinus Problems, Headaches, Fever, Nausea and Vomiting, Menstrual Cramps, Diarrhea, Constipation, Hemorrhoids, Back Pain, Dandruff, Dry and Itchy Skin, Cuts, Scrapes, Sprains, Bruises, and More

Along with Information about Prevention, Self-Care, Choosing a Doctor, Over-the-Counter Medications, Folk Remedies, and Alternative Therapies, and Including a Glossary of Important Terms and a Directory of Resources for Further Help and Information

Edited by Chad T. Kimball. 638 pages. 2001. 0-7808-0435-X. $78.

■

Communication Disorders Sourcebook

Basic Information about Deafness and Hearing Loss, Speech and Language Disorders, Voice Disorders, Balance and Vestibular Disorders, and Disorders of Smell, Taste, and Touch

Edited by Linda M. Ross. 533 pages. 1996. 0-7808-0077-X. $78.

"This is skillfully edited and is a welcome resource for the layperson. It should be found in every public and medical library." — *Booklist Health Sciences Supplement, American Library Association, Oct '97*

■

Congenital Disorders Sourcebook

Basic Information about Disorders Acquired during Gestation, Including Spina Bifida, Hydrocephalus, Cerebral Palsy, Heart Defects, Craniofacial Abnormalities, Fetal Alcohol Syndrome, and More

Along with Current Treatment Options and Statistical Data

Edited by Karen Bellenir. 607 pages. 1997. 0-7808-0205-5. $78.

"Recommended reference source."
— *Booklist, American Library Association, Oct '97*

SEE ALSO *Pregnancy & Birth Sourcebook*

Consumer Issues in Health Care Sourcebook

Basic Information about Health Care Fundamentals and Related Consumer Issues, Including Exams and Screening Tests, Physician Specialties, Choosing a Doctor, Using Prescription and Over-the-Counter Medications Safely, Avoiding Health Scams, Managing Common Health Risks in the Home, Care Options for Chronically or Terminally Ill Patients, and a List of Resources for Obtaining Help and Further Information

Edited by Karen Bellenir. 618 pages. 1998. 0-7808-0221-7. $78.

"Both public and academic libraries will want to have a copy in their collection for readers who are interested in self-education on health issues."
—*American Reference Books Annual, 2000*

"The editor has researched the literature from government agencies and others, saving readers the time and effort of having to do the research themselves. Recommended for public libraries."
—*Reference and User Services Quarterly, American Library Association, Spring '99*

"Recommended reference source."
—*Booklist, American Library Association, Dec '98*

■

Contagious & Non-Contagious Infectious Diseases Sourcebook

Basic Information about Contagious Diseases like Measles, Polio, Hepatitis B, and Infectious Mononucleosis, and Non-Contagious Infectious Diseases like Tetanus and Toxic Shock Syndrome, and Diseases Occurring as Secondary Infections Such as Shingles and Reye Syndrome

Along with Vaccination, Prevention, and Treatment Information, and a Section Describing Emerging Infectious Disease Threats

Edited by Karen Bellenir and Peter D. Dresser. 566 pages. 1996. 0-7808-0075-3. $78.

■

Death & Dying Sourcebook

Basic Consumer Health Information for the Layperson about End-of-Life Care and Related Ethical and Legal Issues, Including Chief Causes of Death, Autopsies, Pain Management for the Terminally Ill, Life Support Systems, Insurance, Euthanasia, Assisted Suicide, Hospice Programs, Living Wills, Funeral Planning, Counseling, Mourning, Organ Donation, and Physician Training

Along with Statistical Data, a Glossary, and Listings of Sources for Further Help and Information

Edited by Annemarie S. Muth. 641 pages. 1999. 0-7808-0230-6. $78.

"Public libraries, medical libraries, and academic libraries will all find this sourcebook a useful addition to their collections."
—*American Reference Books Annual, 2001*

"An extremely useful resource for those concerned with death and dying in the United States."
—*Respiratory Care, Nov '00*

"Recommended reference source."
—*Booklist, American Library Association, Aug '00*

"This book is a definite must for all those involved in end-of-life care." —*Doody's Review Service, 2000*

■

Diabetes Sourcebook, 1st Edition

Basic Information about Insulin-Dependent and Non-insulin-Dependent Diabetes Mellitus, Gestational Diabetes, and Diabetic Complications, Symptoms, Treatment, and Research Results, Including Statistics on Prevalence, Morbidity, and Mortality

Along with Source Listings for Further Help and Information

Edited by Karen Bellenir and Peter D. Dresser. 827 pages. 1994. 1-55888-751-2. $78.

". . . very informative and understandable for the layperson without being simplistic. It provides a comprehensive overview for laypersons who want a general understanding of the disease or who want to focus on various aspects of the disease."
—*Bulletin of the Medical Library Association, Jan '96*

■

Diabetes Sourcebook, 2nd Edition

Basic Consumer Health Information about Type 1 Diabetes (Insulin-Dependent or Juvenile-Onset Diabetes), Type 2 (Noninsulin-Dependent or Adult-Onset Diabetes), Gestational Diabetes, and Related Disorders, Including Diabetes Prevalence Data, Management Issues, the Role of Diet and Exercise in Controlling Diabetes, Insulin and Other Diabetes Medicines, and Complications of Diabetes Such as Eye Diseases, Periodontal Disease, Amputation, and End-Stage Renal Disease

Along with Reports on Current Research Initiatives, a Glossary, and Resource Listings for Further Help and Information

Edited by Karen Bellenir. 688 pages. 1998. 0-7808-0224-1. $78.

"This comprehensive book is an excellent addition for high school, academic, medical, and public libraries. This volume is highly recommended."
—*American Reference Books Annual, 2000*

"An invaluable reference." —*Library Journal, May '00*

Selected as one of the 250 "Best Health Sciences Books of 1999." —*Doody's Rating Service, Mar-Apr 2000*

"Recommended reference source."
—*Booklist, American Library Association, Feb '99*

". . . provides reliable mainstream medical information . . . belongs on the shelves of any library with a consumer health collection." —*E-Streams, Sep '99*

"Provides useful information for the general public."
—*Healthlines, University of Michigan Health Management Research Center, Sep/Oct '99*

Diet & Nutrition Sourcebook, 1st Edition

Basic Information about Nutrition, Including the Dietary Guidelines for Americans, the Food Guide Pyramid, and Their Applications in Daily Diet, Nutritional Advice for Specific Age Groups, Current Nutritional Issues and Controversies, the New Food Label and How to Use It to Promote Healthy Eating, and Recent Developments in Nutritional Research

Edited by Dan R. Harris. 662 pages. 1996. 0-7808-0084-2. $78.

"Useful reference as a food and nutrition sourcebook for the general consumer." — *Booklist Health Sciences Supplement, American Library Association, Oct '97*

"Recommended for public libraries and medical libraries that receive general information requests on nutrition. It is readable and will appeal to those interested in learning more about healthy dietary practices." — *Medical Reference Services Quarterly, Fall '97*

"An abundance of medical and social statistics is translated into readable information geared toward the general reader." — *Bookwatch, Mar '97*

"With dozens of questionable diet books on the market, it is so refreshing to find a reliable and factual reference book. Recommended to aspiring professionals, librarians, and others seeking and giving reliable dietary advice. An excellent compilation." — *Choice, Association of College and Research Libraries, Feb '97*

SEE ALSO *Digestive Diseases & Disorders Sourcebook, Gastrointestinal Diseases & Disorders Sourcebook*

■

Diet & Nutrition Sourcebook, 2nd Edition

Basic Consumer Health Information about Dietary Guidelines, Recommended Daily Intake Values, Vitamins, Minerals, Fiber, Fat, Weight Control, Dietary Supplements, and Food Additives

Along with Special Sections on Nutrition Needs throughout Life and Nutrition for People with Such Specific Medical Concerns as Allergies, High Blood Cholesterol, Hypertension, Diabetes, Celiac Disease, Seizure Disorders, Phenylketonuria (PKU), Cancer, and Eating Disorders, and Including Reports on Current Nutrition Research and Source Listings for Additional Help and Information

Edited by Karen Bellenir. 650 pages. 1999. 0-7808-0228-4. $78.

"This book is an excellent source of basic diet and nutrition information." — *Booklist Health Sciences Supplement, American Library Association, Dec '00*

"This reference document should be in any public library, but it would be a very good guide for beginning students in the health sciences. If the other books in this publisher's series are as good as this, they should all be in the health sciences collections." — *American Reference Books Annual, 2000*

"This book is an excellent general nutrition reference for consumers who desire to take an active role in their health care for prevention. Consumers of all ages who select this book can feel confident they are receiving current and accurate information." — *Journal of Nutrition for the Elderly, Vol. 19, No. 4, '00*

"Recommended reference source." — *Booklist, American Library Association, Dec '99*

SEE ALSO *Digestive Diseases & Disorders Sourcebook, Gastrointestinal Diseases & Disorders Sourcebook*

■

Digestive Diseases & Disorders Sourcebook

Basic Consumer Health Information about Diseases and Disorders that Impact the Upper and Lower Digestive System, Including Celiac Disease, Constipation, Crohn's Disease, Cyclic Vomiting Syndrome, Diarrhea, Diverticulosis and Diverticulitis, Gallstones, Heartburn, Hemorrhoids, Hernias, Indigestion (Dyspepsia), Irritable Bowel Syndrome, Lactose Intolerance, Ulcers, and More

Along with Information about Medications and Other Treatments, Tips for Maintaining a Healthy Digestive Tract, a Glossary, and Directory of Digestive Diseases Organizations

Edited by Karen Bellenir. 335 pages. 1999. 0-7808-0327-2. $48.

"This title would be an excellent addition to all public or patient-research libraries." — *American Reference Books Annual, 2001*

"This title is recommended for public, hospital, and health sciences libraries with consumer health collections." — *E-Streams, Jul-Aug '00*

"Recommended reference source." — *Booklist, American Library Association, May '00*

SEE ALSO *Diet & Nutrition Sourcebook, 1st and 2nd Editions, Gastrointestinal Diseases & Disorders Sourcebook*

■

Disabilities Sourcebook

Basic Consumer Health Information about Physical and Psychiatric Disabilities, Including Descriptions of Major Causes of Disability, Assistive and Adaptive Aids, Workplace Issues, and Accessibility Concerns

Along with Information about the Americans with Disabilities Act, a Glossary, and Resources for Additional Help and Information

Edited by Dawn D. Matthews. 616 pages. 2000. 0-7808-0389-2. $78.

"A much needed addition to the Omnigraphics *Health Reference Series*. A current reference work to provide people with disabilities, their families, caregivers or those who work with them, a broad range of information in one volume, has not been available until now. . . . It is recommended for all public and academic library reference collections." — *E-Streams, May '01*

"An excellent source book in easy-to-read format covering many current topics; highly recommended for all libraries." — *Choice, Association of College and Research Libraries, Jan '01*

"Recommended reference source."
— *Booklist, American Library Association, Jul '00*

"An involving, invaluable handbook."
— *The Bookwatch, May '00*

■

Domestic Violence & Child Abuse Sourcebook

Basic Consumer Health Information about Spousal/Partner, Child, Sibling, Parent, and Elder Abuse, Covering Physical, Emotional, and Sexual Abuse, Teen Dating Violence, and Stalking; Includes Information about Hotlines, Safe Houses, Safety Plans, and Other Resources for Support and Assistance, Community Initiatives, and Reports on Current Directions in Research and Treatment

Along with a Glossary, Sources for Further Reading, and Governmental and Non-Governmental Organizations Contact Information

Edited by Helene Henderson. 1,064 pages. 2000. 0-7808-0235-7. $78.

"Recommended reference source."
— *Booklist, American Library Association, Apr '01*

"Important pick for college-level health reference libraries." — *The Bookwatch, Mar '01*

"Because this problem is so widespread and because this book includes a lot of issues within one volume, this work is recommended for all public libraries." — *American Reference Books Annual, 2001*

■

Drug Abuse Sourcebook

Basic Consumer Health Information about Illicit Substances of Abuse and the Diversion of Prescription Medications, Including Depressants, Hallucinogens, Inhalants, Marijuana, Narcotics, Stimulants, and Anabolic Steroids

Along with Facts about Related Health Risks, Treatment Issues, and Substance Abuse Prevention Programs, a Glossary of Terms, Statistical Data, and Directories of Hotline Services, Self-Help Groups, and Organizations Able to Provide Further Information

Edited by Karen Bellenir. 629 pages. 2000. 0-7808-0242-X. $78.

"Containing a wealth of information, this book will be useful to the college student just beginning to explore the topic of substance abuse. This resource belongs in libraries that serve a lower-division undergraduate or community college clientele as well as the general public." — *Choice, Association of College and Research Libraries, Jun '01*

"Recommended reference source."
— *Booklist, American Library Association, Feb '01*

"Highly recommended." — *The Bookwatch, Jan '01*

"Even though there is a plethora of books on drug abuse, this volume is recommended for school, public, and college libraries."
— *American Reference Books Annual, 2001*

SEE ALSO *Alcoholism Sourcebook, Substance Abuse Sourcebook*

■

Ear, Nose & Throat Disorders Sourcebook

Basic Information about Disorders of the Ears, Nose, Sinus Cavities, Pharynx, and Larynx, Including Ear Infections, Tinnitus, Vestibular Disorders, Allergic and Non-Allergic Rhinitis, Sore Throats, Tonsillitis, and Cancers That Affect the Ears, Nose, Sinuses, and Throat

Along with Reports on Current Research Initiatives, a Glossary of Related Medical Terms, and a Directory of Sources for Further Help and Information

Edited by Karen Bellenir and Linda M. Shin. 576 pages. 1998. 0-7808-0206-3. $78.

"Overall, this sourcebook is helpful for the consumer seeking information on ENT issues. It is recommended for public libraries."
— *American Reference Books Annual, 1999*

"Recommended reference source."
— *Booklist, American Library Association, Dec '98*

■

Eating Disorders Sourcebook

Basic Consumer Health Information about Eating Disorders, Including Information about Anorexia Nervosa, Bulimia Nervosa, Binge Eating, Body Dysmorphic Disorder, Pica, Laxative Abuse, and Night Eating Syndrome

Along with Information about Causes, Adverse Effects, and Treatment and Prevention Issues, and Featuring a Section on Concerns Specific to Children and Adolescents, a Glossary, and Resources for Further Help and Information

Edited by Dawn D. Matthews. 322 pages. 2001. 0-7808-0335-3. $78.

■

Endocrine & Metabolic Disorders Sourcebook

Basic Information for the Layperson about Pancreatic and Insulin-Related Disorders Such as Pancreatitis, Diabetes, and Hypoglycemia; Adrenal Gland Disorders Such as Cushing's Syndrome, Addison's Disease, and Congenital Adrenal Hyperplasia; Pituitary Gland Disorders Such as Growth Hormone Deficiency, Acromegaly, and Pituitary Tumors; Thyroid Disorders Such as Hypothyroidism, Graves' Disease, Hashimoto's Disease, and Goiter; Hyperparathyroidism; and Other Diseases and Syndromes of Hormone Imbalance or Metabolic Dysfunction

Along with Reports on Current Research Initiatives

Edited by Linda M. Shin. 574 pages. 1998. 0-7808-0207-1. $78.

"Omnigraphics has produced another needed resource for health information consumers."
—*American Reference Books Annual, 2000*

"Recommended reference source."
— *Booklist, American Library Association, Dec '98*

■

Environmentally Induced Disorders Sourcebook

Basic Information about Diseases and Syndromes Linked to Exposure to Pollutants and Other Substances in Outdoor and Indoor Environments Such as Lead, Asbestos, Formaldehyde, Mercury, Emissions, Noise, and More

Edited by Allan R. Cook. 620 pages. 1997. 0-7808-0083-4. $78.

"Recommended reference source."
— *Booklist, American Library Association, Sep '98*

"This book will be a useful addition to anyone's library." — *Choice Health Sciences Supplement, Association of College and Research Libraries, May '98*

". . . a good survey of numerous environmentally induced physical disorders . . . a useful addition to anyone's library."
— *Doody's Health Sciences Book Reviews, Jan '98*

". . . provide[s] introductory information from the best authorities around. Since this volume covers topics that potentially affect everyone, it will surely be one of the most frequently consulted volumes in the *Health Reference Series*." — *Rettig on Reference, Nov '97*

■

Ethnic Diseases Sourcebook

Basic Consumer Health Information for Ethnic and Racial Minority Groups in the United States, Including General Health Indicators and Behaviors, Ethnic Diseases, Genetic Testing, the Impact of Chronic Diseases, Women's Health, Mental Health Issues, and Preventive Health Care Services

Along with a Glossary and a Listing of Additional Resources

Edited by Joyce Brennfleck Shannon. 664 pages. 2001. 0-7808-0336-1. $78.

■

Family Planning Sourcebook

Basic Consumer Health Information about Planning for Pregnancy and Contraception, Including Traditional Methods, Barrier Methods, Hormonal Methods, Permanent Methods, Future Methods, Emergency Contraception, and Birth Control Choices for Women at Each Stage of Life

Along with Statistics, a Glossary, and Sources of Additional Information

Edited by Amy Marcaccio Keyzer. 520 pages. 2001. 0-7808-0379-5. $78.

SEE ALSO *Pregnancy & Birth Sourcebook*

Fitness & Exercise Sourcebook, 1st Edition

Basic Information on Fitness and Exercise, Including Fitness Activities for Specific Age Groups, Exercise for People with Specific Medical Conditions, How to Begin a Fitness Program in Running, Walking, Swimming, Cycling, and Other Athletic Activities, and Recent Research in Fitness and Exercise

Edited by Dan R. Harris. 663 pages. 1996. 0-7808-0186-5. $78.

"A good resource for general readers."
— *Choice, Association of College and Research Libraries, Nov '97*

"The perennial popularity of the topic . . . make this an appealing selection for public libraries."
— *Rettig on Reference, Jun/Jul '97*

■

Fitness & Exercise Sourcebook, 2nd Edition

Basic Consumer Health Information about the Fundamentals of Fitness and Exercise, Including How to Begin and Maintain a Fitness Program, Fitness as a Lifestyle, the Link between Fitness and Diet, Advice for Specific Groups of People, Exercise as It Relates to Specific Medical Conditions, and Recent Research in Fitness and Exercise

Along with a Glossary of Important Terms and Resources for Additional Help and Information

Edited by Kristen M. Gledhill. 646 pages. 2001. 0-7808-0334-5. $78.

■

Food & Animal Borne Diseases Sourcebook

Basic Information about Diseases That Can Be Spread to Humans through the Ingestion of Contaminated Food or Water or by Contact with Infected Animals and Insects, Such as Botulism, E. Coli, Hepatitis A, Trichinosis, Lyme Disease, and Rabies

Along with Information Regarding Prevention and Treatment Methods, and Including a Special Section for International Travelers Describing Diseases Such as Cholera, Malaria, Travelers' Diarrhea, and Yellow Fever, and Offering Recommendations for Avoiding Illness

Edited by Karen Bellenir and Peter D. Dresser. 535 pages. 1995. 0-7808-0033-8. $78.

"Targeting general readers and providing them with a single, comprehensive source of information on selected topics, this book continues, with the excellent caliber of its predecessors, to catalog topical information on health matters of general interest. Readable and thorough, this valuable resource is highly recommended for all libraries."
— *Academic Library Book Review, Summer '96*

"A comprehensive collection of authoritative information." — *Emergency Medical Services, Oct '95*

571

Food Safety Sourcebook

Basic Consumer Health Information about the Safe Handling of Meat, Poultry, Seafood, Eggs, Fruit Juices, and Other Food Items, and Facts about Pesticides, Drinking Water, Food Safety Overseas, and the Onset, Duration, and Symptoms of Foodborne Illnesses, Including Types of Pathogenic Bacteria, Parasitic Protozoa, Worms, Viruses, and Natural Toxins

Along with the Role of the Consumer, the Food Handler, and the Government in Food Safety; a Glossary, and Resources for Additional Help and Information

Edited by Dawn D. Matthews. 339 pages. 1999. 0-7808-0326-4. $48.

"This book is recommended for public libraries and universities with home economic and food science programs." — *E-Streams, Nov '00*

"This book takes the complex issues of food safety and foodborne pathogens and presents them in an easily understood manner. [It does] an excellent job of covering a large and often confusing topic."
—*American Reference Books Annual, 2000*

"Recommended reference source."
—*Booklist, American Library Association, May '00*

■

Forensic Medicine Sourcebook

Basic Consumer Information for the Layperson about Forensic Medicine, Including Crime Scene Investigation, Evidence Collection and Analysis, Expert Testimony, Computer-Aided Criminal Identification, Digital Imaging in the Courtroom, DNA Profiling, Accident Reconstruction, Autopsies, Ballistics, Drugs and Explosives Detection, Latent Fingerprints, Product Tampering, and Questioned Document Examination

Along with Statistical Data, a Glossary of Forensics Terminology, and Listings of Sources for Further Help and Information

Edited by Annemarie S. Muth. 574 pages. 1999. 0-7808-0232-2. $78.

"Given the expected widespread interest in its content and its easy to read style, this book is recommended for most public and all college and university libraries." — *E-Streams, Feb '01*

"There are several items that make this book attractive to consumers who are seeking certain forensic data. . . . This is a useful current source for those seeking general forensic medical answers."
—*American Reference Books Annual, 2000*

"Recommended for public libraries."
—*Reference & User Services Quarterly, American Library Association, Spring 2000*

"Recommended reference source."
—*Booklist, American Library Association, Feb '00*

"A wealth of information, useful statistics, references are up-to-date and extremely complete. This wonderful collection of data will help students who are interested in a career in any type of forensic field. It is a great

resource for attorneys who need information about types of expert witnesses needed in a particular case. It also offers useful information for fiction and nonfiction writers whose work involves a crime. A fascinating compilation. All levels." — *Choice, Association of College and Research Libraries, Jan 2000*

■

Gastrointestinal Diseases & Disorders Sourcebook

Basic Information about Gastroesophageal Reflux Disease (Heartburn), Ulcers, Diverticulosis, Irritable Bowel Syndrome, Crohn's Disease, Ulcerative Colitis, Diarrhea, Constipation, Lactose Intolerance, Hemorrhoids, Hepatitis, Cirrhosis, and Other Digestive Problems, Featuring Statistics, Descriptions of Symptoms, and Current Treatment Methods of Interest for Persons Living with Upper and Lower Gastrointestinal Maladies

Edited by Linda M. Ross. 413 pages. 1996. 0-7808-0078-8. $78.

". . . very readable form. The successful editorial work that brought this material together into a useful and understandable reference makes accessible to all readers information that can help them more effectively understand and obtain help for digestive tract problems."
— *Choice, Association of College and Research Libraries, Feb '97*

SEE ALSO *Diet & Nutrition Sourcebook, 1st and 2nd Editions, Digestive Diseases & Disorders Sourcebook*

■

Genetic Disorders Sourcebook, 1st Edition

Basic Information about Heritable Diseases and Disorders Such as Down Syndrome, PKU, Hemophilia, Von Willebrand Disease, Gaucher Disease, Tay-Sachs Disease, and Sickle-Cell Disease, Along with Information about Genetic Screening, Gene Therapy, Home Care, and Including Source Listings for Further Help and Information on More Than 300 Disorders

Edited by Karen Bellenir. 642 pages. 1996. 0-7808-0034-6. $78.

"Recommended for undergraduate libraries or libraries that serve the public." — *Science & Technology Libraries, Vol. 18, No. 1, '99*

"Provides essential medical information to both the general public and those diagnosed with a serious or fatal genetic disease or disorder."
—*Choice, Association of College and Research Libraries, Jan '97*

"Geared toward the lay public. It would be well placed in all public libraries and in those hospital and medical libraries in which access to genetic references is limited." — *Doody's Health Sciences Book Review, Oct '96*

Genetic Disorders Sourcebook, 2nd Edition

Basic Consumer Health Information about Hereditary Diseases and Disorders, Including Cystic Fibrosis, Down Syndrome, Hemophilia, Huntington's Disease, Sickle Cell Anemia, and More; Facts about Genes, Gene Research and Therapy, Genetic Screening, Ethics of Gene Testing, Genetic Counseling, and Advice on Coping and Caring

Along with a Glossary of Genetic Terminology and a Resource List for Help, Support, and Further Information

Edited by Kathy Massimini. 768 pages. 2001. 0-7808-0241-1. $78.

"Recommended for public libraries and medical and hospital libraries with consumer health collections."
— *E-Streams, May '01*

"Recommended reference source."
— *Booklist, American Library Association, Apr '01*

"Important pick for college-level health reference libraries." — *The Bookwatch, Mar '01*

■

Head Trauma Sourcebook

Basic Information for the Layperson about Open-Head and Closed-Head Injuries, Treatment Advances, Recovery, and Rehabilitation

Along with Reports on Current Research Initiatives

Edited by Karen Bellenir. 414 pages. 1997. 0-7808-0208-X. $78.

■

Health Insurance Sourcebook

Basic Information about Managed Care Organizations, Traditional Fee-for-Service Insurance, Insurance Portability and Pre-Existing Conditions Clauses, Medicare, Medicaid, Social Security, and Military Health Care

Along with Information about Insurance Fraud

Edited by Wendy Wilcox. 530 pages. 1997. 0-7808-0222-5. $78.

"Particularly useful because it brings much of this information together in one volume. This book will be a handy reference source in the health sciences library, hospital library, college and university library, and medium to large public library."
— *Medical Reference Services Quarterly, Fall '98*

Awarded "Books of the Year Award"
— *American Journal of Nursing, 1997*

"The layout of the book is particularly helpful as it provides easy access to reference material. A most useful addition to the vast amount of information about health insurance. The use of data from U.S. government agencies is most commendable. Useful in a library or learning center for healthcare professional students."
— *Doody's Health Sciences Book Reviews, Nov '97*

Health Reference Series Cumulative Index 1999

A Comprehensive Index to the Individual Volumes of the Health Reference Series, Including a Subject Index, Name Index, Organization Index, and Publication Index

Along with a Master List of Acronyms and Abbreviations

Edited by Edward J. Prucha, Anne Holmes, and Robert Rudnick. 990 pages. 2000. 0-7808-0382-5. $78.

"This volume will be most helpful in libraries that have a relatively complete collection of the Health Reference Series."
— *American Reference Books Annual, 2001*

"Essential for collections that hold any of the numerous *Health Reference Series* titles."
— *Choice, Association of College and Research Libraries, Nov '00*

■

Healthy Aging Sourcebook

Basic Consumer Health Information about Maintaining Health through the Aging Process, Including Advice on Nutrition, Exercise, and Sleep, Help in Making Decisions about Midlife Issues and Retirement, and Guidance Concerning Practical and Informed Choices in Health Consumerism

Along with Data Concerning the Theories of Aging, Different Experiences in Aging by Minority Groups, and Facts about Aging Now and Aging in the Future; and Featuring a Glossary, a Guide to Consumer Help, Additional Suggested Reading, and Practical Resource Directory

Edited by Jenifer Swanson. 536 pages. 1999. 0-7808-0390-6. $78.

"Recommended reference source."
— *Booklist, American Library Association, Feb '00*

SEE ALSO *Physical & Mental Issues in Aging Sourcebook*

■

Healthy Heart Sourcebook for Women

Basic Consumer Health Information about Cardiac Issues Specific to Women, Including Facts about Major Risk Factors and Prevention, Treatment and Control Strategies, and Important Dietary Issues

Along with a Special Section Regarding the Pros and Cons of Hormone Replacement Therapy and Its Impact on Heart Health, and Additional Help, Including Recipes, a Glossary, and a Directory of Resources

Edited by Dawn D. Matthews. 336 pages. 2000. 0-7808-0329-9. $48.

"A good reference source and recommended for all public, academic, medical, and hospital libraries."
— *Medical Reference Services Quarterly, Summer '01*

573

"Because of the lack of information specific to women on this topic, this book is recommended for public libraries and consumer libraries."
—*American Reference Books Annual, 2001*

"Contains very important information about coronary artery disease that all women should know. The information is current and presented in an easy-to-read format. The book will make a good addition to any library." —*American Medical Writers Association Journal, Summer '00*

"Important, basic reference."
—*Reviewer's Bookwatch, Jul '00*

SEE ALSO *Cardiovascular Diseases & Disorders Sourcebook, 1st Edition, Heart Diseases & Disorders Sourcebook, 2nd Edition, Women's Health Concerns Sourcebook*

■

Heart Diseases & Disorders Sourcebook, 2nd Edition

Basic Consumer Health Information about Heart Attacks, Angina, Rhythm Disorders, Heart Failure, Valve Disease, Congenital Heart Disorders, and More, Including Descriptions of Surgical Procedures and Other Interventions, Medications, Cardiac Rehabilitation, Risk Identification, and Prevention Tips

Along with Statistical Data, Reports on Current Research Initiatives, a Glossary of Cardiovascular Terms, and Resource Directory

Edited by Karen Bellenir. 612 pages. 2000. 0-7808-0238-1. $78.

"This work stands out as an imminently accessible resource for the general public. It is recommended for the reference and circulating shelves of school, public, and academic libraries."
—*American Reference Books Annual, 2001*

"Recommended reference source."
—*Booklist, American Library Association, Dec '00*

"Provides comprehensive coverage of matters related to the heart. This title is recommended for health sciences and public libraries with consumer health collections."
—*E-Streams, Oct '00*

SEE ALSO *Cardiovascular Diseases & Disorders Sourcebook, 1st Edition, Healthy Heart Sourcebook for Women*

■

Immune System Disorders Sourcebook

Basic Information about Lupus, Multiple Sclerosis, Guillain-Barré Syndrome, Chronic Granulomatous Disease, and More

Along with Statistical and Demographic Data and Reports on Current Research Initiatives

Edited by Allan R. Cook. 608 pages. 1997. 0-7808-0209-8. $78.

Infant & Toddler Health Sourcebook

Basic Consumer Health Information about the Physical and Mental Development of Newborns, Infants, and Toddlers, Including Neonatal Concerns, Nutrition Recommendations, Immunization Schedules, Common Pediatric Disorders, Assessments and Milestones, Safety Tips, and Advice for Parents and Other Caregivers

Along with a Glossary of Terms and Resource Listings for Additional Help

Edited by Jenifer Swanson. 585 pages. 2000. 0-7808-0246-2. $78.

"As a reference for the general public, this would be useful in any library." —*E-Streams, May '01*

"Recommended reference source."
—*Booklist, American Library Association, Feb '01*

"This is a good source for general use."
—*American Reference Books Annual, 2001*

■

Kidney & Urinary Tract Diseases & Disorders Sourcebook

Basic Information about Kidney Stones, Urinary Incontinence, Bladder Disease, End Stage Renal Disease, Dialysis, and More

Along with Statistical and Demographic Data and Reports on Current Research Initiatives

Edited by Linda M. Ross. 602 pages. 1997. 0-7808-0079-6. $78.

■

Learning Disabilities Sourcebook

Basic Information about Disorders Such as Dyslexia, Visual and Auditory Processing Deficits, Attention Deficit/Hyperactivity Disorder, and Autism

Along with Statistical and Demographic Data, Reports on Current Research Initiatives, an Explanation of the Assessment Process, and a Special Section for Adults with Learning Disabilities

Edited by Linda M. Shin. 579 pages. 1998. 0-7808-0210-1. $78.

Named "Outstanding Reference Book of 1999."
—*New York Public Library, Feb 2000*

"An excellent candidate for inclusion in a public library reference section. It's a great source of information. Teachers will also find the book useful. Definitely worth reading."
—*Journal of Adolescent & Adult Literacy, Feb 2000*

"Readable . . . provides a solid base of information regarding successful techniques used with individuals who have learning disabilities, as well as practical suggestions for educators and family members. Clear language, concise descriptions, and pertinent information for contacting multiple resources add to the strength of this book as a useful tool."   — *Choice, Association of College and Research Libraries, Feb '99*

"Recommended reference source."
— *Booklist, American Library Association, Sep '98*

"This is a useful resource for libraries and for those who don't have the time to identify and locate the individual publications."
— *Disability Resources Monthly, Sep '98*

■

Liver Disorders Sourcebook

Basic Consumer Health Information about the Liver and How It Works; Liver Diseases, Including Cancer, Cirrhosis, Hepatitis, and Toxic and Drug Related Diseases; Tips for Maintaining a Healthy Liver; Laboratory Tests, Radiology Tests, and Facts about Liver Transplantation

Along with a Section on Support Groups, a Glossary, and Resource Listings

Edited by Joyce Brennfleck Shannon. 591 pages. 2000. 0-7808-0383-3. $78.

"A valuable resource."
— *American Reference Books Annual, 2001*

"This title is recommended for health sciences and public libraries with consumer health collections."
— *E-Streams, Oct '00*

"Recommended reference source."
— *Booklist, American Library Association, Jun '00*

■

Medical Tests Sourcebook

Basic Consumer Health Information about Medical Tests, Including Periodic Health Exams, General Screening Tests, Tests You Can Do at Home, Findings of the U.S. Preventive Services Task Force, X-ray and Radiology Tests, Electrical Tests, Tests of Blood and Other Body Fluids and Tissues, Scope Tests, Lung Tests, Genetic Tests, Pregnancy Tests, Newborn Screening Tests, Sexually Transmitted Disease Tests, and Computer Aided Diagnoses

Along with a Section on Paying for Medical Tests, a Glossary, and Resource Listings

Edited by Joyce Brennfleck Shannon. 691 pages. 1999. 0-7808-0243-8. $78.

"A valuable reference guide."
— *American Reference Books Annual, 2000*

"Recommended for hospital and health sciences libraries with consumer health collections."
— *E-Streams, Mar '00*

"This is an overall excellent reference with a wealth of general knowledge that may aid those who are reluctant to get vital tests performed."
— *Today's Librarian, Jan 2000*

Men's Health Concerns Sourcebook

Basic Information about Health Issues That Affect Men, Featuring Facts about the Top Causes of Death in Men, Including Heart Disease, Stroke, Cancers, Prostate Disorders, Chronic Obstructive Pulmonary Disease, Pneumonia and Influenza, Human Immunodeficiency Virus and Acquired Immune Deficiency Syndrome, Diabetes Mellitus, Stress, Suicide, Accidents and Homicides; and Facts about Common Concerns for Men, Including Impotence, Contraception, Circumcision, Sleep Disorders, Snoring, Hair Loss, Diet, Nutrition, Exercise, Kidney and Urological Disorders, and Backaches

Edited by Allan R. Cook. 738 pages. 1998. 0-7808-0212-8. $78.

"This comprehensive resource and the series are highly recommended."
— *American Reference Books Annual, 2000*

"Recommended reference source."
— *Booklist, American Library Association, Dec '98*

■

Mental Health Disorders Sourcebook, 1st Edition

Basic Information about Schizophrenia, Depression, Bipolar Disorder, Panic Disorder, Obsessive-Compulsive Disorder, Phobias and Other Anxiety Disorders, Paranoia and Other Personality Disorders, Eating Disorders, and Sleep Disorders

Along with Information about Treatment and Therapies

Edited by Karen Bellenir. 548 pages. 1995. 0-7808-0040-0. $78.

"This is an excellent new book . . . written in easy-to-understand language."
— *Booklist Health Sciences Supplement, American Library Association, Oct '97*

". . . useful for public and academic libraries and consumer health collections."
— *Medical Reference Services Quarterly, Spring '97*

"The great strengths of the book are its readability and its inclusion of places to find more information. Especially recommended."   — *Reference Quarterly, American Library Association, Winter '96*

". . . a good resource for a consumer health library."
— *Bulletin of the Medical Library Association, Oct '96*

"The information is data-based and couched in brief, concise language that avoids jargon. . . . a useful reference source."   — *Readings, Sep '96*

"The text is well organized and adequately written for its target audience."   — *Choice, Association of College and Research Libraries, Jun '96*

". . . provides information on a wide range of mental disorders, presented in nontechnical language."
— *Exceptional Child Education Resources, Spring '96*

"Recommended for public and academic libraries."
— *Reference Book Review, 1996*

Mental Health Disorders Sourcebook, 2nd Edition

Basic Consumer Health Information about Anxiety Disorders, Depression and Other Mood Disorders, Eating Disorders, Personality Disorders, Schizophrenia, and More, Including Disease Descriptions, Treatment Options, and Reports on Current Research Initiatives

Along with Statistical Data, Tips for Maintaining Mental Health, a Glossary, and Directory of Sources for Additional Help and Information

Edited by Karen Bellenir. 605 pages. 2000. 0-7808-0240-3. $78.

"Well organized and well written."
— *American Reference Books Annual, 2001*

"Recommended reference source."
— *Booklist, American Library Association, Jun '00*

■

Mental Retardation Sourcebook

Basic Consumer Health Information about Mental Retardation and Its Causes, Including Down Syndrome, Fetal Alcohol Syndrome, Fragile X Syndrome, Genetic Conditions, Injury, and Environmental Sources

Along with Preventive Strategies, Parenting Issues, Educational Implications, Health Care Needs, Employment and Economic Matters, Legal Issues, a Glossary, and a Resource Listing for Additional Help and Information

Edited by Joyce Brennfleck Shannon. 642 pages. 2000. 0-7808-0377-9. $78.

"Public libraries will find the book useful for reference and as a beginning research point for students, parents, and caregivers."
— *American Reference Books Annual, 2001*

"The strength of this work is that it compiles many basic fact sheets and addresses for further information in one volume. It is intended and suitable for the general public. The sourcebook is relevant to any collection providing health information to the general public."
— *E-Streams, Nov '00*

"From preventing retardation to parenting and family challenges, this covers health, social and legal issues and will prove an invaluable overview."
— *Reviewer's Bookwatch, Jul '00*

■

Obesity Sourcebook

Basic Consumer Health Information about Diseases and Other Problems Associated with Obesity, and Including Facts about Risk Factors, Prevention Issues, and Management Approaches

Along with Statistical and Demographic Data, Information about Special Populations, Research Updates, a Glossary, and Source Listings for Further Help and Information

Edited by Wilma Caldwell and Chad T. Kimball. 376 pages. 2001. 0-7808-0333-7. $48.

" Recommended pick both for specialty health library collections and any general consumer health reference collection."
— *The Bookwatch, Apr '01*

"Recommended reference source."
— *Booklist, American Library Association, Apr '01*

■

Ophthalmic Disorders Sourcebook

Basic Information about Glaucoma, Cataracts, Macular Degeneration, Strabismus, Refractive Disorders, and More

Along with Statistical and Demographic Data and Reports on Current Research Initiatives

Edited by Linda M. Ross. 631 pages. 1996. 0-7808-0081-8. $78.

■

Oral Health Sourcebook

Basic Information about Diseases and Conditions Affecting Oral Health, Including Cavities, Gum Disease, Dry Mouth, Oral Cancers, Fever Blisters, Canker Sores, Oral Thrush, Bad Breath, Temporomandibular Disorders, and other Craniofacial Syndromes

Along with Statistical Data on the Oral Health of Americans, Oral Hygiene, Emergency First Aid, Information on Treatment Procedures and Methods of Replacing Lost Teeth

Edited by Allan R. Cook. 558 pages. 1997. 0-7808-0082-6. $78.

"Unique source which will fill a gap in dental sources for patients and the lay public. A valuable reference tool even in a library with thousands of books on dentistry. Comprehensive, clear, inexpensive, and easy to read and use. It fills an enormous gap in the health care literature."
— *Reference and User Services Quarterly, American Library Association, Summer '98*

"Recommended reference source."
— *Booklist, American Library Association, Dec '97*

■

Osteoporosis Sourcebook

Basic Consumer Health Information about Primary and Secondary Osteoporosis and Juvenile Osteoporosis and Related Conditions, Including Fibrous Dysplasia, Gaucher Disease, Hyperthyroidism, Hypophosphatasia, Myeloma, Osteopetrosis, Osteogenesis Imperfecta, and Paget's Disease

Along with Information about Risk Factors, Treatments, Traditional and Non-Traditional Pain Management, a Glossary of Related Terms, and a Directory of Resources

Edited by Allan R. Cook. 584 pages. 2001. 0-7808-0239-X. $78.

SEE ALSO *Women's Health Concerns Sourcebook*

Pain Sourcebook

Basic Information about Specific Forms of Acute and Chronic Pain, Including Headaches, Back Pain, Muscular Pain, Neuralgia, Surgical Pain, and Cancer Pain

Along with Pain Relief Options Such as Analgesics, Narcotics, Nerve Blocks, Transcutaneous Nerve Stimulation, and Alternative Forms of Pain Control, Including Biofeedback, Imaging, Behavior Modification, and Relaxation Techniques

Edited by Allan R. Cook. 667 pages. 1997. 0-7808-0213-6. $78.

"**The text is readable, easily understood, and well indexed. This excellent volume belongs in all patient education libraries, consumer health sections of public libraries, and many personal collections.**"
— American Reference Books Annual, 1999

"**A beneficial reference.**" *— Booklist Health Sciences Supplement, American Library Association, Oct '98*

"**The information is basic in terms of scholarship and is appropriate for general readers. Written in journalistic style . . . intended for non-professionals. Quite thorough in its coverage of different pain conditions and summarizes the latest clinical information regarding pain treatment.**" *— Choice, Association of College and Research Libraries, Jun '98*

"**Recommended reference source.**"
— Booklist, American Library Association, Mar '98

Pediatric Cancer Sourcebook

Basic Consumer Health Information about Leukemias, Brain Tumors, Sarcomas, Lymphomas, and Other Cancers in Infants, Children, and Adolescents, Including Descriptions of Cancers, Treatments, and Coping Strategies

Along with Suggestions for Parents, Caregivers, and Concerned Relatives, a Glossary of Cancer Terms, and Resource Listings

Edited by Edward J. Prucha. 587 pages. 1999. 0-7808-0245-4. $78.

"**A valuable addition to all libraries specializing in health services and many public libraries.**"
— American Reference Books Annual, 2000

"**Recommended reference source.**"
— Booklist, American Library Association, Feb '00

"**An excellent source of information. Recommended for public, hospital, and health science libraries with consumer health collections.**" *— E-Streams, Jun '00*

Physical & Mental Issues in Aging Sourcebook

Basic Consumer Health Information on Physical and Mental Disorders Associated with the Aging Process, Including Concerns about Cardiovascular Disease, Pulmonary Disease, Oral Health, Digestive Disorders,

Musculoskeletal and Skin Disorders, Metabolic Changes, Sexual and Reproductive Issues, and Changes in Vision, Hearing, and Other Senses

Along with Data about Longevity and Causes of Death, Information on Acute and Chronic Pain, Descriptions of Mental Concerns, a Glossary of Terms, and Resource Listings for Additional Help

Edited by Jenifer Swanson. 660 pages. 1999. 0-7808-0233-0. $78.

"**Recommended for public libraries.**"
— American Reference Books Annual, 2000

"**This is a treasure of health information for the layperson.**" *— Choice Health Sciences Supplement, Association of College & Research Libraries, May 2000*

"**Recommended reference source.**"
— Booklist, American Library Association, Oct '99

SEE ALSO *Healthy Aging Sourcebook*

Podiatry Sourcebook

Basic Consumer Health Information about Foot Conditions, Diseases, and Injuries, Including Bunions, Corns, Calluses, Athlete's Foot, Plantar Warts, Hammertoes and Clawtoes, Clubfoot, Heel Pain, Gout, and More

Along with Facts about Foot Care, Disease Prevention, Foot Safety, Choosing a Foot Care Specialist, a Glossary of Terms, and Resource Listings for Additional Information

Edited by M. Lisa Weatherford. 400 pages. 2001. 0-7808-0215-2. $78.

Pregnancy & Birth Sourcebook

Basic Information about Planning for Pregnancy, Maternal Health, Fetal Growth and Development, Labor and Delivery, Postpartum and Perinatal Care, Pregnancy in Mothers with Special Concerns, and Disorders of Pregnancy, Including Genetic Counseling, Nutrition and Exercise, Obstetrical Tests, Pregnancy Discomfort, Multiple Births, Cesarean Sections, Medical Testing of Newborns, Breastfeeding, Gestational Diabetes, and Ectopic Pregnancy

Edited by Heather E. Aldred. 737 pages. 1997. 0-7808-0216-0. $78.

"**A well-organized handbook. Recommended.**"
— Choice, Association of College and Research Libraries, Apr '98

"**Recommended reference source.**"
— Booklist, American Library Association, Mar '98

"**Recommended for public libraries.**"
— American Reference Books Annual, 1998

SEE ALSO *Congenital Disorders Sourcebook, Family Planning Sourcebook*

Prostate Cancer Sourcebook

Basic Consumer Health Information about Prostate Cancer, Including Information about the Associated Risk Factors, Detection, Diagnosis, and Treatment of Prostate Cancer

Along with Information on Non-Malignant Prostate Conditions, and Featuring a Section Listing Support and Treatment Centers and a Glossary of Related Terms

Edited by Dawn D. Matthews. 300 pages. 2001. 0-7808-0324-8. $78.

■

Public Health Sourcebook

Basic Information about Government Health Agencies, Including National Health Statistics and Trends, Healthy People 2000 Program Goals and Objectives, the Centers for Disease Control and Prevention, the Food and Drug Administration, and the National Institutes of Health

Along with Full Contact Information for Each Agency

Edited by Wendy Wilcox. 698 pages. 1998. 0-7808-0220-9. $78.

"Recommended reference source."
—*Booklist, American Library Association, Sep '98*

"This consumer guide provides welcome assistance in navigating the maze of federal health agencies and their data on public health concerns."
—*SciTech Book News, Sep '98*

■

Reconstructive & Cosmetic Surgery Sourcebook

Basic Consumer Health Information on Cosmetic and Reconstructive Plastic Surgery, Including Statistical Information about Different Surgical Procedures, Things to Consider Prior to Surgery, Plastic Surgery Techniques and Tools, Emotional and Psychological Considerations, and Procedure-Specific Information

Along with a Glossary of Terms and a Listing of Resources for Additional Help and Information

Edited by M. Lisa Weatherford. 374 pages. 2001. 0-7808-0214-4. $48.

■

Rehabilitation Sourcebook

Basic Consumer Health Information about Rehabilitation for People Recovering from Heart Surgery, Spinal Cord Injury, Stroke, Orthopedic Impairments, Amputation, Pulmonary Impairments, Traumatic Injury, and More, Including Physical Therapy, Occupational Therapy, Speech/ Language Therapy, Massage Therapy, Dance Therapy, Art Therapy, and Recreational Therapy

Along with Information on Assistive and Adaptive Devices, a Glossary, and Resources for Additional Help and Information

Edited by Dawn D. Matthews. 531 pages. 1999. 0-7808-0236-5. $78.

"This is an excellent resource for public library reference and health collections."
—*American Reference Books Annual, 2001*

"Recommended reference source."
—*Booklist, American Library Association, May '00*

■

Respiratory Diseases & Disorders Sourcebook

Basic Information about Respiratory Diseases and Disorders, Including Asthma, Cystic Fibrosis, Pneumonia, the Common Cold, Influenza, and Others, Featuring Facts about the Respiratory System, Statistical and Demographic Data, Treatments, Self-Help Management Suggestions, and Current Research Initiatives

Edited by Allan R. Cook and Peter D. Dresser. 771 pages. 1995. 0-7808-0037-0. $78.

"Designed for the layperson and for patients and their families coping with respiratory illness. . . . an extensive array of information on diagnosis, treatment, management, and prevention of respiratory illnesses for the general reader."
—*Choice, Association of College and Research Libraries, Jun '96*

"A highly recommended text for all collections. It is a comforting reminder of the power of knowledge that good books carry between their covers."
—*Academic Library Book Review, Spring '96*

"A comprehensive collection of authoritative information presented in a nontechnical, humanitarian style for patients, families, and caregivers."
—*Association of Operating Room Nurses, Sep/Oct '95*

■

Sexually Transmitted Diseases Sourcebook, 1st Edition

Basic Information about Herpes, Chlamydia, Gonorrhea, Hepatitis, Nongonoccocal Urethritis, Pelvic Inflammatory Disease, Syphilis, AIDS, and More

Along with Current Data on Treatments and Preventions

Edited by Linda M. Ross. 550 pages. 1997. 0-7808-0217-9. $78.

Sexually Transmitted Diseases Sourcebook, 2nd Edition

Basic Consumer Health Information about Sexually Transmitted Diseases, Including Information on the Diagnosis and Treatment of Chlamydia, Gonorrhea, Hepatitis, Herpes, HIV, Mononucleosis, Syphilis, and Others

Along with Information on Prevention, Such as Condom Use, Vaccines, and STD Education; And Featuring a Section on Issues Related to Youth and Adolescents, a Glossary, and Resources for Additional Help and Information

Edited by Dawn D. Matthews. 538 pages. 2001. 0-7808-0249-7. $78.

"Recommended pick both for specialty health library collections and any general consumer health reference collection." *— The Bookwatch, Apr '01*

"Recommended reference source."
— Booklist, American Library Association, Apr '01

■

Skin Disorders Sourcebook

Basic Information about Common Skin and Scalp Conditions Caused by Aging, Allergies, Immune Reactions, Sun Exposure, Infectious Organisms, Parasites, Cosmetics, and Skin Traumas, Including Abrasions, Cuts, and Pressure Sores

Along with Information on Prevention and Treatment

Edited by Allan R. Cook. 647 pages. 1997. 0-7808-0080-X. $78.

". . . comprehensive, easily read reference book."
— Doody's Health Sciences Book Reviews, Oct '97

SEE ALSO Burns Sourcebook

■

Sleep Disorders Sourcebook

Basic Consumer Health Information about Sleep and Its Disorders, Including Insomnia, Sleepwalking, Sleep Apnea, Restless Leg Syndrome, and Narcolepsy

Along with Data about Shiftwork and Its Effects, Information on the Societal Costs of Sleep Deprivation, Descriptions of Treatment Options, a Glossary of Terms, and Resource Listings for Additional Help

Edited by Jenifer Swanson. 439 pages. 1998. 0-7808-0234-9. $78.

"This text will complement any home or medical library. It is user-friendly and ideal for the adult reader."
—American Reference Books Annual, 2000

"Recommended reference source."
— Booklist, American Library Association, Feb '99

"A useful resource that provides accurate, relevant, and accessible information on sleep to the general public. Health care providers who deal with sleep disorders patients may also find it helpful in being prepared to answer some of the questions patients ask."
— Respiratory Care, Jul '99

Sports Injuries Sourcebook

Basic Consumer Health Information about Common Sports Injuries, Prevention of Injury in Specific Sports, Tips for Training, and Rehabilitation from Injury

Along with Information about Special Concerns for Children, Young Girls in Athletic Training Programs, Senior Athletes, and Women Athletes, and a Directory of Resources for Further Help and Information

Edited by Heather E. Aldred. 624 pages. 1999. 0-7808-0218-7. $78.

"Public libraries and undergraduate academic libraries will find this book useful for its nontechnical language." *—American Reference Books Annual, 2000*

"While this easy-to-read book is recommended for all libraries, it should prove to be especially useful for public, high school, and academic libraries; certainly it should be on the bookshelf of every school gymnasium." *—E-Streams, Mar '00*

■

Substance Abuse Sourcebook

Basic Health-Related Information about the Abuse of Legal and Illegal Substances Such as Alcohol, Tobacco, Prescription Drugs, Marijuana, Cocaine, and Heroin; and Including Facts about Substance Abuse Prevention Strategies, Intervention Methods, Treatment and Recovery Programs, and a Section Addressing the Special Problems Related to Substance Abuse during Pregnancy

Edited by Karen Bellenir. 573 pages. 1996. 0-7808-0038-9. $78.

"A valuable addition to any health reference section. Highly recommended."
— The Book Report, Mar/Apr '97

". . . a comprehensive collection of substance abuse information that's both highly readable and compact. Families and caregivers of substance abusers will find the information enlightening and helpful, while teachers, social workers and journalists should benefit from the concise format. Recommended."
— Drug Abuse Update, Winter '96/'97

SEE ALSO Alcoholism Sourcebook, Drug Abuse Sourcebook

■

Transplantation Sourcebook

Basic Consumer Health Information about Organ and Tissue Transplantation, Including Physical and Financial Preparations, Procedures and Issues Relating to Specific Solid Organ and Tissue Transplants, Rehabilitation, Pediatric Transplant Information, the Future of Transplantation, and Organ and Tissue Donation

Along with a Glossary and Listings of Additional Resources

Edited by Joyce Brennfleck Shannon. 600 pages. 2001. 0-7808-0322-1. $78.

Traveler's Health Sourcebook

Basic Consumer Health Information for Travelers, Including Physical and Medical Preparations, Transportation Health and Safety, Essential Information about Food and Water, Sun Exposure, Insect and Snake Bites, Camping and Wilderness Medicine, and Travel with Physical or Medical Disabilities

Along with International Travel Tips, Vaccination Recommendations, Geographical Health Issues, Disease Risks, a Glossary, and a Listing of Additional Resources

Edited by Joyce Brennfleck Shannon. 613 pages. 2000. 0-7808-0384-1. $78.

"Recommended reference source."
— *Booklist, American Library Association, Feb '01*

"This book is recommended for any public library, any travel collection, and especially any collection for the physically disabled."
— *American Reference Books Annual, 2001*

■

Women's Health Concerns Sourcebook

Basic Information about Health Issues That Affect Women, Featuring Facts about Menstruation and Other Gynecological Concerns, Including Endometriosis, Fibroids, Menopause, and Vaginitis; Reproductive Concerns, Including Birth Control, Infertility, and Abortion; and Facts about Additional Physical, Emotional, and Mental Health Concerns Prevalent among Women Such as Osteoporosis, Urinary Tract Disorders, Eating Disorders, and Depression

Along with Tips for Maintaining a Healthy Lifestyle

Edited by Heather E. Aldred. 567 pages. 1997. 0-7808-0219-5. $78.

"Handy compilation. There is an impressive range of diseases, devices, disorders, procedures, and other physical and emotional issues covered . . . well organized, illustrated, and indexed." — *Choice, Association of College and Research Libraries, Jan '98*

SEE ALSO *Breast Cancer Sourcebook, Cancer Sourcebook for Women, 1st and 2nd Editions, Healthy Heart Sourcebook for Women, Osteoporosis Sourcebook*

Workplace Health & Safety Sourcebook

Basic Consumer Health Information about Workplace Health and Safety, Including the Effect of Workplace Hazards on the Lungs, Skin, Heart, Ears, Eyes, Brain, Reproductive Organs, Musculoskeletal System, and Other Organs and Body Parts

Along with Information about Occupational Cancer, Personal Protective Equipment, Toxic and Hazardous Chemicals, Child Labor, Stress, and Workplace Violence

Edited by Chad T. Kimball. 626 pages. 2000. 0-7808-0231-4. $78.

"Provides helpful information for primary care physicians and other caregivers interested in occupational medicine. . . . General readers; professionals."
— *Choice, Association of College and Research Libraries, May '01*

"Recommended reference source."
— *Booklist, American Library Association, Feb '01*

"Highly recommended." — *The Bookwatch, Jan '01*

■

Worldwide Health Sourcebook

Basic Information about Global Health Issues, Including Malnutrition, Reproductive Health, Disease Dispersion and Prevention, Emerging Diseases, Risky Health Behaviors, and the Leading Causes of Death

Along with Global Health Concerns for Children, Women, and the Elderly, Mental Health Issues, Research and Technology Advancements, and Economic, Environmental, and Political Health Implications, a Glossary, and a Resource Listing for Additional Help and Information

Edited by Joyce Brennfleck Shannon. 614 pages. 2001. 0-7808-0330-2. $78.